T0263362

Geriatric Urology

Editor

TOMAS LINDOR GRIEBLING

CLINICS IN
GERIATRIC MEDICINE

www.geriatric.theclinics.com

November 2015 • Volume 31 • Number 4

ELSEVIER

1600 John F. Kennedy Boulevard • Suite 1800 • Philadelphia, Pennsylvania, 19103-2899

http://www.theclinics.com

CLINICS IN GERIATRIC MEDICINE Volume 31, Number 4
November 2015 ISSN 0749–0690, ISBN-13: 978-0-323-39334-8

Editor: Jessica McCool
Developmental Editor: Colleen Viola

Clinics in Geriatric Medicine (ISSN 0749-0690) is published quarterly by Elsevier Inc., 360 Park Avenue South, New York, NY 10010-1710. Months of issue are February, May, August, and November. Business and Editorial Offices: 1600 John F. Kennedy Blvd., Suite 1800, Philadelphia, PA 191023-2899. Periodicals postage paid at New York, NY, and additional mailing offices. Subscription prices are $280.00 per year (US individuals), $498.00 per year (US institutions), $145.00 per year (US student/resident), $370.00 per year (Canadian individuals), $632.00 per year (Canadian institutions), $195.00 per year (Canadian student/resident), $390.00 per year (international individuals), $632.00 per year (international institutions), and $195.00 per year (international student/resident). Foreign air speed delivery is included in all *Clinics* subscription prices. All prices are subject to change without notice. POSTMASTER: Send address changes to *Clinics in Geriatric Medicine*, Elsevier Health Sciences Division, Subscription Customer Service, 3251 Riverport Lane, Maryland Heights, MO 63043. **Telephone: 1-800-654-2452 (U.S. and Canada); 314-447-8871 (outside U.S. and Canada). Fax: 314-447-8029. E-mail:** journalscustomerservice-usa@elsevier.com **(for print support) or** journalsonlinesupport-usa@elsevier.com **(for online support).**

Reprints. For copies of 100 or more, of articles in this publication, please contact the Commercial Reprints Department, Elsevier Inc., 360 Park Avenue South, New York, New York 10010-1710. Tel.: 212-633-3874; Fax: 212-633-3820, E-mail: reprints@elsevier.com.

Clinics in Geriatric Medicine is covered in *MEDLINE/PubMed (Index Medicus)*, *EMBASE/Excerpta Medica*, *Current Contents/Clinical Medicine (CC/CM)*, and the *Cumulative Index to Nursing & Allied Health Literature*.

Contributors

EDITOR

TOMAS LINDOR GRIEBLING, MD, MPH
John P. Wolf 33rd-Degree Masonic Distinguished Professor of Urology; Professor, Vice-Chair and Residency Program Director, Department of Urology; Faculty Associate, The Landon Center on Aging; Assistant Dean for Student Affairs, School of Medicine, The University of Kansas, Kansas City, Kansas

AUTHORS

KARL-ERIK ANDERSSON, MD, PhD
Professor, Department of Urology, Institute for Regenerative Medicine, Wake Forest Baptist Medical Center, Wake Forest University School of Medicine, Winston Salem, North Carolina; Professor, Aarhus Institute of Advanced Studies, Aarhus University, Aarhus C, Denmark

RAJIB K. BHATTACHARYA, MD, FACE
Associate Professor of Endocrinology and Metabolism, Co-Director of the Renal/Endocrine Module, University of Kansas School of Medicine, Kansas City, Kansas

SHELLEY B. BHATTACHARYA, DO, MPH
Associate Professor of Geriatric Medicine, Department of Family Medicine; Assistant Dean of Student Affairs, University of Kansas School of Medicine, Kansas City, Kansas

LORI ANN BIRDER, PhD
Professor, Renal-Electrolyte Division, Medicine Department; Professor, Pharmacology and Chemical Biology, University of Pittsburgh School of Medicine, Pittsburgh, Pennsylvania

MICHAEL B. CHANCELLOR, MD
Department of Urology, Aikens Neurourology Research Center, Oakland University William Beaumont School of Medicine, Royal Oak, Michigan

YAO-CHI CHUANG, MD
Department of Urology, Kaohsiung Chang Gung Memorial Hospital, Chung Shan Medical University Institute of Medicine, Kaohsiung, Taiwan

MARISA M. CLIFTON, MD
Department of Urology, Center for Female Pelvic Medicine and Reconstructive Surgery, The Cleveland Clinic, Cleveland, Ohio

WILLIAM DALE, MD, PhD
Chief, Section of Geriatrics and Palliative Medicine; Director, Specialized Oncology Care and Research in the Elderly (SOCARE) Clinic, Department of Medicine, University of Chicago, Chicago, Illinois

DAVID R. ELLINGTON, MD, FACOG
Assistant Professor, Division of Urogynecology and Pelvic Reconstructive Surgery, University of Alabama at Birmingham, Birmingham, Alabama

ELISABETH A. EREKSON, MD, MPH, FACOG
Assistant Professor, Division of Female Pelvic Medicine and Reconstructive Surgery, The Geisel School of Medicine at Dartmouth, Lebanon, New Hampshire

HOWARD B. GOLDMAN, MD
Department of Urology, Center for Female Pelvic Medicine and Reconstructive Surgery, The Cleveland Clinic, Cleveland, Ohio

E. ANN GORMLEY, MD
Professor, Section of Urology, Department of Surgery, Dartmouth-Hitchcock Medical Center, Lebanon, New Hampshire

TOMAS LINDOR GRIEBLING, MD, MPH
John P. Wolf 33rd-Degree Masonic Distinguished Professor of Urology; Professor, Vice-Chair and Residency Program Director, Department of Urology; Faculty Associate, The Landon Center on Aging; Assistant Dean for Student Affairs, School of Medicine, The University of Kansas, Kansas City, Kansas

DEREK GRIFFITHS, PhD
Visiting Professor of Geriatric Medicine (retired), Department of Medicine, University of Pittsburgh, Pittsburgh, Pennsylvania

PETROS D. GRIVAS, MD, PhD
Associate Staff, Department of Hematology/Oncology, Taussig Cancer Institute, The Cleveland Clinic, Cleveland, Ohio

JESSICA L. KALENDER-RICH, MD
Assistant Professor of Medicine, Geriatric Medicine, Palliative Medicine, Internal Medicine, Landon Center on Aging, University of Kansas School of Medicine, Kansas City, Kansas

GEORGE A. KUCHEL, MD
Professor of Medicine, Division of Geriatrics, UConn Center on Aging, University of Connecticut Health, Farmington, Connecticut

FLORENTA AURA KULLMANN, PhD
Research Assistant Professor, Renal-Electrolyte Division, Medicine Department, University of Pittsburgh School of Medicine, Pittsburgh, Pennsylvania

LAURA E. LAMB, PhD
Department of Urology, Aikens Neurourology Research Center, Oakland University William Beaumont School of Medicine, Royal Oak, Michigan

MOBEN MIRZA, MD, FACS
Assistant Professor, Division of Urologic Oncology, Department of Urology, University of Kansas, Kansas City, Kansas

SUPRIYA G. MOHILE, MD, MS
Division of Hematology/Oncology, Department of Medicine, Wilmot Cancer Institute, University of Rochester, Rochester, New York

GREGORY M. OUELLET, MD
Department of Medicine, Yale University School of Medicine, New Haven, Connecticut

WILLIAM P. PARKER, MD
Department of Urology, The Landon Center on Aging, School of Medicine, The University of Kansas, Kansas City, Kansas

JAVIER PIZARRO-BERDICHEVSKY, MD
Department of Urology, Center for Female Pelvic Medicine and Reconstructive Surgery, The Cleveland Clinic, Cleveland, Ohio; Urogynecology Unit, Dr. Sotero del Rio Hospital; Division de Obstetricia y Ginecologia, Pontificia Universidad Catolica de Chile, Santiago, Chile

MAURICIO PLATA, MD
Department of Urology, Fundación Santa Fe de Bogotá University Hospital, Universidad de los Andes School of Medicine, Bogotá, Colombia

KARIN PORTER-WILLIAMSON, MD
Associate Professor and Division Director, Palliative Medicine; Medical Director for Palliative Care Services, Kansas University Hospital; Medical Director, KS-MO TPOPP Coalition, Kansas City, Kansas

HOLLY E. RICHTER, PhD, MD, FACOG, FACS
Professor and J. Marion Sims Endowed Chair, Division Director, Division of Urogynecology and Pelvic Reconstructive Surgery, University of Alabama at Birmingham, Birmingham, Alabama

THOMAS N. ROBINSON, MD, MS, FACS
Department of Surgery, University of Colorado, Aurora, Colorado

BRETON ROUSSEL, BS
Robert Wood Johnson Medical School, Rutgers University, New Brunswick, New Jersey

CHRISTIAN T. SINCLAIR, MD
Assistant Professor, Division of Palliative Medicine, University of Kansas School of Medicine, Kansas City, Kansas

PHILLIP P. SMITH, MD
Associate Professor of Urology and Gynecology, Department of Surgery, UConn Center on Aging, University of Connecticut Health, Farmington, Connecticut

CARA TANNENBAUM, MD, MSc
Professor of Medicine and Pharmacy, Division of Geriatric Medicine, Université de Montréal, Montreal, Quebec, Canada

NICOLE T. TOWNSEND, MD
Department of Surgery, University of Colorado, Aurora, Colorado

JOSEPH E. YARED, MD
Resident, Section of Urology, Department of Surgery, Dartmouth-Hitchcock Medical Center, Lebanon, New Hampshire

BO ZHAO, MD
Clinical Fellow, Department of Hematology/Oncology, Taussig Cancer Institute, The Cleveland Clinic, Cleveland, Ohio

Contents

Urinary incontinence is a prevalent condition in elderly women with significant associated morbidity. Incontinence can by grouped into several types: stress incontinence, urgency incontinence, overflow incontinence, functional incontinence, and mixed urinary incontinence. Careful evaluation, including history and physical examination, is critical to making the correct diagnosis and guiding therapy. A variety of nonsurgical treatments, including behavioral therapies, pelvic floor muscle exercise, medications, and other treatments, are available; can be successful for many older women; and may preclude the need for surgery. Working closely with the patient, understanding her goals of care, and targeting treatments accordingly are essential for success.

As population demographics continue to evolve, specifics on age-related outcomes of stress urinary incontinence interventions will be critical to patient counseling and management planning. Understanding medical factors unique to older women and their lower urinary tract conditions will allow caregivers to optimize surgical outcomes, both physical and functional, and minimize complications within this population.

Pelvic organ prolapse is a common disease in elderly patients. The most important symptom is vaginal bulge (bulge sensation or the sensation of something coming down through the vaginal introitus). This symptom is not different than in the general population. Diagnosis can be confirmed using just vaginal examinations to identify the presence of protrusion beyond the hymen, and is not different than in the general population. Different treatment options are available, including observation, nonsurgical, and surgical techniques. Pessaries and colpocleisis are the treatment options used more often in elderly patients than in the general population.

Overactive bladder is one of the most common bladder problems, but an estimated 20 million Americans have underactive bladder (UAB), which makes going to the bathroom difficult, increases the risk of urinary tract infections, and even leads to institutionalization. This article provides an overview of UAB in older adults, and discusses the prevalence, predisposing factors, cause, clinical investigations, and treatments. At present, there is no effective therapy for UAB. A great deal of work still needs to be done on understanding the pathogenesis and the development of effective therapies.

Age-related lower urinary tract (LUT) dysfunctions result from complex processes controlled by multiple genetic, epigenetic, and environmental factors and account for high costs of health care. This article discusses risk factors that may play a role in age-related LUT dysfunction and presents available data comparing structural and functional changes that occur with aging in the bladder of humans and animal models. A better understanding of factors and mechanisms underlying LUT symptoms in the older population may lead to therapeutic interventions to reduce these dysfunctions.

Brain abnormalities may contribute to the increased prevalence of urinary dysfunction such as overactive bladder and urge incontinence in older individuals. Functional brain imaging suggests that three independent neural circuits (frontal, midcingulate, and subcortical) control voiding by suppressing the voiding reflex in the brainstem periaqueductal gray. Damage to the connecting pathways subserving these circuits (white matter hyperintensities) increases with age and is associated both with severity of urge incontinence and changes in brain function. Multicomponent therapies targeting structural and functional neural abnormalities may be more effective than any single treatment focused on the bladder.

Urodynamic testing is the study of the function of the bladder and its outlet. Geriatric patients are at greater risk for lower urinary tract dysfunction owing to age or neurologic disease, such as Parkinson disease or stroke. Although urodynamic testing may best diagnose an individual patient's bladder storage and emptying function, the tests should be tailored to answer the question being asked, and the test should only be done when the outcome of the test is going to impact decision-making regarding management or treatment.

Fifty percent of sexually active older men and women complain of one or more sexual problems. Sexual dysfunction involves a complex interplay of partner factors, relationship factors, individual factors, concomitant mental health disorders, life stressors, medical comorbidity, and medication intake. Although lower urinary tract symptoms are associated with decreased sexual activity, it is unclear whether the relationship is causal or influenced by shared risk factors, or the presence of overall poor health and function. Taking a complete sexual history in patients with lower urinary tract symptoms is the first step toward detection and possible treatment.

Almost two-thirds of urology operations are performed in patients 65 years and older. Older adults are at higher risk for complications and mortality compared with their younger counterparts. There are two primary methods to quantify surgical risk in these patients: frailty measurement and organ/comorbidity-based surgical risk calculators. A frailty assessment can be used to independently forecast the risk of postoperative complications. A paradigm shift in the preoperative assessment of the geriatric patient has occurred, which emphasizes the evaluation of frailty over more traditional surgical risk assessment, which uses comorbidities and single end-organ dysfunction to define risk.

Small renal masses in older adults are common and usually found incidentally. Although many small renal masses are benign, most are malignant. In older patients, the small renal mass poses a challenge because the treatment paradigm has to strike the balance between competing comorbidities and a lethal cancer. Partial nephrectomy, mainly via robot-assisted technique, has gained favor over radical nephrectomy as the intervention of choice. Cryoablation and radiofrequency ablation are also viable treatment options and have a role to play in patients who desire treatment but either are not suitable surgical candidates or prefer not to have a surgical intervention.

Prostate cancer (PCa) is a common medical condition in the United States, with an estimated 16% of men receiving a diagnosis during their lifetime. Although it is the second leading cause of cancer-specific deaths among men, PCa will not be the cause of death for most men who are diagnosed with it. Although there are notable improvements recently, the relative dearth of high-quality data concerning PCa screening and treatment in older men calls for a thoughtful approach to evaluating such men for screening, diagnosis, and treatment options. This article offers guidance to an approach here.

Late-onset hypogonadism is an underdiagnosed and easily-treated condition defined by low serum testosterone levels in men older than 65 years.

When treated, a significant improvement in quality of life may be reached in this rapidly rising sector of the population. During the evaluation, laboratory tests and a full medication review should be performed to exclude other illnesses or adverse effects from medications. The major goal of treatment in this population is treating the symptoms related to hypogonadism. There has not been clear evidence supporting universally giving older men with low serum testosterone levels and hypogonadal symptoms testosterone replacement therapy.

Current data on systemic therapy in geriatric populations with genitourinary malignancies are largely derived from retrospective analyses of prospectively conducted trials or retrospective reviews. Although extrapolation of these data to real-world patients should be cautious, patients aged 65 years or older with good functional status and minimal comorbidities seem to enjoy similar survival benefit from therapy as their younger counterparts. Chronologic age alone should generally not be used to guide management decisions. Comprehensive geriatric assessment tools and prospective studies in older adults integrating comprehensive geriatric assessment can shed light on the optimal management of urologic malignancies in this population.

This article focuses on the issues facing patients with advanced and terminal urologic illness, from the framework of care planning based on defining patient-specific and family-specific goals of care, to palliative management strategies for common symptoms and syndromes that these patients and their families experience. This article also focuses on the management of common urologic issues that may arise in the course of care for all patients at the end of life, as well as the impact of these conditions on caregivers.

CLINICS IN GERIATRIC MEDICINE

ISSUE OF RELATED INTEREST

Urologic Clinics of North America, August 2015 (Vol. 42, No. 3)
Testicular Cancer
Daniel W. Lin, MD, *Editor*
http://www.urologic.theclinics.com

THE CLINICS ARE AVAILABLE ONLINE!
Access your subscription at:
www.theclinics.com

Preface

Urologic Issues in Geriatric Health Care

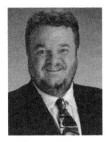

Tomas Lindor Griebling, MD, MPH
Editor

Analysis of demographic trends reveals that the world population is rapidly expanding, and the fastest overall growth is occurring among elderly people. This has led to an increased need for enhanced knowledge and expertise among practitioners across essentially all specialties. Urology is clearly at the forefront of this trend. Most urologists in general practice estimate that approximately 70% of their patients are over 65 years of age. In fact, Urology consistently ranks in the top three among all medical and surgical specialties in terms of the total volume of care provided to geriatric patients. Only Ophthalmology and Cardiology provide more total geriatrics care.

Many of the most common genitourinary conditions, such as urinary incontinence, pelvic organ prolapse, urinary tract infections, sexual dysfunction, hypogonadism, and most of the urologic malignancies, occur with increasing incidence and prevalence with advancing age. Although some urologic health issues present with an acute onset and can be effectively treated with a short course of therapy, many genitourinary conditions are chronic in nature and are associated with ongoing health care needs. In many cases, the choice of treatments is influenced in part by age, but more by associated comorbidities seen in older adults. Urologic care must be provided within the context of overall health and tailored to the unique needs of each patient.

This issue of *Clinics in Geriatric Medicine* focuses on some of the most common urologic conditions seen in elderly patients. Each of the articles presents a highly current state-of-the-art assessment of current thinking, research, and practice on the topics. New research has led to increased options for many of these clinical entities treated both medically and surgically. In addition, there is expanding understanding of the role of urology in palliative medicine and end-of-life care for older adults.

I have enjoyed the opportunity to serve as editor, and I am most grateful to all of the authors who have contributed material to this issue. Many are long-time friends and colleagues, and several have been mentors to me throughout my career. They are all truly experts in their fields and have generously shared their time and expertise to

Clin Geriatr Med 31 (2015) xiii–xiv
http://dx.doi.org/10.1016/j.cger.2015.08.013
0749-0690/15/$ – see front matter © 2015 Published by Elsevier Inc.   **geriatric.theclinics.com**

create a resource with the most current information for each topic. I am also indebted to my colleagues, Jessica McCool, Colleen Viola, and Palani Murugesan from Elsevier, who provided outstanding assistance with the development and editorial aspects of this project. Finally, I thank my partner, Michael A. Miklovic, for his unflagging support. His gentle guidance and patience during my many hours spent at the computer writing and editing are sincerely appreciated.

Tomas Lindor Griebling, MD, MPH
Department of Urology
The Landon Center on Aging
School of Medicine
The University of Kansas
Kansas City, KS 66160, USA

E-mail address:
tgriebling@kumc.edu

Nonsurgical Treatment of Urinary Incontinence in Elderly Women

William P. Parker, MD, Tomas Lindor Griebling, MD, MPH*

KEYWORDS

- Urinary incontinence • Geriatrics • Elderly women • Nonsurgical • Treatments

KEY POINTS

- Incontinence can be divided into broad categories: stress, urgency, mixed, overflow, and function incontinence, which are used to guide treatment.
- Review of medications, comorbid conditions, and pelvic examination is essential in the initial assessment of the incontinent patient.
- Numerous treatment options exist for urgency urinary incontinence but must be used selectively in the elder patient.
- Behavioral modification and strengthening exercises should be offered before pharmacologic intervention and can result in meaningful outcomes.
- Reassessment should be performed at 8 to 12 weeks with the use of validated questionnaires to guide follow-up.

INTRODUCTION

Urinary incontinence (UI) is a common problem in elderly women, with a prevalence of 17% to 24% in women over the age of 65,[1,2] increasing to approximately 75% in women greater than 75 years of age.[3] Notably, 6% of nursing home admissions can be attributed to UI[4] with an annual cost of $66 billion.[5] UI can be subdivided into broad categories based on symptoms that are classified according to the International Continence Society and the International Urogynecological Association. The most prevalent include stress urinary incontinence (SUI) and urgency urinary incontinence (UUI), although others exist (**Table 1**). According to these guidelines, SUI is defined as the involuntary loss of urine with activity[6] and is the dominant form of UI in the overall female population, representing 42% of patients with UI in a large meta-analysis.[7] Conversely, UUI is defined as the loss of urine accompanied by or immediately

Department of Urology, The Landon Center on Aging, School of Medicine, The University of Kansas, 3901 Rainbow Boulevard, Kansas City, KS 66160, USA
* Corresponding author.
E-mail address: tgriebling@kumc.edu

Clin Geriatr Med 31 (2015) 471–485
http://dx.doi.org/10.1016/j.cger.2015.07.003
0749-0690/15/$ – see front matter © 2015 Elsevier Inc. All rights reserved.

Table 1
Types of urinary incontinence

Type of Incontinence	Manifestation	Pathophysiology
Stress incontinence	Leakage of urine with activity	Inadequate bladder outlet resistance to counteract increases in intra-abdominal pressure
Urgency incontinence	Leakage of urine with sensation of need to void	Bladder muscle (detrusor) overactivity leading to loss of urine
Mixed UI	Leakage of urine with activity and desire to void	A combination of the above 2 pathologic conditions
Overflow incontinence	Leakage due to retained urine	Leakage as a result of retained urine volume
Functional incontinence	Incontinence as a result of barriers to voiding	Impaired cognition/alertness, mobility impairment, inadequate access to toilet, and so on

preceded by the urgency to void.[8] It is the most common form of UI seen among older adults.

Continence relies on adequate and coordinated function of the bladder muscle (detrusor) and the bladder outlet (sphincter and pelvic floor). As such, incontinence can result from perturbation of any of these mechanisms. Simplified, SUI can be thought of as an outlet failure during times of increased bladder pressure,[9] whereas UUI is related to a storage failure from detrusor overactivity.[6] Overflow incontinence results from retention of urine to the point of capacity, at which point urine leakage occurs. Often overflow incontinence is related to neurologic causes as opposed to mechanical obstruction. Finally, functional incontinence is incontinence as a result of situation, either a failure to recognize the need to void or an inability to reach the toilet, and is a problem that is of unique importance in the elderly population.[10] In the current review, the evaluation and nonsurgical management of the incontinent older adult woman are discussed.

MANAGEMENT GOALS

- Initial evaluation and recognition of type of incontinence
- Reduction in incontinent episodes
- Improvement in quality of life

CLINICAL EVALUATION

The evaluation of the incontinent patient begins with a careful history and physical examination. Up to 50% of patients with UI will not report this symptom to physicians.[11] Initial screening for incontinence in older adults can be facilitated through the use of validated questionnaires.[8] There are several available questionnaires, the simplest of which is the 3IQ, representing 3 questions[12]; however, numerous questionnaires exist with increasing complexity that address not only the type of incontinence but also the degree of bother caused by the symptoms, all of which have been validated for the use in elderly patients.[13] Although the authors do not recommend one questionnaire more than any other, they do recommend familiarity with available options and selection of an instrument that is most applicable to the individual practice and population. The duration and frequency of the incontinence should be carefully assessed, because acute onset or transient incontinence is often managed differently than chronic worsening incontinence. Common causes of transient incontinence include urinary tract infection, atrophic vaginitis, fecal impaction, delirium, medications, polyuria, reduced mobility, urinary retention, cognitive impairment, or psychological factors. As incontinence is related to fluid status and micturition, the patient's dietary intake should be assessed in the initial management. Identification of bladder irritants such as caffeine or alcohol is an important component of this part of the assessment and is a potentially modifiable risk factor for UI.

Careful evaluation of the patient's past medical history and current medications should be performed, particularly in the elderly patient. Certain conditions can exacerbate existing incontinence and should be optimized in the management of the condition. For example, the patient with chronic obstructive pulmonary disease (COPD) may suffer from recurrent cough, which in turn exposes them to increased episodes of SUI. In addition, neurologic conditions, which can impair sensation, not only can worsen existing incontinence but also can be a source of incontinence. Specific comorbid conditions will not be discussed in the present review; however, all efforts should be made to optimize the patient during the management of their incontinence. Polypharmacy can be a significant problem in geriatric patients[14] and specific medication adjustments are discussed separately.

Examination can be difficult in the frail patient. However, pelvic examination should be performed as a routine part of the evaluation.[8] Examination should include a visual assessment of the vaginal mucosa, a strength assessment of the pelvic floor musculature, sensory evaluation of the perineum, the presence and degree of pelvic organ prolapse, and the degree of incontinence on a cough stress test.[8,15,16] Urinalysis should be performed to assess for other underlying conditions and comorbidities, such as urinary tract infection or hematuria. Increased urinary glucose could indicate underling diabetes, and proteinuria may be a hallmark of renal disease. In addition, a measurement of postvoid bladder volume should be obtained to rule out incomplete bladder emptying and overflow UI. Each component of the examination can identify potential sources of incontinence, from atrophic vaginitis to neurologic compromise or muscular dysfunction of the pelvic floor.

PHARMACOLOGIC THERAPIES
General Principles

Initial medical management of the incontinent older patient involves a careful evaluation of currently used medications. There are several commonly used medications that can exacerbate UI and should be adjusted, if possible, during treatment (**Table 2**). After evaluating for potentially modifiable medications, addition of medications in the management of incontinence in elderly patients must be done cautiously.[14]

Urgency Urinary Incontinence

The treatment of UUI lends itself to pharmacologic intervention. The main pharmacologic targets in UUI are the M2 and M3 acetylcholine receptors[17] and the β_3-adrenergic receptor.[18] There are numerous options available that target these receptors and that are summarized in **Table 3**.

Anticholinergic Agents

Anticholinergic medications work through the inhibition of muscarinic receptors in the bladder.[34] As a class, these medications can result in a significant improvement in incontinent episodes. Currently available anticholinergic medications are listed in

Table 2		
Medications that can contribute to urinary incontinence		
Medication	**Effect**	**Potential Result**
Alcohol	Polyuria and sedation	Functional incontinence, increased urgency
α-Adrenergic agonists (nonprescription cold medications)	Increase bladder outlet tone	Urinary retention/ overflow incontinence
α-Adrenergic antagonists	Decrease sphincter tone	Stress urinary incontinence
Angiotensin-converting enzyme inhibitors	Can increase cough	Stress urinary incontinence
Anticholinergic medications (tricyclic antidepressants, antihistamines, muscle relaxants, antipsychotics)	Inhibit bladder smooth muscle, can result in urinary retention	Urinary retention/overflow incontinence
Antiparkinsonian medications	Cholinergic stimulation	Urgency/urge urinary incontinence
β-Adrenergic agonists	Relaxation of the bladder	Urinary retention/overflow incontinence
Caffeiee	Stimulates detrusor contraction	Urgency/urge urinary incontinence
Calcium-channel blockers	Inhibit bladder smooth muscle	Urinary retention/overflow incontinence
Diuretics	Increase urine output, leading to polyuria	Functional incontinence, increased urgency
NSAIDs	Increase fluid retention	Nocturnal enuresis
Sedatives	Impair cognition	Functional incontinence

Abbreviation: NSAIDs, nonsteroidal anti-inflammatory drugs.

Adapted from Frank C, Szlanta A. Office management of urinary incontinence among elderly patients. Can Fam Physician 2010;56:1115–20; and Erdem N, Chu FM. Management of overactive bladder and urge urinary incontinence in the elderly patient. Am J Med 2006;119:29–36.

Table 3. There is a paucity of data regarding comparative efficacy of various anticholinergic medications, and currently, the only meta-analysis addressing this topic compares 4 of the currently available agents (oxybutynin, tolterodine, fesoterodine, and solfenacin).[35] In the authors' practice, they initiate anticholinergic medications based largely on the potential side-effect profile, competing risks of unique comorbid conditions, and the insurance profile of the patient, which can substantially influence out-of-pocket costs.

Cholinergic receptors are ubiquitous in the human body, and as such, this class of medications is associated with a wide side-effect profile. The most common side effects include dry mouth, constipation, and blurred vision.[18,36] Certainly, these are bothersome side effects; however, the most concerning side effects come from inhibition of the M1-receptor in the central nervous system and can result in cognitive decline.[37,38] Despite this fact, there is evidence supporting the safety of these medications in the elderly population with regard to cognition.[30,32,39] The authors recommend careful monitoring of patient's cognition during initiation of these

Table 3
Selected medications used in the treatment of urgency urinary incontinence

Medication (Trade Name)	Formulations	Dosing	Evidence	Special Consideration in Geriatrics
Oxybutynin (Ditropan/Ditropan XL/Oxytrol/Gelnique)	Immediate release	5 mg Tablets 1–3 times daily	Level Ia: 52% Reduction in incontinent episodes, 33% reduction in frequency of voids[19]	70% Rate of side effects; most commonly dry mouth, blurred vision, and constipation[19]
	Extended release	10 mg, 15 mg daily	Level Ia: Similar improvement in incontinence to oxybutynin IR[20]	Reduced side-effect profile; 29.3% dry mouth[20]
	Transdermal patch	3.9 mg/patch every 3–4 d	Level Ia: 75% Reduction in incontinent episodes, 18% reduction in frequency of voids[21]	7% Dry mouth. Must ensure routine patch changes; 14%–16% rate of puritis and local skin reaction from adhesive[21,22]
	Topical gel	3% gel (84 mg) Daily	Level Ia: 46.7% Reduction in incontinent episodes; 23.2% reduction in frequency of voids[23]	12.1% Dry mouth; 3.7% rate of skin reaction[23]
Tolterodine (Detrol/Detrol LA)	Immediate release / Extended release	2 mg Twice daily or 2–4 mg Daily (LA)	Level Ia: 69.5% Reduction in incontinent episodes; 26.2% reduction in frequency of voids[24,25]	10%–22.3% Rate of dry mouth,[24,25] metabolized by CYP2D6: 10%–20% of patients are deficient in enzyme → sleep disturbances[26]
Fesoteroodine (Toviaz)	Extended release	4–8 mg Daily	Level Ia: 75%–83% Reduction in incontinent episodes; 15%–17% reduction in frequency of voids[27]	19%–35% Dry mouth, 6% rate of constipation[27]
Tropsium (Sanctura/Sanctura XR)	Immediate release / Extended release	20 mg Twice daily or 60 mg (XR)	Level Ia: 50% Reduction in incontinent episodes; 33% reduction in frequency of voids[28]	33% dry mouth, 7% constipation; renal clearance, reduced central nervous system affinity[28]
Darifenacin (Enablex)	Extended release	7.5–15 mg Daily	Level Ia: 67.7%–72.8% Reduction in incontinent episodes; 16% change in frequency of voids[29]	31.3% Dry mouth, 13.9% constipation, selective anticholinergic agent; no effect on cognition[30]
Solifenacin (Vesicare)	Extended release	5–10 mg Daily	Level Ia: 60.7% Reduction in incontinent episodes; 21.9% reduction in frequency of voids[31]	23.1% Dry mouth, 9.1% constipation,[31] no effect on cognition in elderly adults[32]
Mirabegron (Myrbetric)	Extended release	25–50 mg Daily	Level Ia: 53.4% Reduction in incontinent episodes; 30.1% reduction in frequency of voids[33]	No anticholinergic side effects; hypertension (10.7%) and nasopharyngitis (5.7%)[33]

Data from Refs.[19–33]

medications. In addition, they recommend counseling patients on the need for medication compliance for at least 8 to 12 weeks before symptom reassessment in order to adequately evaluate medication success. The current guidelines from the American Geriatrics Society recommend against the routine use of these agents unless no other alternatives exist,[14] and contraindications to the use of anticholinergic medications include dementia, urinary retention, intestinal obstruction, chronic constipation, and poorly controlled narrow-angle glaucoma.[40]

β_3-Agonists

Although anticholinergic mediations function through the inhibition of detrusor contraction, β-adrenergic agents target the storage phase of bladder function. Specifically, β_3 stimulation leads to an active bladder relaxation.[41] The only currently available pharmacologic target of the β_3 receptor is mirabegron. Compared with placebo, mirabegron has been shown to have significant reductions in the number of incontinent episodes and the number of voids in a 24-hour period at all available doses.[42] Specific to the geriatric population, mirabegron has been shown to be effective and safe, with the most common adverse events being hypertension, nasopharyngitis, and urinary tract infection.[43] Most importantly, compared with the traditionally used anticholinergic medications, β_3-agonism results in a significantly lower rate of dry mouth, constipation, and cognitive decline.

Estrogen

The role of estrogen in the relief of UUI is poorly understood. Initial data from large observational studies suggested that estrogen replacement resulted in worsening of urinary symptoms.[44–46] However, a meta-analysis of 11 randomized controlled trials (RCTs) of estrogen therapy found that estrogen replacement resulted in a significant improvement in frequency, urgency, nocturia, and UUI episodes,[47] with the greatest effect seen through the use of transvaginal topical estrogen replacement. The authors currently recommend the use of vaginal estrogen in the setting of vaginal mucosal atrophy without prior history of hormonally sensitive malignancy.

Other Medications

Several other medication classes have been proposed or used for the treatment of UUI. Specifically, duloxetine, a serotonin and norepinephrine reuptake inhibitor, and imipramine have been studied for the treatment of incontinence. Duloxetine, which has compelling evidence for use, is not currently approved for this indication in the United States, and as such will not be discussed. In addition, imipramine, which has been used for many years for the treatment of UI, has not been studied in RCTs. It has potential risks in vulnerable populations, particularly with regard to anticholinergic effects. The authors do not recommend its routine use, particularly in elderly patients.

Stress Urinary Incontinence

Because SUI is a manifestation of decreased outlet resistance, the target of pharmacotherapy is aimed at increasing bladder outlet resistance. The pharmacology of the lower urinary react offers several potential targets for the treatment of SUI. Pharmacologic options toward this end are limited, and results of trials targeting outlet resistance have generated mixed results. The International Consultation on Incontinence (ICI) does not recommend any medications for the treatment of SUI,[8] and no medications are currently approved in the United States for this purpose.

NONPHARMACOLOGIC STRATEGIES
Pelvic Floor Muscle Training

In the nonoperative management of UI, pelvic floor muscle training (PFMT) has been long considered a mainstay of therapy. Initially described in 1948, Kegel exercises were used to restore pelvic floor strength in an effort to reduce UI and included the use of biofeedback through a perineometer.[48] Today, PFMT is a broad term used to describe any program of pelvic floor strengthening where the aim is to reduce incontinence.

Women with UI often have pelvic floor dysfunction,[49–51] and the goal of PFMT is to strengthen the pelvic floor support. The literature supporting the success of PFMT is varied largely because of the heterogeneity in the patient groups, types of PFMT used, and the metrics used to measure success. Despite this variability, a *Cochrane Review* performed to evaluate the effect of PFMT demonstrated significant improvements in voiding (1 fewer incontinent episode and 3 fewer voids per day) and quality of life.[52] Although there is clearly a benefit to PFMT, the effectiveness of the training and compliance with regimens is paramount to success. Patients must be carefully selected for PFMT based on ability to participate in training programs. This consideration is particularly important in the geriatric population, where cognitive decline may make treatment adherence a challenge. However, there is evidence supporting its use in the motivated elder patient.[53]

Types of training used vary widely, and in the *Cochrane Review* previously mentioned, techniques used included clinician observed training, strength training, motor relearning exercises, and endurance training.[54] The current recommendations from the ICI[55] are that PFMT be offered as first-line therapy in the management of UI (grade A) and that it should be performed under the direction of a clinician. Although there is no standardized method of performing PFMT, a program suggested by Hay-Smith and colleagues[55] is to perform 8 to 12 contractions of 6- to 8-second duration 5 times per day. The investigator suggests that each set be concluded with a series of 5 to 10 rapid contractions. In addition, in patients with a predominate urge symptom, instructions are made to perform several fast pelvic floor contractions, called quick flicks, at the time of urgency to suppress the micturition reflex.[56]

Regardless of the PFMT technique used, the initial training should be performed by a clinician. However, despite adequate education, not all women will be able to consistently reproduce the exercises as taught,[57] and through referral to a trained physical therapist, meaningful improvement can occur.[58,59] In addition, biofeedback may be used either with clinician feedback during examination or with mechanical devices in order to reinforce exercises,[60–62] the use of which has been shown to improve outcomes even in the incontinent elder patient.[63] In a meta-analysis of PFMT with and without biofeedback, there was a significant improvement in subjective outcomes in women treated with biofeedback, particularly those where the clinician was involved.[64] Currently, the ICI does not advocate the routine use of biofeedback in the application of PFMT.[55] However, in the authors' experience, biofeedback, particularly under the direction of a trained physical therapist, can result in excellent outcomes in the motivated older patient whereby a more active treatment program is useful.

Mechanical Devices

Although initially described for use in pelvic organ prolapse, pessaries have excellent data regarding their utility in the incontinent patient. Traditional pessary use in women with pelvic organ prolapse and concomitant incontinence is associated with significant improvements in incontinent episodes.[65] Based on these data, incontinence-specific pessaries have been created, such as Uresta, and in small trials have excellent effectiveness on incontinence outcomes.[66]

Important in the utilization of a pessary for incontinence is patient selection and understanding of the device sizing. Patients must be selected by their understanding of the importance of pessary removal[67] and must have adequate hand dexterity for replacement. In the authors' practice, they pretreat all postmenopausal women who have vaginal atrophy with estrogen cream unless there is a contraindication because of prior breast or uterine cancer. They additionally instruct women to come to the fitting session with a moderately full bladder, which allows testing of the efficacy of the pessary. Women are asked to mimic vigorous activity in the clinic area, such as brisk walking, jumping jacks, squatting, or straining, to ensure that the device is effective and comfortable, and that it does not come out with physical activity.

Other devices for UI exist, which include disposable urethral inserts and urethral patches.[68,69] Currently, the only product available in the United States is the Fem-Soft,[70] a urethral insert, which in prospective study demonstrated significant reduction in incontinent episodes, pad weights, and improvements in quality-of-life scores. The disadvantage to this device is the relatively high rate of urinary tract infection at 31%. Patients best suited for this device are those who can prospectively identify times of incontinence, such as with exercise, and require adequate dexterity for placement.

Catheters

Although some physicians use catheters for the control of incontinence, the authors generally only recommend their use in temporizing situations where perineal dryness, such as when treating a decubitus ulcer is required, or in cases where essentially no other option is feasible because of body habitus or other situations.

SELF-MANAGEMENT STRATEGIES
General Principles

Patients who are willing and able to modify behaviors should be counseled on options that may reduce incontinent episodes (**Table 4**). After identification of potentially modifiable behaviors, plans should be relayed to not only the patient but also caregivers. This communication is especially important in the setting of patients residing in a residential or long-term care facility and is of particular importance in the setting of functional incontinence, where careful attention to reduction of barriers to the voiding process can result in substantial improvements in the voiding pattern of these patients. Commonly used strategies in this setting include prompted voiding, bedside commodes, and use of nonrestrictive clothing.

Table 4
Self-management strategies for urinary incontinence

Risk Factor	Modification	Type of Incontinence	Level of Evidence
Voiding pattern	Timed and double voiding	All types	Level II
Smoking	Cessation	UUI and SUI	Level III
Caffeine intake	Reduction in caffeine intake	UUI	Level III
Fluid intake	Reduction in excess fluid intake	All types	Level III
Obesity	Weight reduction	SUI	Level Ib
Constipation	Improved fecal function	All types	Level III

Voiding Hygiene

Disturbed voiding patterns are a common finding in the incontinent adult. Although there is a paucity of evidence regarding the appropriate approach to retraining the bladder, current guidelines from the ICI recommend voiding hygiene with a grade A recommendation as first line in the management of the incontinent adult.[55] The approach to bladder retraining varies in the literature. The authors recommend counseling patients and caregivers on the need for a maximal voiding interval of 2 to 3 hours with an emphasis on ensuring complete emptying through double-voiding, defined as attempting a second void immediately following the initial void.

Smoking Cessation

Smoking as a modifiable target for incontinence control has been assessed in numerous studies[71–74] with mixed results and has led to an inability of the ICI to make a recommendation regarding smoking cessation.[55] Despite this, there is evidence supporting an increased risk of SUI and urgent urinary symptoms in women who smoke,[73,74] and progression to COPD is associated with a 2-fold increase in SUI.[75] As such, the authors routinely recommend smoking cessation in women with UI.

Dietary Modifications

Caffeine

Caffeine acts as a diuretic and a stimulant that exerts an effect on voiding through multiple pathways.[76] Cross-sectional studies have demonstrated an increased risk of incontinence in women who consume caffeine,[77,78] and studies assessing the effect of caffeine reduction have shown a concomitant decrease in incontinent episodes.[79]

Fluid intake

Voiding frequency is dependent on the volume of fluid intake. Many patients self-restrict fluid intake in an effort to reduce frequency of voids and incontinent episodes; however, there is a theoretic risk of increased urgency with concentrated urine.[80] Testing this effect of fluid intake, Hashim and Abrams[81] performed a crossover trial of fluid reduction and fluid increase and found that a reduction of 25% resulted in improvements in urinary urgency and frequency. However, using the Nurses' Health Study data, Townsend and colleagues[82] found no association with fluid intake and number of incontinent episodes, suggesting that although fluid intake is important, there is no absolute volume cutoff to use in counseling patients. The authors recommend an assessment of fluid intake using a frequency-volume chart and carefully adjust fluid intake based on associated comorbid conditions.

Weight loss

Obesity is a well-documented risk factor for incontinence,[83] with body mass index related to the degree of urinary leakage.[84] In addition, weight gain has been shown to be associated with the development of incontinence.[85] Most notable is that although obesity and weight gain are associated with the risk of incontinence, weight loss has been shown to result in significant improvements of continence in randomized controlled clinical trials.[86] This finding seems to be durable over long follow-up times.[87]

Bowel habits

The anatomy and neural control of the pelvis are complex and closely interconnected. This relationship becomes important when evaluating the incontinent patient with fecal symptoms. In correlative studies, there is an association between constipation and

UI.[88,89] Urodynamic studies of patients with constipation revealed lower bladder volumes; however, this finding did not reveal an effect on UI.[90] Although the literature regarding this topic does not implicate fecal symptoms as causative of UI, addressing fecal symptoms at the time of urinary evaluation may potentially lead to improvements in urinary control and overall quality of life.

CLINICAL FOLLOW-UP

After introduction of an intervention for UI, follow-up evaluation should be arranged 8 to 12 weeks later.[8] During follow-up, voiding diaries and validated questionnaires can be useful in the assessment of treatment response. Importantly, the authors recommend assessment of treatment adherence before alteration of treatment plan during follow-up. The treatment of incontinence is often a lengthy process, and it is important to stress to patients that several visits may be required to garner a significant improvement in symptoms. However, it is reasonable to offer referral to a specialist in the setting of persistent treatment failure or patient dissatisfaction.

SUMMARY AND RECOMMENDATIONS

UI is a prevalent problem in the geriatric population, which is made more complex by comorbid conditions and polypharmacy. Physicians caring for elderly patients should be cognizant of the multifactorial nature of incontinence and the options available for the treatment of these patients. The authors recommend the following:

- Careful history and physical examination
- Optimization of comorbid conditions and chronic medications
- Behavioral modification early in the management of incontinence
- Judicious use of pharmacotherapy
- Follow-up assessment after 8 to 12 weeks of attempted treatment with the use of validated questionnaires and voiding diaries
- Selective referral to specialists in the treatment of female UI when
  - Managing the complex incontinent patient
  - Treatment failure occurs

REFERENCES

1. Bresee C, Dubina ED, Khan AA, et al. Prevalence and correlates of urinary incontinence among older community-dwelling women. Female Pelvic Med Reconstr Surg 2014;20(6):328–33.
2. Hung KJ, Awtrey CS, Tsai AC. Urinary incontinence, depression, and economic outcomes in a cohort of women between the ages of 54 and 65 years. Obstet Gynecol 2014;123:822–7.
3. Sampselle CM, Harlow SD, Skurnick J, et al. Urinary incontinence predictors and life impact in ethnically diverse perimenopausal women. Obstet Gynecol 2002; 100:1230–8.
4. Morrison A, Levy R. Fraction of nursing home admission attributable to urinary incontinence. Value Health 2006;9:272.
5. Coyne KS, Wein A, Nicholson S. Economic burden of urgency urinary incontinence in the United States: a systematic review. J Manag Care Pharm 2014;20:130–40.
6. Haylen BT, de Ridder D, Freeman RM, et al. International Urogynecological Association, International Continence Society: an International Urogynecological

Association (IUGA)/International Continence Society (ICS) joint report on the terminology for female pelvic floor dysfunction. Neurourol Urodyn 2010;29:4–20.

7. van Leijsen SA, Hoogstad-van Evert JS, Mol BW, et al. The correlation between clinical and urodynamic diagnosis in classifying the type of urinary incontinence in women. A systematic review of the literature. Neurourol Urodyn 2011;30: 495–502.

8. Abrams P, Andersson KE, Birder L, et al. Fourth International Consultation on Incontinence Recommendations of the International Scientific Committee: evaluation and treatment of urinary incontinence, pelvic organ prolapse, and fecal incontinence. Neurourol Urodyn 2010;29:213–40.

9. Abrams P, Cardozo L, Khoury S, et al. International Consultation on Incontinence. 3rd edition. Plymouth (UK): Health Publications Ltd; 2005.

10. Gibbs CF, Johnson TM, Ouslander JG. Office management of geriatric incontinence. Am J Med 2007;120:211–20.

11. Griffiths AN, Makam A, Edwards GJ. Should we actively screen for urinary and anal incontinence in the general gynaecology outpatient setting? A prospective observational study. J Obstet Gynaecol 2006;26:442–4.

12. Brown JS, Bradley CS, Subak LL. The sensitivity and specificity of a simple test to distinguish between urge and stress urinary incontinence. Ann Intern Med 2006; 144(10):715–23.

13. Kirschner-Hermanns R, Scherr PA, Branch LG. Accuracy of survey questions for geriatric urinary incontinence. J Urol 1998;159(6):1903–8.

14. American Geriatrics Society 2012 Beers Criteria Update Expert Panel. American Geriatrics Society updated Beers Criteria for potentially inappropriate medication use in older adults. J Am Geriatr Soc 2012;60(4):616–31.

15. Goode PS, Burgio KL, Richter HS. Incontinence in older women. JAMA 2010; 303(21):2172–81.

16. Wood LN, Anger JT. Urinary incontinence in women. BMJ 2014;349:g4531.

17. DeMaagd G. Urinary incontinence: treatment update with a focus on pharmacologic management. US Pharm 2007;32(6):1257–62.

18. Maman K, Aballea S, Nazir J. Comparative efficacy and safety of medical treatments for the management of overactive bladder: a systematic literature review and mixed treatment comparison. Eur Urol 2014;65:755–65.

19. Thüroff JW, Chartier E, Corcus J, et al. Medical treatment and medical side effects in urinary incontinence in the elderly. World J Urol 1998;16(Suppl 1):S48–61.

20. Gupta SK, Sathyan G. Pharmacokinetics of an oral once a day controlled-release oxybutynin formulation compared with immediate-release oxybutynin. J Clin Pharmacol 1999;39:289–96.

21. Dmochowski RR, Nitti V, Staskin D, et al. Transdermal oxybutynin in the treatment of adults with overactive bladder: combined results of two randomized clinical trials. World J Urol 2005;23:263–70.

22. Pizzi LT, Talati A, Gemmen E, et al. Impact of transdermal oxybutynin on work productivity in patients with overactive bladder: results from the MATRIX study. Pharmacoeconomics 2009;27:329–39.

23. Goldfischer ER, Sand PK, Thomas H, et al. Efficacy and safety of oxybutynin topical gel 3% in patients with urgency and/or mixed urinary incontinence: a randomized, double-blind placebo controlled study. Neurourol Urodyn 2013;34(1): 37–43.

24. Elinoff V, Bavendam T, Glasser DB, et al. Symptom-specific efficacy of tolterodine extended release in patients with overactive bladder: the IMPACT trial. Int J Clin Pract 2006;60:745–51.

25. Diokno AC, Appell RA, Sand PK, et al, OPERA Study Group. Prospective, randomized, double-blind study of the efficacy and tolerability of the extended-release formulations of oxybutynin and tolterodine for overactive bladder: results of the OPERA trial. Mayo Clin Proc 2003;78:687–95.

26. Diefenbach K, Jaeger K, Wollny A, et al. Effect of tolterodine on sleep structure modulated by CYP2D6 genotype. Sleep Med 2008;9:579–82.

27. Khullar V, Rovner ES, Dmochowski R, et al. Fesoterodine dose response in subjects with overactive bladder syndrome. Urology 2008;71:839–43.

28. Halaska M, Ralph G, Wiedemann A, et al. Controlled, double-blind, multicenter clinical trial to investigate long-term tolerability and efficacy of trospium chloride in patients with detrusor instability. World J Urol 2003;20:392–9.

29. Haab F, Stewart L, Dwyer P. Darifenacin, an M3 selective receptor antagonist, is an effective and well tolerated once daily treatment for overactive bladder. Eur Urol 2004;45:420–9.

30. Lipton RB, Kolodner K, Wesnes K. Assessment of cognitive function of the elderly population: effects of darifenacin. J Urol 2005;173:493–8.

31. Cardozo L, Lisec M, Millard R, et al. Randomized, double-blind placebo controlled trial of the once daily antimuscarinic agent solifenacin succinate in patients with overactive bladder. J Urol 2004;172(pt 1):1919–24.

32. Wagg A, Dale M, Tretter R, et al. Randomised, multicentre, placebo-controlled, double-blind crossover study investigating the effect of solifenacin and oxybutynin in elderly people with mild cognitive impairment: the SENIOR Study. Eur Urol 2013;64(1):74–81.

33. Herschorn S, Barkin J, Castro-Diaz D, et al. A phase III, randomized, double-blind, parallel-group, placebo-controlled, multicentre study to assess the efficacy and safety of the β_3 adrenoceptor agonist, mirabegron, in patients with symptoms of overactive bladder. Urology 2013;82(2):313–20.

34. Smith AL, Wein AJ. Urinary incontinence: pharmacotherapy options. Ann Med 2011;43:461–76.

35. Madhurvata P, Cody JD, Ellis G, et al. Which anticholinergic drug for overactive bladder symptoms in adults. Cochrane Database Syst Rev 2012;(1):CD005429.

36. Benner JS, Nichol MB, Rovner ES. Patient-reported reasons for discontinuing overactive bladder medication. BJU Int 2010;105:1276–82.

37. Guay DR. Clinical pharmacokinetics of drugs used to treat urge incontinence. Clin Pharmacokinet 2003;42:1243–85.

38. Tsao JW, Heilman KM. Transient memory impairment and hallucinations associated with tolterodine use. N Engl J Med 2003;349:2274–5.

39. Debeau CE, Kraus SR, Griebling TL. Effect of fesoterodine in vulnerable elderly subjects with urgency incontinence: a double-blind placebo controlled trial. J Urol 2014;191(2):395–404.

40. Hersch L, Salzman B. Clinical management of urinary incontinence in women. Am Fam Physician 2013;87:634–40.

41. Imran M, Najmi AK, Tabrez S. Mirabegron for overactive bladder: a novel, first-in-class beta3-agonist therapy. Urol J 2013;10(3):935–40.

42. Bridgeman MB, Friia NJ, Taft C, et al. Mirabegron: B_3-adrenergic receptor agonist for the treatment of overactive bladder. Ann Pharmacother 2013;47:1029–38.

43. Wagg A, Cardozo L, Nitti VW, et al. The efficacy and tolerability of the beta3-adrenoceptor agonist mirabegron for the treatment of symptoms of overactive bladder in older patients. Age Ageing 2014;43(5):666–75.

44. Grady D, Brown JS, Vittinghoff E, et al. Postmenopausal hormones and incontinence: the Heart and Estrogen/Progestin Replacement Study. Obstet Gynecol 2001;97:116–20.
45. Grodstein F, Lifford K, Resnick NM, et al. Postmenopausal hormone therapy and risk of developing urinary incontinence. Obstet Gynecol 2004;103:254–60.
46. Hendrix SL, Cochrane BB, Nygaard IE, et al. Effects of estrogen with and without progestin on urinary incontinence. JAMA 2005;293:935–48.
47. Cardozo L, Lose G, McClish D, et al. A systematic review of the effects of estrogens for symptoms suggestive of overactive bladder. Acta Obstet Gynecol Scand 2004;83:892–7.
48. Kegel AH. Progressive resistance exercise in the function and restoration of the perineal muscles. Am J Obstet Gynecol 1948;56:238.
49. Gunnarsson M, Teleman P, Mattiasson A, et al. Effects of pelvic floor exercises in middle aged women with a history of naïve urinary incontinence: a population based study. Eur Urol 2002;41:556–61.
50. Teleman PM, Mattiasson A. Urethral pressure response patterns induced by squeeze in continent and incontinent women. Int Urogynecol J Pelvic Floor Dysfunct 2007;18:1027–31.
51. Shishido K, Peng Q, Jones R, et al. Influence of pelvic floor muscle contraction on the profile of vaginal closure pressure in continent and stress urinary incontinent women. J Urol 2008;179:1917–22.
52. Dumoulin C, Hay-Smith J. Pelvic floor muscle training versus no treatment, or inactive control treatments, for urinary incontinence in women. Cochrane Database Syst Rev 2010;(1):CD005654.
53. Betschart C, Mol SE, Lütolf-Keller B, et al. Pelvic floor muscle training for urinary incontinence: a comparison of outcomes in premenopausal versus postmenopausal women. Female Pelvic Med Reconstr Surg 2013;19:219–24.
54. Dumoulin C, Glazener C, Jenkinson D. Determining the optimal pelvic floor muscle training regimen for women with stress urinary incontinence. Neurourol Urodyn 2011;30:746–53.
55. Hay-Smith J, Berghmans B, Burgio K. Adult conservative management. In: Abrams P, Cardozo L, Khoury S, et al, editors. Incontinence. 4th edition. Plymouth (United Kingdom): Health Publications, Ltd; 2009. p. 1025–120.
56. Burgio KL. Update on behavioral and physical therapies for incontinence and overactive bladder: the role of pelvic floor muscle training. Curr Urol Rep 2013;14:457–64.
57. Sampselle C, Messer KL, Seng JS, et al. Learning outcomes of a group behavioral modification program to prevent urinary incontinence. Int Urogynecol J 2005;16:441–6.
58. Zanetti MR, Castro Rde A, Rotta AL, et al. Impact of supervised physiotherapeutic pelvic floor exercises for treating female stress urinary incontinence. Sao Paulo Med J 2007;125:265–9.
59. Felicíssimo MF, Carneiro MM, Saleme CS, et al. Intensive supervised versus unsupervised pelvic floor muscle training for the treatment of stress urinary incontinence: a randomized comparative trial. Int Urogynecol J 2010;21:835–40.
60. Doumouchtis SK, Jeffrey S, Fynes M. Female voiding dysfunction. Obstet Gynecol Surv 2008;63:519–26.
61. Pages IH, Jahr S, Schaufele MK, et al. Comparative analysis of biofeedback and physical therapy for treatment of urinary stress incontinence in women. Am J Phys Med Rehabil 2001;80:494–502.

62. Aukee P, Immonen P, Laaksonen D, et al. The effect of home biofeedback training on stress incontinence. Acta Obstet Gynecol Scand 2004;83:973–7.

63. Burgio KL, Goode PS, Locher JL, et al. Behavioral training with and without biofeedback in the treatment of urge incontinence in older women: a randomized controlled trial. JAMA 2002;288:2293–9.

64. Herderschee R, Hay-Smith EJ, Herbison GP, et al. Feedback or biofeedback to augment pelvic floor muscle training for urinary incontinence in women. Cochrane Database Syst Rev 2011;(7):CD009252.

65. Noblett KL, McKinney A, Lane FL. Effects of the incontinence dish pessary on urethral support and urodynamic parameters. Am J Obstet Gynecol 2008;198:592.

66. Farrell SA, Baydock S, Baharak A, et al. Effectiveness of new self-positioning pessary for the management of urinary incontinence in women. Am J Obstet Gynecol 2007;196:474.e1–8.

67. Wu V, Farrell SA, Baskett TF, et al. A simplified protocol for pessary management. Obstet Gynecol 1997;90:990–4.

68. Robinson H, Schulz J, Flood C, et al. A randomized controlled trial of the NEAT expandable tip continence device. Int Urogynecol J Pelvic Floor Dysfunct 2002;14:199–203.

69. Versi E, Griffiths DJ, Harvey M. A new external urethral occlusive device for female urinary incontinence. Obstet Gynecol 1998;92:286–91.

70. Sirls LT, Foote JE, Kaufman JM, et al. Long-term results of the FemSoft urethral insert for the management of female stress urinary incontinence. Int Urogynecol J Pelvic Floor Dysfunct 2002;13:88–95.

71. Luber KM. The definition, prevalence, and risk factors for stress urinary incontinence. Rev Urol 2004;6(Suppl 3):S3–9.

72. Minassian VA, Stewart WF, Wood GC. Urinary incontinence in women: variation in prevalence estimates and risk factors. Obstet Gynecol 2008;111:324–31.

73. Richter HE, Burgio KL, Brubaker L, et al. Factors associated with incontinence frequency in a surgical cohort of stress incontinent women. Am J Obstet Gynecol 2005;193:2088–93.

74. Dallosso HM, McGrother CW, Matthews RJ, et al. The association of diet and other lifestyle factors with overactive bladder and stress incontinence: a longitudinal study in women. BJU Int 2003;92:69–77.

75. Hrisanfow E, Hagglund D. The prevalence of urinary incontinence among women and men with chronic obstructive pulmonary disease in Sweden. J Clin Nurs 2011;20:1895–905.

76. Cho YS, Ko GK, Kim SE, et al. Caffeine enhances micturition through neuronal activation in micturition centers. Mol Med Rep 2014;10:2931–6.

77. Gleason JL, Richter HE, Redden DT, et al. Caffeine and urinary incontinence in US women. Int Urogynecol J 2013;24:295–302.

78. Jura YH, Townsend MK, Curham GC, et al. Caffeine intake and the risk of stress, urgency, and mixed urinary incontinence. J Urol 2011;185:1775–80.

79. Tomlinson BU, Dougherty MC, Pendergast JF, et al. Dietary caffeine, fluid intake and urinary incontinence in older rural women. Int Urogynecol J Pelvic Floor Dysfunct 1999;10:22–8.

80. Juszczak J, Ziomber A, Wyczółkowski M, et al. Hyperosmolarity alters micturition: a comparison of urinary bladder motor activity in hyperosmolar and cyclophosphamide-induced models of overactive bladder. Can J Physiol Pharmacol 2010;89(9):899–906.

81. Hashim H, Abrams P. How should patients with an overactive bladder manipulate their fluid intake? BJU Int 2008;102:62–6.

82. Townsend MK, Jura YH, Curhan GC, et al. Fluid intake and the risk of stress, urgency, and mixed urinary incontinence. Am J Obstet Gynecol 2011;205(1): 73.e1–6.
83. Melville JL, Katon W, Delaney K, et al. Urinary incontinence in US women. Arch Intern Med 2005;165:537–42.
84. Hannestad YS, Rortveit G, Daltveit AK, et al. Are smoking and other lifestyle factors associated with female urinary incontinence? The Norwegian EPINCONT Study. Br J Obstet Gynaecol 2003;110:247–54.
85. Townsend MK, Danforth KN, Rosner B, et al. Body mass index, weight gain, and incident urinary incontinence in middle-aged women. Obstet Gynecol 2007;110: 346–53.
86. Subak LL, Wing R, West DS, et al. Weight loss to treat urinary incontinence in overweight and obese women. N Engl J Med 2009;360:481–90.
87. Wing RR, West DS, Grady D, et al. Effect of weight loss on urinary incontinence in overweight and obese women: results at 12 and 18 months. J Urol 2010;184: 1005–10.
88. Raza-Khan F, Cunkelman J, Lowenstein L, et al. Prevalence of bowel symptoms in women with pelvic floor disorders. Int Urogynecol J 2010;21:933–8.
89. Spence-Jones C, Kamm MA, Henry MM, et al. Bowel dysfunction: a pathogenic factor in uterovaginal prolapse and urinary stress incontinence. Br J Obstet Gynaecol 1994;101:147–52.
90. Panayi DC, Khullar V, Digesu GA, et al. Rectal distension: the effect on bladder function. Neurourol Urodyn 2011;30:344–7.

Outcomes of Surgery for Stress Urinary Incontinence in the Older Woman

David R. Ellington, MD[a], Elisabeth A. Erekson, MD, MPH[b],
Holly E. Richter, PhD, MD[a],*

KEYWORDS

- Age-related outcomes • Stress urinary incontinence • Older women
- Urogynecology • Urology • Counseling

KEY POINTS

- Women aged 65 years and older have many unique age-related concerns that are critical to optimizing patient care and surgical outcomes.
- Older women may have increased comorbidities, resulting in decreased physical reserve. Careful preoperative evaluation is paramount to avoid adverse geriatric postoperative outcomes that often include falls, disability, nursing home admission, and mortality.
- Several minimally invasive surgical interventions exist for the treatment of stress urinary incontinence (SUI) and are well tolerated in older women. Balancing the risks and benefits of each of these management options is imperative.
- Differences in surgical outcomes between older and younger women may reflect changing physiology with aging. Robust patient counseling regarding available data may inform to patient expectations of outcomes.
- As the population of older women continues to expand, robust data on age-related outcomes of SUI interventions are needed to enhance patient counseling and outcomes.

CRITICAL NEED FOR AGE-RELATED OUTCOMES
Introduction: Context for Understanding Age-Related Surgical Outcomes

Prevalence rates of urinary incontinence (UI) increase with age. A large secondary analysis of the National Health and Nutrition Examination study revealed that the proportion of women who reported UI symptoms increased from 6.9% (95% confidence

[a] Division of Urogynecology and Pelvic Reconstructive Surgery, University of Alabama at Birmingham, 176 F Suite 10382, 619 19th Street South, Birmingham, AL 35249-7333, USA; [b] Division of Female Pelvic Medicine and Reconstructive Surgery, The Geisel School of Medicine at Dartmouth, 1 Medical Center Drive, Lebanon, NH 03756, USA
* Corresponding author.
E-mail address: hrichter@uabmc.edu

Clin Geriatr Med 31 (2015) 487–505
http://dx.doi.org/10.1016/j.cger.2015.06.006
0749-0690/15/$ – see front matter © 2015 Elsevier Inc. All rights reserved.
geriatric.theclinics.com

interval [CI], 4.9%–9.0%) in women aged 20 to 39 years, to 17.2% (95% CI, 13.9%–20.5%) in women aged 40 to 59 years, to 23.3% (95% CI, 17.0%–29.7%) in women aged 60 to 79 years, and to 31.7% (95% CI, 22.3%–41.2%; P<.001) in women aged 80 years or older.[1] Furthermore, as the US population aged 65 years and older continues to increase, women will be seeking surgical care for this condition in increasing numbers.[2–5]

Older women (aged ≥65 years) have many more concerns with respect to undergoing SUI surgery compared with younger women. Increasing medical morbidities including cardiac arrhythmias, use of blood thinners, diabetes, and hypertension require optimization before surgery. Older women have an increased risk of postoperative morbidity and mortality compared with the younger woman.[6] Risk of perioperative complications were also noted to be higher in women aged 80 years or older compared with the younger woman (odds ratio [OR], 1.4; 95% CI, 1.3–1.5). Attention to cognitive and functional outcomes as well as quality of life are also important to consider in this population.

Bladder physiology and function also changes with age.[7,8] In a recent study of 2 large cohorts of women undergoing SUI surgery, noninvasive maximum urinary flow decreased significantly with age (26.2 vs 22 mL/s, P = .002). Noninvasive flow voiding time increased by 2.7 seconds for each 10-year age increment, and detrusor pressure at maximum flow decreased by 2.1 cm H_2O for each 10-year increase in age (each P = .003). Hypocontractility was more likely in women aged 65 years or older (OR, 2.89; 95% CI, 1.59–5.27). The bladder contractility index was inversely related to age, decreasing by a mean ± standard deviation of 7.68 ± 1.96 cm H_2O for each 10-year age increase (P<.001). These observed changes in voiding parameters suggest that detrusor contractility and efficiency decrease with age and will have implications for management of postoperative voiding function.

In the older woman, outcomes of surgery reflect all these considerations and not just a negative result of cough stress test. This review discusses outcomes and other important considerations in the setting of SUI surgery in the older woman.

PERIOPERATIVE CONSIDERATIONS AND EVALUATION IN OLDER WOMEN
Pathophysiological Changes to the Lower Urinary Tract

Urinary symptoms, including urinary frequency, urinary urgency, nocturia, and UI are common conditions in older women and increase dramatically with age. The underlying cause for the age-related onset of urinary symptoms is not completely understood, but it is likely multifactorial, resulting from sensory changes in the aging detrusor muscle, muscle loss of the levator ani muscle and urethral sphincter, physiologic changes in urine production, concurrent medications, and coexisting neurologic disease.[9] As women age, bladder capacity, detrusor contraction pressure during micturition, functional urethral length, and maximal urethral closure pressure decrease, whereas postvoid residual nocturnal urine production increases.[10–12]

Increased UI in the older woman is often not only due to sensory and muscle loss in the lower urinary tract but also due to a combination of systemic disease and functional decline affecting the lower urinary tract. Decreased mobility also affects urinary symptoms. Functional UI is "from physical or cognitive limitations [that prevent a person from] reaching or using the toilet" and common in older women.[13]

UI in older women is often considered a geriatric syndrome.[14] Geriatric syndromes are highly prevalent multifactorial health conditions that have substantial morbidity and are associated with adverse outcomes of aging in older adults including disability, nursing home admission, and mortality. Other common geriatric syndromes include delirium, falls, dizziness, and frailty. UI and functional dependence share many common risk factors, and functional dependence has been demonstrated to be highly prevalent among older women with UI.[15,16] Studies examining adverse outcomes of aging demonstrate UI to be associated with increased mortality; however, after adjusting for other comorbid conditions, incontinence was not demonstrated to be an independent predictor of mortality.[17] Because UI is not an independent predictor of mortality, incontinence is unique compared with other geriatric syndromes directly linked with increased mortality.

Preoperative Evaluation of the Lower Urinary Tract

Evaluation of women presenting with symptoms of SUI should include questions about the type of incontinence (leakage with stress maneuvers, urgency, continuous leakage, or leakage without awareness) (**Table 1**). Precipitating events, frequency of occurrence, severity, pad use, the impact of symptoms on activities of daily living (ADL), and prior antiincontinence procedures should be documented. Physical examination should include demonstration of urine leakage with visualization of leakage from the urethra with stress maneuvers/cough termed a cough stress test.[18]

Evaluation should also include assessment for pelvic organ prolapse past the vaginal introitus, assessment for urethral mobility, postvoid residual, and urine analysis/urine culture to evaluate for the presence of hematuria and/or infection. Careful history and examination, especially a thorough review of patient medications, can determine if women have uncomplicated or complicated SUI (**Table 2**).

Women with uncomplicated SUI without hematuria do not generally require urodynamic testing before considering surgical options.[19] Women with complicated SUI may benefit from additional testing including urodynamic testing or cystoscopy and upper urinary tract imaging if microscopic hematuria is present.[20]

Preoperative Evaluation of the Geriatric Patient

Preoperative medical risk assessments should include a comprehensive cardiac history and can help to identify patients who will benefit from preoperative cardiac testing (stress test or coronary angiography) and perioperative β-blocker use. The exact timing of initiation and duration of therapy is still under debate.[21,22] Medical evaluation to optimize medical comorbidities and identify modifiable risk factors is recommended.[23] Interventions to this effect include polypharmacy reduction, substance abuse interventions, smoking cessation, nutritional improvement, and preoperative activity increase to increase aerobic capacity before anesthesia.

There is a growing body of evidence demonstrating that combining measurements of frailty, functional status, mobility, and cognitive function are important predictors of surgical outcomes and have increased prognostic ability to predict postoperative complications after surgery better than medical comorbidities or American Society of Anesthesiologists status alone.[24–29] Frailty is a common biological syndrome of decreased reserve and resistance to stressors that increases with age.[30] Markers of frailty can be measured before an overt functional disability (decline in functional status and increased functional dependence) is evident.[24,30] A joint best practice guideline statement from the American College of Surgeons and the American Geriatrics Society recommends that, in addition to routine assessment and optimization of medical conditions, all older adults undergoing surgical procedures should be assessed for frailty, cognitive ability, and functional status in the preoperative period.[23]

To streamline geriatric preoperative assessment, Robinson and colleagues[27] developed a simple predictive tool combining clinical measures of frailty with cognitive status and functional disability. This preoperative assessment tool includes 6

Table 1
Basic evaluation findings for uncomplicated versus complicated SUI

Evaluation	Findings	
	Uncomplicated	Complicated
History[a]	UI associated with involuntary loss of urine on effort, physical exertion, sneezing, or coughing	Symptoms of urgency, incomplete emptying, incontinence associated with chronic urinary retention, functional impairment, or continuous leakage
	Absence of recurrent urinary tract infection	Recurrent urinary tract infection[b]
	No prior extensive pelvic surgery No prior surgery for SUI	Previous extensive or radical pelvic surgery (eg, radical hysterectomy)
	—	Prior antiincontinence surgery or complex urethral surgery (eg, urethral diverticulectomy or urethrovaginal fistula repair)
	Absence of voiding symptoms	Presence of voiding symptoms: hesitancy, slow stream, intermittency, straining to void, spraying or urinary stream, feeling of incomplete voiding, need to immediately revoid, postmicturition leakage, position-dependent micturition, and dysuria
	Absence of medical conditions that can affect lower urinary tract function	Presence of neurologic disease, poorly controlled diabetes mellitus, or dementia
Physical examination	Absence of vaginal bulge beyond the hymen on examination Absence of urethral abnormality	Symptoms of vaginal bulge or known pelvic organ prolapse beyond the hymen confirmed by physical examination, presence of genitourinary fistula, or urethral diverticulum
Urethral mobility assessment	Presence of urethral mobility	Absence of urethral mobility
Postvoid residual urine volume	<150 mL	≥150 mL
Urinalysis/urine culture	Negative result for urinary tract infection or hematuria	—

[a] A complete list of the patient's medications (including nonprescription medications) should be obtained to determine whether individual drugs may be influencing the function of the bladder or urethra, which leads to urinary incontinence or voiding difficulties.
[b] Recurrent urinary tract infection is defined as 3 documented infections in 12 months or 2 documented infections in 6 months.
Adapted from American College of Obstetricians and Gynecologists and American Urogynecologic Society. Committee opinion: evaluation of uncomplicated stress urinary incontinence in women before surgical treatment. Number 603. Female Pelvic Med Reconstr Surg 2014;20(5):248–51; with permission.

measurements: Mini-Cog score, Charlson comorbidity index, functional disability, history of falls, preoperative serum albumin, and preoperative serum hematocrit. The Mini-Cog is a simple cognitive screening test that combines clock drawing with 3-object recall.[31] To assess for mobility, the Timed Get-Up-and-Go test has been

Table 2 Medications that can affect lower urinary tract function	
Type of Medication	**Lower Urinary Tract Effects**
Diuretics	Polyuria, frequency, urgency
Caffeine	Frequency, urgency
Alcohol	Sedation, impaired mobility, diuresis
Narcotic analgesics	Urinary retention, fecal impaction, sedation, delirium
Anticholinergic agents	Urinary retention, voiding difficulty
Antihistamines	Anticholinergic actions, sedation
Psychotropic agents	
Antidepressants	Anticholinergic actions, sedation
Antipsychotics	Anticholinergic actions, sedation
Sedatives and hypnotics	Sedation, muscle relaxation, confusion
α-adrenergic blockers	Stress incontinence
α-adrenergic agonists	Urinary retention, voiding difficulty
Calcium channel blockers	Urinary retention, voiding difficulty

Adapted from American College of Obstetricians and Gynecologists. Practice bulletin: urinary incontinence in women. Number 63. Obstet Gynecol 2005;105(6):1533–45; with permission.

advocated as a preferred measure and demonstrated by Robinson and colleagues[32] to be an effective predictor of postoperative complications (**Table 3**).[33] These simple screening tools have been proven to be impactful in vascular surgery, general surgery, and colorectal surgery.[25,26,32,34,35] More research needs to determine the impact of preoperative geriatric screening in older women undergoing surgery for UI on outcomes, both immediate postoperative complications and overall quality of life.

SURGICAL INTERVENTIONS AND OUTCOMES
Urethral Bulking Agents

Injectable agents, either injected transurethrally or periurethrally, to add bulk to the proximal urethra have been documented to improve SUI symptoms in women who either do not want to undergo more invasive surgery or who are not surgical candidates because of medical comorbidity. Advantages of injectable urethral bulking agents, especially in older women, include that this is a procedure easily performed in the office setting, that many women tolerate well without anesthesia, and that anticoagulation does not always need to be stopped before injections. Injectable agents are divided into 2 categories: collagen, which degrades over a 6- to 12-month period requiring repeat injections, and nondegradable synthetic agents. These synthetic agents are usually beads or particles of varying sizes and include silicone particles, calcium hydroxyapatite, carbon spheres, ethylene vinyl alcohol, and dextranomer hyaluronic acid.[36,37]

The American Urological Association review on efficacy of urethral bulking agents concluded that treatment efficacy for these agents was present but declined over time, with the anticipated efficacy of collagen injection being 48% at 12 to 23 months, decreasing to 32% at 24 to 47 months.[20]

Complications of bulking agents include urinary retention and urinary tract infection. The chances of allergic reaction to collagen is 4%, and skin testing to evaluate for possible allergic reaction is recommended before collagen injection.[20] Collagen is

Table 3
Preoperative assessments: the Robinson frailty index

Frailty Characteristic	Scale Explanation	Score	Cutoff Value	Points
Mini-Cog	3-item recall (1 point per item) paired with clock drawing test (2 points)	Scores range from 0 (impaired cognition) to 5 (normal cognition)	<4	1
Katz ADL score	1 point for each of the 6 basic ADLs that the patient is able to perform independently (bathing, dressing, toileting, transferring in or out of bed, walking, and feeding)	Scores range from 0 (totally dependent) to 6 (independent)	<6	1
Charlson comorbidity index	16-item medical comorbidity assessment	Scores range from 0 (no comorbid conditions) to 33 (severe comorbidity)	≥3	1
History of falls	Recorded answer to the question "How many times have you fallen in the last 6 mo"?	—	≥1 fall	1
Preoperative serum albumin	Indicative of poor nutritional status	—	≤3.3 g/dL	1
Preoperative serum hematocrit	Indicative of anemia of chronic disease	—	<35%	1
Timed-Up-and-Go test[a]	Patient sits in an armless chair and is timed to: 1. Rise from chair 2. Walk 10 ft 3. Turn around 4. Walk 10 ft 5. Sit back down in chair	≤10 s (fast) 11–14 s (intermediate) ≥15 s (slow)	≥15 s	—

[a] Walking aids are allowed, and no instructions are given to the patient about the use of their arms.

Adapted from Ferrucci L, Guralnik JM, Studenski S, et al. Designing randomized, controlled trials aimed at preventing or delaying functional decline and disability in frail, older persons: a consensus report. J Am Geriatr Soc 2004;52(4):625–34; and Robinson TN, Wu DS, Sauaia A, et al. Slower walking speed forecasts increased postoperative morbidity and 1-year mortality across surgical specialties. Ann Surg 2013;258(4):582–8; [discussion: 588–90].

currently not manufactured for use in the United States. There are also complications unique to nondegradable synthetic agents including bead migration with rare events such as distant arterial thrombosis reported, vaginal and urethral erosion, and periurethral abscess.[36–40] These complications vary depending on the properties of the nondegradable injection agent being used.

Burch Colposuspension and Pubovaginal (Autologous Rectus Fascia) Sling

Before the advent of today's minimally invasive midurethral sling (MUS) techniques, 2 of the most common surgical intervention options for the treatment of SUI were the Burch colposuspension and the pubovaginal sling. The Burch colposuspension was first described in the early 1960s and reported cure rates of almost 90%.[41,42] This procedure has been modified over the years, and currently, it involves the suspension of the anterior wall, at the level of the bladder neck, to the iliopectineal ligament.[43] In the pubovaginal sling, a strip of rectus fascia is harvested and positioned at the proximal urethra transvaginally. The upper portion of the sling is then secured to the rectus fascia with permanent sutures.[44] Both procedures have reported long-term cure rates of 70% to 85%.[45,46] The Stress Incontinence Surgical Treatment Efficacy Trial (SISTEr), a multicenter, randomized trial of women with uncomplicated SUI, compared the Burch colposuspension with the pubovaginal sling (autologous rectus fascia). The primary outcomes were success in terms of overall incontinence measures including a negative result of pad test, no UI on a 3-day diary, negative results of cough and Valsalva stress tests, and no re-treatment of the condition. At 24 months, success rates for women who underwent the pubovaginal sling operation were higher than those for women who underwent Burch colposuspension for the category-specific stress incontinence (66% vs 49%, $P<.01$); however, more women in the pubovaginal trial arm had urinary tract infections, difficulty voiding, and postoperative urgency urinary incontinence (UUI).[47]

Regarding age-related outcomes for these procedures, Carr and colleagues[48] reported a retrospective cohort of 19 women (aged >70 years) undergoing a modified pubovaginal (autologous rectus fascia) sling compared with 77 younger women with a mean follow-up of 22 months.[49] There were no reported differences in outcomes between the older-aged and control groups. A more robust study involving a planned secondary analysis of the SISTEr evaluated 2-year outcomes in older women (aged ≥65 years) versus younger women and revealed that older women were more likely to have a positive result of stress test at follow-up (OR, 3.7; 95% CI, 1.70–7.97; $P = .001$) and less subjective improvement in SUI and UUI measured by the Medical and Epidemiologic Social Aspects of Aging questionnaire.[50,51] In addition, there was no difference in postoperative adverse events, but older women were more likely to undergo surgical re-treatment for SUI.[50]

Despite the effectiveness of these minimally invasive MUS procedures, both the transvaginal, retropubic, tension-free vaginal tape (TVT) and the transobturator vaginal tape (TOT) are increasingly recognized as the gold standard of care for the surgical intervention and treatment of SUI. For the purposes of this review, the authors restrict the remaining portion of this discussion to these procedures.[52,53]

Midurethral Sling

MUSs using synthetic material for the treatment of female SUI were first described in 1996 by Ulmsten and colleagues.[52] These minimally invasive surgical procedures involve placement of a permanent mesh of knitted polypropylene by tactile sensation through the retropubic space at the level of the midurethra and eliminating the need for full dissection of the retropubic space or harvesting autologous fascia. The decreased dissection results in decreased surgical time and surgical site morbidity compared with other antiincontinence procedures. In 2001, an alternative route involving placement of the synthetic mesh through the obturator foramen was first described.[53] The rationale of the transobturator approach was to minimize the potential of inadvertent bladder and bowel perforation. A large randomized controlled equivalence trial of the retropubic and transobturator sling routes demonstrated equivalence of efficacy and safety of these 2 approaches.[54] Furthermore, in a large noninferiority randomized controlled trial (RCT), the results of the transobturator approach were noninferior to those of the retropubic sling.[55] Both of these MUS routes use minimal dissection and can be performed as outpatient procedures.

Long-term efficacy data exist for both MUS routes. A recent analysis of health care claims data within the United States over a 9-year period, which included 127, 848 sling surgeries (including pubovaginal slings), revealed that the cumulative incidence of repeat surgery was relatively low (13.0%; 95% CI, 11.7–14.3).[56] A recent report of 10-year subjective outcome from a retrospective cohort of 54 women who underwent retropubic (TVT) surgery for urodynamically confirmed SUI revealed that 65% of women in this cohort considered their condition cured.[57] In contrast, a cohort of 69 women who had undergone TVT for primary SUI reported subjective cure at 77%. The remainder of the cohort reported their condition as improved (20%), and only 3% regarded the operation as a failure.[58]

The minimally invasive nature of the MUS has increased the number of women, especially older women, who may be considered surgical candidates for antiincontinence procedures. Multiple retrospective and prospective cohorts have reported on favorable outcomes of older women undergoing these procedures (**Table 4**).

There are increasing numbers of age-related outcomes data for women undergoing MUS procedures for SUI. Recently, Stav and colleagues[71] reported a prospective trial of women undergoing MUS procedures for SUI, comparing 96 patients (aged ≥80 years) to a cohort of 1016 patients (aged <80 years). In this study, there was no difference in overall cure rate between the older and younger women. Although hospitalization time was significantly longer in the older women cohort, major perioperative complications were uncommon (1%) and the rate of bladder perforation, long-term voiding difficulty, and de novo UUI was similar between the groups. Similarly, for the TOT approach, Groutz and colleagues[62] reported age-related outcomes for a prospective study of 97 patients (aged ≥70 years) versus 256 younger women, undergoing surgery for SUI. In this study, the TOT approach was noted to be safe and efficient for both cohorts, but older women were noted to have increased risks for perioperative recurrent urinary tract infections as well as de novo overactive bladder. An additional prospective study evaluating the TOT approach included 60 patients older than 70 years and 121 patients younger than 70 years. There were no differences observed between the 2 groups in terms of cure rates or complications. A recent study compared primary MUS outcomes in 160 women (aged ≥70 years) with those in 536 woman (aged <70 years). Multivariable analysis revealed no differences in SUI failure rates between the older and younger cohort (adjusted OR, 1.7; 95% CI, 0.9–3.1). Despite similar SUI outcomes, older women had greater persistent UUI and worse impression of improvement.[67]

AGE-RELATED SURGICAL OUTCOMES

There is conflicting information in the peer-reviewed literature on the impact of age on surgical outcomes.[75] Large data sets demonstrate age as an independent predictor of adverse outcomes after surgery. Sung and colleagues[6] demonstrated that increasing

Table 4
TVT—outcomes in the older woman

References	Study Details	Outcomes	Comments
Allahdin et al,[59] 2004	179 patients in 3 age cohorts: 30–49, 50–69, and 70–90 y; TVT for SUI; prospective	1-y subjective cure rate 84.9, 81.3, and 85.3% in the 3 cohorts, respectively	Higher incidence of postoperative urgency in the older cohort (9.5%)
Centinel et al,[60] 2004	75 patients, median age 51.2 y (range 33–69 y), predictors for continence after TVT, prospective	Subjective and objective outcome measures, mean follow-up 21.6 mo, cure rate 95.9 vs 76.9% in patients aged <55 y vs >55 y, respectively	The only statistically significant parameter affecting cure rate was age >55 y
Gordon et al,[61] 2005	123 patients aged ≥70 vs 208 patients aged <70 y (control group), TVT, prospective	Objective follow-up, mean ± SD follow-up 26 ± 13 mo, persistent SUI 7% in older group vs 6% in younger group	De novo postoperative urge UI more common in older group (18 vs 4%), older group with 2 cases of pulmonary thromboembolism, 1 case of DVT, 2 cases of cardiac arrhythmia, and 1 case of pneumonia
Groutz et al,[62] 2011	97 patients (aged ≥70 y) vs 256 younger women, TVT-O, prospective	Mean follow-up 30 ± 17 mo (3–58 mo), early and late postoperative morbidity was similar in both groups, incidence of persistent SUI was similar in both age groups	More recurrent UTIs among elderly women (13.7% vs 6.2%) De novo OAB was more common in elderly patients (11.9% vs 4.7%, P<.05)
Hellberg et al,[63] 2007	113 patients aged ≥75 y vs younger cohort, TVT, retrospective	Mean follow-up 5.7 y, cure rate 55.7 vs 79.7% in older vs younger cohort, respectively	Mixed UI, UTI, and previous surgery not related to outcomes
Karantais et al,[64] 2004	34 patients aged ≥65 y vs younger group, case-control study	Follow-up 6–23 mo, subjective continence cure rate 45 vs 73% and satisfaction rate 90 vs 100% in older vs younger patients, respectively	Older group had lower outcome satisfaction, equivalent postoperative urge symptoms

(continued on next page)

Table 4
(continued)

References	Study Details	Outcomes	Comments
Ku et al,[65] 2006	60 patients (aged ≥65 y) vs 206 younger women (aged 45–64 y), TVT and SPARC, retrospective	Objective and subjective outcome measures, mean follow-up 10.4 mo, no significant difference in cure rate	No significant differences between the groups for the rates of postoperative UUI
Liapis et al,[66] 2006	51 patients aged ≥65 y, TVT	Objective follow-up >12 mo, 76% dry	Better outcome with preoperative hypermobile urethra
Malek et al,[67] 2015	160 women (aged ≥70 y) vs 536 younger women, TVT and TOT, retrospective	Subjective outcome measures, mean follow-up 38 mo, no difference in SUI failure rates between older and younger women	Older women had more persistent UUI and worse impression of improvement than younger women
Pugsley et al,[68] 2005	34 patients aged ≥70 y vs 192 younger controls, colposuspension vs TVT, retrospective	Subjective measure, 3-month postoperative cure or improvement for TVT was 77.3 vs 89.3% and for colposuspension was 81.8 vs 89.4% in older vs younger patients, respectively	Postoperative voiding dysfunction, UTI, and irritative symptoms more common in older group with either surgery
Sevestre et al,[69] 2003	76 patients aged ≥70 y	Subjective and objective measures, mean follow-up 24.6 mo, 67% cured, 82% satisfied	De novo urgency rate 21%, preoperative urgency cured in 46%
Serati et al,[70] 2013	60 patients aged >70 y vs 121 younger patients, comparing TVT-O, prospective	Subjective and objective measures, mean follow-up 26 mo, no differences in cure rate	No differences in postoperative voiding dysfunction, vaginal erosion, or de novo overactive bladder

Study	Patients	Outcome measures	Results
Stav et al,[71] 2010	96 patients aged ≥80 y vs 1016 younger patients, comparing TVT to TOT	Subjective measure, 6 wk, and 6, 12, 18, and 24 mo using validated measures. Overall subjective cure rate was 85% (elderly group 81%, young group 85%, P = .32). There was no difference between TVT and TOT approaches for the elderly group	The rate of de novo urgency was similar between the 2 groups. 37% of older women failed their first voiding trial compared with 9% in the younger cohort (P<.001). Patient's age was not found to be an independent risk factor for sling failure
Sung et al,[72] 2007	81 patients aged ≥60 y vs 168 younger women, comparing QOL outcomes, retrospective	Subjective outcomes, mean follow-up 11.8 mo, improved QOL in both cohorts	Older women had lower mean baseline subjective QOL scores but there was no difference in improved QOL postoperatively
Touloupidis,et al,[73] 2007	51 patients aged ≥65 y, TVT, retrospective	SUI cure rate 96%, follow-up 35.6 mo (range 14–60 mo), mailed questionnaire	9.8% de novo urgency, maximum urine flow rate unchanged before vs after surgery
Walsh et al,[74] 2004	21 patients aged ≥70 y vs 46 patients aged <70 y (control group), prospective	Significant improvement of SUI, UUI, frequency, and urgency in both groups on King's Health Questionnaire, mean follow-up 9–12 mo	Younger cohort had better improvement scores, older cohort had more previous surgical procedures for SUI

Abbreviations: DVT, deep vein thrombosis; OAB, overactive bladder; QOL, quality of life; SD, standard deviation; SPARC, suprapubic arc procedure; TVT-O, tension-free vaginal tape-obturator; UTI, urinary tract infection.

Adapted from Gerten KA, Markland AD, Lloyd KL, et al. Prolapse and incontinence surgery in older women. J Urol 2008;179:2114; with permission.

age is associated with very small increases in absolute risks of complications in older women after surgery for UI and other pelvic floor disorders. However, the relative risk of complications in older women was significantly increased compared with their younger counterparts. This is consistent with studies reporting on postoperative complications analyzing large data sets from general, colorectal, vascular, and gynecologic surgery demonstrating that increasing age, especially age greater than 80 years, is associated with increased complications. However, many single-institution cases series have reported excellent surgical results with well-selected octogenarians and nanogenarians undergoing surgeries for incontinence and other pelvic floor disorders.[76–78] The findings of these case series should be considered with caution because they tend to describe healthy well-selected older women undergoing procedures at specialized centers. The true risk of surgery in older women is likely higher. Considering medical comorbidities, frailty, and functional status in addition to age will help surgeons better lead discussions with women on their individual risk of complications after surgery.

Treatment Failure After Midurethral Sling

Risk factors for treatment failure of MUS at 12 months have been examined and noted to be prior antiincontinence surgery, an immobile urethra (with urethral mobility documented at <30°), and indicators of incontinence severity including increased symptom bother on validated surveys and increased pad weight on 24-hour pad tests.[79]

Postoperative Complications

Overall, TOT and TVT MUS procedures are considered safe and effective procedures; however, there are several surgically related complications that must be carefully considered. Bladder and vaginal perforation; hematoma formation; neurologic symptoms, including numbness and weakness, pain, and mesh exposure; as well as complications specific to the lower urinary tract, including voiding dysfunction and new-onset and persistent UUI, are well documented. In a recent systematic review, Novara and colleagues[80] compared TVT and TOT sling complications, reviewing 27 RCTs (4224 patients) reporting bladder/vaginal perforations, and noted an OR of 2.5 (95% CI, 1.75–3.57) favoring the TOT approach. Regarding vascular complications, the same systematic review evaluated 19 RCTs (2927 patients) reporting hematoma formation after MUS with an OR of 2.62 (95% CI, 1.35–5.08) favoring the TOT approach. For mesh complications, a review of 25 RCTs (3837 patients) reporting vaginal erosion revealed an OR of 0.64 (95% CI, 0.41–0.97) favoring TVT. In the most recent, aforementioned, large, equivalence RCTs comparing the TVT and TOT sling routes, there were no differences in mesh exposure rates or surgical site infections but there were higher rates of vascular events in the TVT arm when compared with the TOT arm (6.0% vs 2.3%, $P = .03$). Regarding neurologic symptoms, patients undergoing the TOT approach reported a higher incidence of complications (9.4% vs 4.0%, $P = .01$). There were no differences in pain between the groups. Lower urinary tract complications, including voiding dysfunction, new UUI, and persistent UUI were similar between the study groups.[54]

Age-related risk of other specific complications of incontinence surgery is not well delineated in the medical literature, and attention to general postoperative complications within the geriatric population is prudent. Despite limited data that address age-related risk specifically for incontinence surgery, Anger and colleagues[81] analyzed the 1999–2001 Medicare Public Use Files and reported on 1356 female Medicare beneficiaries (aged ≥65 years and older) undergoing sling surgery and noted high rates of urinary tract infections (33.6%) in the early postoperative period and 49.7% infections at 1 year. In addition, 9.4% of subjects reported new-onset pelvic pain. Regarding complications specific to the lower urinary tract, there were high incidences of new-onset UUI and outlet obstruction (**Table 5**).[81] Of note, multivariate analysis revealed that patient race, age, and comorbidities each had a significant influence on outcomes.

Geriatric Postoperative Considerations

Common geriatric postoperative medical complications that should be considered in all older women undergoing surgery are falls, delirium, and surgical site infections.[82] As antiincontinence procedures are commonly considered outpatient procedures by Medicare, women are often not discharged to skilled nursing facilities. The rates of discharge to skilled nursing facilities, 30-day readmissions, and 2-year postoperative mortality are not well described in the peer-reviewed literature.

- Postoperative falls are common, although the true prevalence of postoperative falls is not known. Almost 30% of community-dwelling adults older than 65 years fall every year and 10% of these falls result in major injury or sequelae including fracture, serious soft tissue injury, traumatic brain injury, dehydration, pressure ulcers, and rhabdomyolysis.[83] Risk factors predisposing older adults to falls include previous fall, balance impairment, gait disturbances, decreased muscle strength, visual impairments (including cataracts), polypharmacy (>4 medications), functional impairment for ADLs, depression, low body mass index, age greater than 80 years, female gender, and cognitive impairments.[83] In the postoperative period, narcotic use, dehydration, and urinary tract infections may all contribute to falls in older women undergoing surgery for incontinence.
- Delirium is a state of acute confusion and is a common complication reported in 9% of older adults undergoing major surgery. Unfortunately, 50% to 80% of acute episodes of delirium in hospitalized patients go unrecognized because patients are often not screened postoperatively. Risk factors for postoperative delirium after surgery are well defined and include age greater than or equal to

Table 5
Surgical outcomes among Medicare beneficiaries

Characteristics	Treatment Failure (Repeat Incontinence Procedure)	New Diagnosis of Urgency Urinary Incontinence	Diagnosis of Urinary Obstruction	Management of Outlet Obstruction
Nonwhite (vs white)	1.81 (0.84–3.87)[a]	1.46 (0.75–2.84)	2.30 (1.07–4.91)[b]	1.78 (0.84–3.78)
Ages 65–69 y (vs >75 y)	0.53 (0.32–0.87)[b]	0.44 (0.29–0.65)[b]	0.60 (0.34–1.03)	0.58 (0.36–0.94)
Ages 70–74 y (vs >75 y)	0.76 (0.48–1.22)	0.84 (0.58–1.20)	1.0 (0.60–1.65)	0.58 (0.35–0.95)[b]
Charlson ≥1 (vs 0)[c]	1.09 (0.71–1.66)	1.26 (0.91–1.74)	0.74 (0.46–1.21)	1.23 (0.81–1.88)

Data are expressed as ORs (95% CI).
[a] $.05 < P < .10$.
[b] $P < .05$.
[c] Charlson comorbidity index score.
Adapted from Anger JT, Litwin MS, Wang Q. Complications of sling surgery among female Medicare beneficiaries. Obstet Gynecol 2007;109:712; with permission.

70 years, alcohol abuse, preoperative cognitive impairment, preoperative physical impairment, and abnormal levels of serum sodium (<130 or >150 mmol/L), potassium (<3.0 or >16.7 mmol/L), or glucose (<60 or >300 mg/dL).[84] In a study of women older than 60 years undergoing gynecologic surgery, age greater than 70 years, taking more than 5 medications, and additional narcotic dosing to supplement intravenous patient-controlled analgesia were identified as independent predictors of postoperative delirium.[85] The National Institute for Health and Clinical Excellence from the United Kingdom has published recommendations for the prevention of delirium. These recommendations include assessing patients on admission for their risk factors for developing delirium and screening patients for incident delirium by assessing for changes in cognitive function.

- Surgical site infections have long been associated with increasing age. Impaired functional status for ADLs has emerged as an important independent predictor of surgical site infection, especially methicillin-resistant *Staphylococcus aureus* infections, even after stratifying patients by age.[86] There are 2 hypotheses to explain this: (1) decreased nutritional status in dependent patients predisposes to infection and poor wound healing and (2) this could be due to health care workers spreading infections between dependent patients requiring increased wound care.

SUMMARY/NEED FOR FURTHER INVESTIGATION

Surgery has been proved to be highly effective for the treatment of SUI in women participating in large clinical trials but carries risks of postoperative complications. Well-selected older women have been demonstrated to do well with antiincontinence surgery and have significant gains in QOL. Major gaps in our knowledge exist about which surgical treatments will benefit individual women who may not have been represented in clinical trials because of age, multiple comorbidities, functional disability, or cognitive impairment. Research to identify which treatments for UI are most appropriate in real-world settings for different older women is needed.

As antiincontinence procedures are commonly considered outpatient procedures by Medicare, women are often not discharged to skilled nursing facilities. Common geriatric complications including the rates of postoperative delirium, discharge to skilled nursing facilities, 30-day readmissions, 30-day falls, and 2-year postoperative mortality after antiincontinence surgery and surgery for pelvic floor disorders are not well described in the peer-reviewed literature. Research that includes preoperative geriatric assessments, such as the Robinson Predictive tool and the Timed Get-Up-and-Go test, in prospective surgical trials of older women undergoing surgical procedures for UI coupled with measurements of postoperative geriatric morbidity will help to establish the actual risk of these complications in older women, resulting in improved patient counseling and surveillance.

REFERENCES

1. Nygaard I, Barber MD, Burgio KL, et al. Prevalence of symptomatic pelvic floor disorders in US women. JAMA 2008;300:1311–6.
2. Vincent GK, Velkoff VA. The next four decades, the older population in the United States: 2010 to 2050. Washington, DC: US Census Bureau; 2010.
3. Wu J, Matthews CA, Conover MM, et al. Lifetime risk of stress urinary incontinence or pelvic organ prolapse surgery. Obstet Gynecol 2014;123:1201–6.

4. Oliphant SS, Wang L, Bunker CH, et al. Trends in stress urinary incontinence inpatient procedures in the United States, 1979–2004. Am J Obstet Gynecol 2009;200:521.e1–6.
5. Erekson EA, Lopes VV, Raker CA, et al. Ambulatory procedures for female pelvic floor disorders in the United States. Am J Obstet Gynecol 2010;203:497.e1–5.
6. Sung VW, Weitzen S, Sokol ER, et al. Effect of patient age on increasing morbidity and mortality following urogynecologic surgery. Am J Obstet Gynecol 2006; 194(5):1411–7.
7. Dubeau CE. The aging lower urinary tract. J Urol 2006;175(3 Pt 2):S11–5.
8. Zimmern P, Litman HJ, Nager CW, et al. Effect of aging on storage and voiding function in women with stress predominant urinary incontinence. J Urol 2014; 192:464–8.
9. DuBeau CE, Kuchel GA, Johnson T 2nd, et al, Fourth International Consultation on Incontinence. Incontinence in the frail elderly: report from the 4th International Consultation on Incontinence. Neurourol Urodyn 2010;29(1):165–78.
10. Dolan LM, Smith AR, Hosker GL. Opening detrusor pressure and the influence of age on success following colposuspension. Neurourol Urodyn 2004;23(1):10–5.
11. Rud T. Urethral pressure profile in continent women from childhood to old age. Acta Obstet Gynecol Scand 1980;59(4):331–5.
12. Madersbacher S, Pycha A, Schatzl G, et al. The aging lower urinary tract: a comparative urodynamic study of men and women. Urology 1998;51(2):206–12.
13. Elkadry E. Functional urinary incontinence in women. Female Pelvic Med Reconstr Surg 2006;12(1):1–13.
14. Inouye SK, Studenski S, Tinetti ME, et al. Geriatric syndromes: clinical, research, and policy implications of a core geriatric concept. J Am Geriatr Soc 2007;55(5): 780–91.
15. Tinetti ME, Inouye SK, Gill TM, et al. Shared risk factors for falls, incontinence, and functional dependence. Unifying the approach to geriatric syndromes. JAMA 1995;273(17):1348–53.
16. Erekson EA, Ciarleglio MM, Hanissian PD, et al. Functional disability and compromised mobility among older women with urinary incontinence. Female Pelvic Med Reconstr Surg 2015;21(3):170–5.
17. Johnson TM 2nd, Bernard SL, Kincade JE, et al. Urinary incontinence and risk of death among community-living elderly people: results from the National Survey on Self-Care and Aging. J Aging Health 2000;12(1):25–46.
18. Nager CW. The urethra is a reliable witness: simplifying the diagnosis of stress urinary incontinence. Int Urogynecol J 2012;23(12):1649–51.
19. Nager CW, Brubaker L, Litman HJ, et al. A randomized trial of urodynamic testing before stress-incontinence surgery. N Engl J Med 2012;366(21):1987–97.
20. Dmochowski RR, Blaivas JM, Gormley EA, et al. Update of AUA guideline on the surgical management of female stress urinary incontinence. J Urol 2010;183(5): 1906–14.
21. Eagle KA, Berger PB, Calkins H, et al. ACC/AHA guideline update for perioperative cardiovascular evaluation for noncardiac surgery—executive summary a report of the American College of Cardiology/American Heart Association task force on practice guidelines (committee to update the 1996 guidelines on perioperative cardiovascular evaluation for noncardiac surgery). Circulation 2002; 105(10):1257–67.
22. Fleisher LA, Beckman JA, Brown KA, et al. 2009 ACCF/AHA focused update on perioperative beta blockade incorporated into the ACC/AHA 2007 guidelines on perioperative cardiovascular evaluation and care for noncardiac surgery: a report

of the American College of Cardiology Foundation/American Heart Association Task Force on Practice Guidelines. Circulation 2009;120(21):e169–276.

23. Chow WB, Rosenthal RA, American College of Surgeons National Surgical Quality Improvement Program, et al. Optimal preoperative assessment of the geriatric surgical patient: a best practices guideline from the American College of Surgeons National Surgical Quality Improvement Program and the American Geriatrics Society. J Am Coll Surg 2012;215(4):453–66.

24. Dasgupta M, Rolfson DB, Stolee P, et al. Frailty is associated with postoperative complications in older adults with medical problems. Arch Gerontol Geriatr 2009; 48(1):78–83.

25. Robinson TN, Wallace JI, Wu DS, et al. Accumulated frailty characteristics predict postoperative discharge institutionalization in the geriatric patient. J Am Coll Surg 2011;213(1):37–42 [discussion: 42–4].

26. Robinson TN, Wu DS, Stiegmann GV, et al. Frailty predicts increased hospital and six-month healthcare cost following colorectal surgery in older adults. Am J Surg 2011;202(5):511–4.

27. Robinson TN, Eiseman B, Wallace JI, et al. Redefining geriatric preoperative assessment using frailty, disability and co-morbidity. Ann Surg 2009;250(3): 449–55.

28. Makary MA, Segev DL, Pronovost PJ, et al. Frailty as a predictor of surgical outcomes in older patients. J Am Coll Surg 2010;210(6):901–8.

29. Hamel MB, Henderson WG, Khuri SF, et al. Surgical outcomes for patients aged 80 and older: morbidity and mortality from major noncardiac surgery. J Am Geriatr Soc 2005;53(3):424–9.

30. Fried LP, Tangen CM, Walston J, et al. Frailty in older adults: evidence for a phenotype. J Gerontol A Biol Sci Med Sci 2001;56(3):M146–56.

31. Borson S, Scanlan JM, Chen P, et al. The Mini-Cog as a screen for dementia: validation in a population-based sample. J Am Geriatr Soc 2003;51(10):1451–4.

32. Robinson TN, Wu DS, Sauaia A, et al. Slower walking speed forecasts increased postoperative morbidity and 1-year mortality across surgical specialties. Ann Surg 2013;258(4):582–8 [discussion: 588–90].

33. Ferrucci L, Guralnik JM, Studenski S, et al. Designing randomized, controlled trials aimed at preventing or delaying functional decline and disability in frail, older persons: a consensus report. J Am Geriatr Soc 2004;52(4):625–34.

34. Gajdos C, Hawn MT, Kile D, et al. Risk of major nonemergent inpatient general surgical procedures in patients on long-term dialysis. JAMA Surg 2013;148:1–7.

35. Robinson TN, Wu DS, Pointer LF, et al. Preoperative cognitive dysfunction is related to adverse postoperative outcomes in the elderly. J Am Coll Surg 2012; 215(1):12–7 [discussion: 17–8].

36. Zoorob D, Karram M. Bulking agents: a urogynecology perspective. Urol Clin North Am 2012;39(3):273–7.

37. Kirchin V, Page T, Keegan PE, et al. Urethral injection therapy for urinary incontinence in women. Cochrane Database Syst Rev 2012;(2):CD003881.

38. Erekson EA, Sung VW, Rardin CR, et al. Ethylene vinyl alcohol copolymer erosions after use as a urethral bulking agent. Obstet Gynecol 2007;109(2 Pt2):490–2.

39. Hurtado EA, McCrery RJ, Appell RA. Complications of ethylene vinyl alcohol copolymer as an intraurethral bulking agent in men with stress urinary incontinence. Urology 2008;71(4):662–5.

40. Lai HH, Hurtado EA, Appell RA. Large urethral prolapse formation after calcium hydroxylapatite (Coaptite) injection. Int Urogynecol J Pelvic Floor Dysfunct 2008; 19(9):1315–7.

41. Burch JC. Urethrovaginal fixation to Cooper's ligament for correction of stress incontinence, cystocele, and prolapse. Am J Obstet Gynecol 1961;81:281–90.

42. Jarvis GJ. Surgery for genuine stress incontinence in women. Br J Obstet Gynaecol 1994;101(5):371–4.

43. Tanagho EA. Colpocystourethropexy: the way we do it. J Urol 1976;116:751–3.

44. McGuire EJ, Lytton B. Pubovaginal sling procedure for stress urinary incontinence. J Urol 2002;167:1120–3.

45. Bezerra CA, Bruschini H, Cody DJ. Traditional suburethral sling operations for urinary incontinence in women. Cochrane Database Syst Rev 2005;(3):CD001754.

46. Lapitan MC, Cody DJ, Grant AM. Open retropubic colposuspension for urinary incontinence in women. Cochrane Database Syst Rev 2005;(3):CD002912.

47. Albo ME, Richter HE, Brubaker L, et al. Burch colposuspension versus fascial sling to reduce urinary stress incontinence. N Engl J Med 2007;356(21):2143–55.

48. Carr LK, Walsh PJ, Abraham VE, et al. Favorable outcome of pubovaginal slings for geriatric women with stress incontinence. J Urol 1997;157:125–8.

49. Blaivas JG, Jacobs BZ. Pubovaginal fascial sling for the treatment of complicated stress urinary incontinence. J Urol 1991;145:1214.

50. Richter HE, Goode PS, Brubaker L, et al. Two-year outcomes after surgery for stress incontinence in older compared to younger women. Obstet Gynecol 2008;112:621–9.

51. Herzog A, Diokno A, Brown M, et al. Two year incidence, remission, and change patterns, of urinary incontinence in no institutionalized older adults. J Gerontol 1990;45:67–74.

52. Ulmsten U, Henriksson L, Johnson P, et al. An ambulatory surgical procedure under local anesthesia for treatment of female urinary incontinence. Int Urogynecol J Pelvic Floor Dysfunct 1996;7(2):81–5 [discussion: 85–6].

53. Delorme E. Transobturator urethral suspension: mini-invasive procedure in the treatment of stress urinary incontinence in women. Prog Urol 2001;11(6):1306–13.

54. Richter HE, Albo ME, Zyczynski HM, et al. Retropubic versus transobturator midurethral slings for stress incontinence. N Engl J Med 2010;362(22):2066–76.

55. Barber MD, Kleeman S, Karram MM, et al. Transobturator tape compared with tension-free vaginal tape for the treatment of stress urinary incontinence: a randomized controlled trial. Obstet Gynecol 2008;111(3):611–21.

56. Funk MJ, Siddiqui NY, Kawasaki A, et al. Long-term outcomes after stress urinary incontinence surgery. Obstet Gynecol 2012;120:83–90.

57. Groutz A, Rosen G, Cohen A, et al. Ten-year subjective outcome results of the retropubic tension-free vaginal tape for treatment of stress urinary incontinence. J Minim Invasive Gynecol 2011;18(6):726–9.

58. Nilsson CG, Palva K, Rezapour M, et al. Eleven years prospective follow-up of the tension-free vaginal tape procedure for the treatment of stress urinary incontinence. Int Urogynecol J 2008;19:1043–7.

59. Allahdin S, McKinely CA, Mahmood TA, et al. Tension-free vaginal tape: a procedure for all ages. Acta Obstet Gynecol Scand 2004;83:937.

60. Centinel B, Oktay D, Bulent O, et al. Are there any factors predicting the cure and complication rates of tension-free vaginal tape? Int Urogynecol J Pelvic Floor Dysfunct 2004;15:188.

61. Gordon G, Gold R, Pauzner D, et al. Tension-free vaginal tape in the elderly: is it a safe procedure? Urology 2005;65:479.

62. Groutz A, Cohen A, Gold R, et al. The safety and efficacy of the "inside-out" transobturator TVT in elderly versus younger stress-incontinent women: a prospective study of 353 consecutive patients. Neurourol Urodyn 2011;30:380–3.

63. Hellberg D, Homgren C, Lanner L, et al. The very obese and the very old woman: tension-free vaginal tape for the treatment of stress urinary incontinence. Int Urogynecol J Pelvic Floor Dysfunct 2007;18:423.

64. Karantais E, Fynes MM, Stanton SL, et al. The tension-free vaginal tape in older women. BJOG 2004;111:837.

65. Ku JH, Oh JG, Shin JW, et al. Age is not a limiting factor for midurethral sling procedures in the elderly with urinary incontinence. Gynecol Obstet Invest 2006;61: 194–9.

66. Liapis A, Panagiotis B, Giner M, et al. Tension-free vaginal tape versus tension-free vaginal tape obturator in women with stress incontinence. Gynecol Obstet Invest 2006;62:160–4.

67. Malek JM, Ellington DR, Jauk V, et al. The effect of age on stress and urgency urinary incontinence outcomes in women undergoing primary midurethral sling. Int Urogynecol J 2015;26(6):831–5.

68. Pugsley H, Barbrook C, Mayne CJ, et al. Morbidity of incontinence surgery in women over 70 years old; a retrospective cohort study. BJOG 2005;1112:786.

69. Sevestre S, Ciofu C, Deval B, et al. Results of tension-free vaginal tape technique in the elderly. Eur Urol 2003;44:128.

70. Serati M, Braga A, Cattoni E, et al. Transobturator vaginal tape for the treatment of stress urinary incontinence in elderly women without concomitant pelvic organ prolapse: is it effective and safe? Eur J Obstet Gynecol Reprod Biol 2013;166: 107–10.

71. Stav K, Dwyer PL, Rosamilia A, et al. Midurethral sling procedures for stress urinary incontinence in women over 80 years. Neurourol Urodyn 2010;29:1262–6.

72. Sung VW, Glasgow BA, Wohlrab KJ, et al. Impact of age on perioperative and postoperative urinary incontinence quality of life. Am J Obstet Gynecol 2007; 197:680.e1–5.

73. Touloupidis S, Papatsoris AG, Thanopoulos C, et al. Tension-free vaginal tape for the treatment of stress urinary incontinence in geriatric patients. Gerontology 2007;53:125.

74. Walsh K, Generao SE, White MJ, et al. The influence of age on quality of life outcomes in women following a tension-free vaginal tape procedure. J Urol 2004; 171:1185.

75. Robinson TN, Finlayson E. How to best forecast adverse outcomes following geriatric trauma: an ageless question? JAMA Surg 2014;149(8):773.

76. Stepp KJ, Barber MD, Yoo EH, et al. Incidence of perioperative complications of urogynecologic surgery in elderly women. Am J Obstet Gynecol 2005;192(5): 1630–6.

77. Parker DY, Burke JJ 2nd, Gallup DG. Gynecological surgery in octogenarians and nonagenarians. Am J Obstet Gynecol 2004;190(5):1401–3.

78. Toglia MR, Nolan TE. Morbidity and mortality rates of elective gynecologic surgery in the elderly woman. Am J Obstet Gynecol 2003;189(6):1584–7 [discussion: 1587–9].

79. Richter HE, Litman HJ, Lukacz ES, et al. Demographic and clinical predictors of treatment failure one year after midurethral sling surgery. Obstet Gynecol 2011; 117(4):913–21.

80. Novara G, Artibani W, Barber MD, et al. Updated systematic review and meta-analysis of the comparative data on colposuspensions, pubovaginal slings, and midurethral tapes in the surgical treatment of female stress urinary incontinence. Eur Urol 2010;58:218–38.

81. Anger JT, Litwin MS, Wang Q. Complications of sling surgery among female Medicare beneficiaries. Obstet Gynecol 2007;109:707–14.
82. Erekson EA, Ratner ES, Walke LM, et al. Gynecologic surgery in the geriatric patient. Obstet Gynecol 2012;119(6):1262–9.
83. Tinetti ME, Kumar C. The patient who falls: "It's always a trade-off". JAMA 2010; 303(3):258–66.
84. Marcantonio ER, Goldman L, Mangione CM, et al. A clinical prediction rule for delirium after elective noncardiac surgery. JAMA 1994;271(2):134–9.
85. McAlpine JN, Hodgson EJ, Abramowitz S, et al. The incidence and risk factors associated with postoperative delirium in geriatric patients undergoing surgery for suspected gynecologic malignancies. Gynecol Oncol 2008;109(2):296–302.
86. Chen TY, Anderson DJ, Chopra T, et al. Poor functional status is an independent predictor of surgical site infections due to methicillin-resistant staphylococcus aureus in older adults. J Am Geriatr Soc 2010;58(3):527–32.

Evaluation and Management of Pelvic Organ Prolapse in Elderly Women

Javier Pizarro-Berdichevsky, MD[a,b,c,*], Marisa M. Clifton, MD[a],
Howard B. Goldman, MD[a]

KEYWORDS

• Pelvic organ • Prolapse • Elderly women • Vaginal bulge

KEY POINTS

• Pelvic organ prolapse is a common disease in elderly patients.
• The most important symptom is vaginal bulge (bulge sensation or the sensation of something coming down through the vaginal introitus). This symptom is not different than in the general population.
• Diagnosis can be confirmed with vaginal examination to identify the presence of protrusion beyond the hymen, and is not different than in the general population.
• Different treatment options are available, including observation, nonsurgical interventions, and surgical techniques.
• Pessaries and colpocleisis are the treatment options used more often in elderly patients than in the general population.

INTRODUCTION

The number of women aged 65 years or older in the United States in 2010 was estimated to be 22.9 million, which represents 7.4% of the total US population. By 2030, there will be approximately 39.9 million women in this age group, with a rate of growth almost double that of the general population. Overall, individuals aged 65 years and older will represent 19% of the population by 2030, compared with 12.4% of the population in 2000.[1] In addition, women more than 80 years of age are the fastest growing segment of society. As both the incidence and prevalence of prolapse surgery increase with age, pelvic organ prolapse (POP) becomes an increasingly bothersome disorder in this patient population.[1]

[a] Department of Urology, Center for Female Pelvic Medicine and Reconstructive Surgery, The Cleveland Clinic, 9500 Euclid Avenue, Cleveland, OH 44195, USA; [b] Urogynecology Unit, Dr. Sotero del Rio Hospital, Av Concha y Toro 3459, Santiago 8207257, Chile; [c] Division de Obstetricia y Ginecologia, Pontificia Universidad Catolica de Chile, Avenida Libertador Bernardo O Higgins 340, Santiago 8331150, Chile
* Corresponding author. Department of Urology, Center for Female Pelvic Medicine and Reconstructive Surgery, The Cleveland Clinic, 9500 Euclid Avenue, Cleveland, OH 44195.
E-mail addresses: jpizarro@med.puc.cl; PIZARRJ@ccf.org

Clin Geriatr Med 31 (2015) 507–521
http://dx.doi.org/10.1016/j.cger.2015.06.008
0749-0690/15/$ – see front matter © 2015 Elsevier Inc. All rights reserved.

In the subgroup of patients 80 years of age or older, the prevalence has been reported to be 37%.[2] Studies have shown that older age and increased parity are important risk factors for the development POP.[3–5] Recently, the lifetime risk of undergoing prolapse repair has been reported as 12%,[6] which implies that there will be more than 4.5 million POP surgeries performed in the United States by 2030. POP may impair quality of life (QoL) via physical activity limitations, depression, poor self-image, as well as an impairment of participation in social activities.[7,8] The physiologic effects of POP may include bladder, bowel, and sexual symptoms. These symptoms often present together and are associated with worse QoL.[7,9] Studies have shown that the impact of POP on QoL is significant, regardless of the stage of POP.[10] For all of these reasons, POP currently is, and will continue to be, one of the major health concerns in the older female population.

PATIENT EVALUATION
Patient History

The history of present illness is critical in the evaluation of prolapse in the older female population. In general, the evaluation is similar to that of the general population with several additional focused questions.[11] The most common POP symptoms with their respective descriptions are shown in **Table 1**.

- Symptoms of vaginal bulge: bulge symptoms may worsen toward the end of the day and improve when the patient is supine.[12–15] Studies have shown that a physical bulge is the most frequent symptom in patients with POP, with a high sensitivity and specificity for clinically relevant POP.[12] For these reasons, the single question "Do you feel a vaginal bulge that is bothersome?" should be used as a screening tool. Some patients may complain of a full sensation in the pelvis or a low backache that worsens in the evening. With a large prolapse, a patient may experience dyspareunia or difficulty with penetration.[16] Occasionally, patients may have vaginal bleeding secondary to irritation of the vaginal bulge.[17]
- Lower urinary tract symptoms:
  ○ Stress urinary incontinence (SUI) symptoms should be addressed. This leakage is the result of increased intra-abdominal pressure, which can result from cough, sneeze, lifting, and other activities. Often this symptom improves as POP worsens because of kinking of the urethrovesical junction. Thus, this symptom may worsen with prolapse treatment. It may also require additional treatment at the time of surgery if the patient is an appropriate surgical candidate.

Table 1
Most common prolapse symptoms and description

Symptom	Description
Vaginal bulge	Bulge sensation or something coming down through the vaginal introitus
Pelvic pressure	Complaint of increased heaviness or dragging in the suprapubic area
Bleeding, discharge, infection	Vaginal bleeding, discharge, or infection related to dependent ulceration of the prolapse
Splinting/digitation	Complaint of the need to digitally replace the prolapse or to otherwise apply manual pressure; eg, to the vagina or perineum (splinting), or to the vagina or rectum (digitation) to assist voiding or defecation
Low backache	Complaint of low, sacral (or similar to menstrual period pain) backache associated temporally with POP

- o Urgency incontinence symptoms should also be elicited. This leakage is the result of urgency and can be sensed before the leakage episode. Importantly, these symptoms may or may not improve with treatment of POP.
- o Obstructive urinary symptoms, such as hesitancy, terminal dribbling, and weak urinary stream, should also be discussed. These patients may have incomplete bladder emptying and increased postvoid residuals. Patients may need to manually reduce the bladder (splinting) in order to empty successfully. Recurrent urinary tract infections could occur in these patients secondary to incomplete bladder emptying. Occasionally, patients with significant POP may even experience renal dysfunction caused by ureteral kinking. Although up to 8% of patients may have hydroureteronephrosis at the time of surgery for prolapse, less than 1% have severe hydroureteronephrosis.[18,19]
- Bowel symptoms: patients may experience obstructive defecatory symptoms that require reduction of their prolapse to effectively defecate. Occasionally, patients have to digitally remove stool. It is important to inquire whether a patient experiences fecal incontinence as well.
- Sexual activity status: a review of a patient's sexual activity should be made because this may determine the particular treatment a patient wishes to pursue. For instance, there are particular pessaries that do not allow for sexual intercourse and there are surgical options that preclude vaginal penetration.
- Uterine disorder: postmenopausal bleeding and Pap smear status should be determined before proceeding with any surgical interventions
- Medical comorbidities: it is important to query patients on their medical history. For instance, some patients may not be appropriate surgical candidates because of medical issues, or may not be able to discontinue anticoagulant medications. In addition, conditions that cause increased abdominal pressure, such as chronic cough or significant constipation, may lead to an increased risk of failure after surgical intervention.
- Surgical history must be determined as well. Surgical approaches vary significantly if in patients who have had a hysterectomy. In addition, whether or not patients have a history of extensive intra-abdominal surgery may affect whether the abdominal or vaginal route of surgery is preferred.

The most important factor in determining how to manage most women with POP is the degree of bother it causes the patient. If a patient does not have any bothersome symptoms associated with her prolapse, it rarely requires any treatment.

Physical Examination

- In general, the physical examination of the older female population is not significantly different than that of the general population.
- o General appearance: it is important to determine the overall physical status of the patient. If she is frail and has limited mobility, an aggressive intra-abdominal surgery may not be in her best interest.
- o Abdominal examination: special attention should be paid to any incisions on the abdomen or any evidence of tumor. If the patient has extensive abdominal incisions, she may not be a candidate for an abdominal approach. If there are symptomatic hernias, they may need repair at the time of surgery.
- o Pelvic examination:
  - If the patient has a positive answer to the question "Do you feel any bothersome sensation of a vaginal bulge?" she should undergo a pelvic examination to rule out POP.

- The gold standard measurement of pelvic organ prolapse is the POP-Q (POP Quantification) examination, which is used extensively in the literature.[20] However, in the context of a nonsubspeciality clinic this evaluation is not routinely needed.
- POP evaluation should be done with an empty bladder (and if possible an empty rectum) in a supine position. However, if POP is not noted in lithotomy position in a patient complaining of vaginal bulge, the examination should be repeated in a standing position.
- It is important to identify the pelvic organ compartment when determining treatment of POP: anterior (cystocele; **Fig. 1**), posterior (rectocele; **Fig. 2**), and apical (hysterocele/uterine prolapse or vaginal vault prolapse; **Fig. 3**). The compartment can commonly be determined by using a half speculum. With the speculum on the posterior vaginal wall, the patient should Valsalva. This maneuver unmasks an anterior prolapse (cystocele). Attention should then be directed at the cervix/cuff descent. Using the half speculum, the cervix/cuff is identified and the patient is asked again to Valsalva. The speculum should then follow the downward movement of the cervix/cuff to fully identify the degree of apical prolapse. In addition, the speculum is pulled out, inverted, and reinserted to hold the anterior vaginal wall. The same maneuver is repeated to unmask a posterior prolapse (rectocele).
- The most relevant finding during the pelvic examination for prolapse is the presence of protrusion beyond the hymen.
- There are 4 stages of POP. However, a clinically relevant POP that often needs to be treated is prolapsed tissue that extends beyond the hymen (stage $\geq$II).
- In addition, the patient is assessed for occult SUI. A cost-effective, office-based option to evaluate SUI is to instill at least 200 mL of fluid into the bladder and then ask the patient to cough or Valsalva while her POP is reduced with a half speculum. This technique unmasks stress urinary leakage. This method was determined to be noninferior to urodynamic testing in patients without POP with pure SUI.[21] At present, there is no such comparison for patients with POP in the literature.
- A cervical examination should also be performed to rule out malignancy. If surgery is being considered, a recent PAP smear is needed.

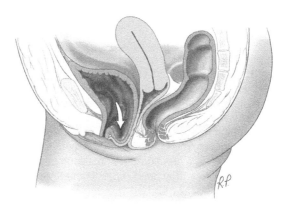

Fig. 1. Anterior compartment prolapse: cystocele. (*Reprinted* with permission, Cleveland Clinic Center for Medical Art & Photography © 2015. All Rights Reserved.)

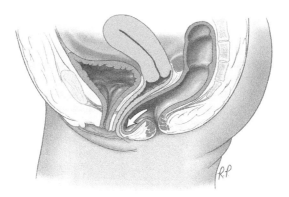

Fig. 2. Posterior compartment prolapse: rectocele. (*Reprinted* with permission, Cleveland Clinic Center for Medical Art & Photography © 2015. All Rights Reserved.)

- ▪ Importantly, the neurologic status of the pelvic floor should be assessed, including a rectal examination assessing sphincter tone.
- • Again, the main determinant to proceed with surgery is symptoms of a vaginal bulge with a pelvic examination consistent with prolapse at any point below the hymenal ring.[12] Is also important to know that there are many asymptomatic elderly patients with significant anatomic POP. Those patients may not need any treatment.

PELVIC ORGAN PROLAPSE TREATMENT OPTIONS
Nonpharmacologic Pelvic Organ Prolapse Treatment Options

Natural evolution of prolapse
Information regarding the exact evolution of POP is scarce and conflicting. Incidence of significant POP in the literature ranges between 15% and 50% (**Fig. 4**).[12] In addition, Bland and colleagues[22] and Gilchrist and colleagues[23] described progression of prolapse in women over time, whereas Bradley and colleagues[24] and Handa and colleagues[25] showed that regression of symptomatic prolapse may also be possible.

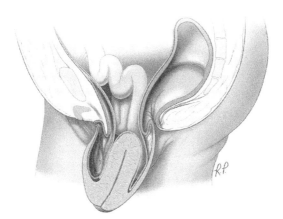

Fig. 3. Apical compartment prolapse: genital procidentia. (*Reprinted* with permission, Cleveland Clinic Center for Medical Art & Photography © 2015. All Rights Reserved.)

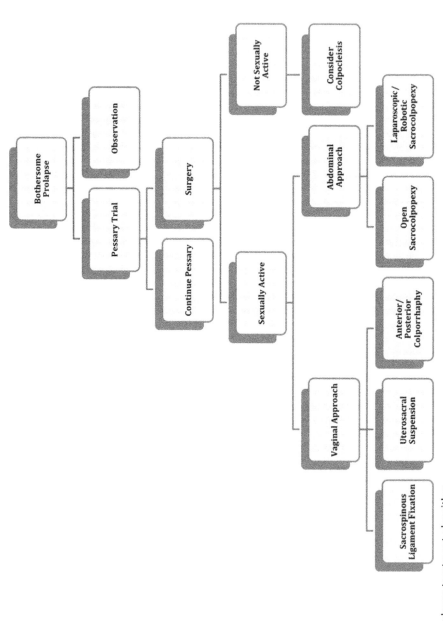

Fig. 4. Prolapse treatment algorithm.

However, this literature must be interpreted with caution because patients included in these studies were not actively seeking treatment or decided not to undergo any treatment of their POP. Therefore, it may be inferred that these patients may be less symptomatic and did not wish to undergo treatment. With this perspective, index patients with POP may not be adequately described by these studies. Pizarro-Berdichevsky and colleagues[26] recently reported a 47.5% progression rate in patients with symptomatic POP actively seeking treatment. In that report, they identified that, when the leading edge is beyond the hymen, the chance of prolapse progression is increased 2-fold.

- Nonsurgical treatments:
  - Physical therapy: the least invasive POP treatment option is pelvic floor physical therapy (PFPT). When therapy is directed by a PFPT specialized therapist, there are data suggesting some anatomic improvement in the POP.[27] PFPT may also improve POP symptoms when patients undergo 1 preoperative and 6 postoperative PFPT sessions at 12 months after surgery compared with usual care (no PFPT).[28] However, it is important not to overestimate the effect of PFPT. In the opinion of the authors, PFPT may be useful for patients with mild to moderate POP, but it is difficult to support the utility of PFPT in patients with severe POP (stage III or IV).
  - Pessaries: these are passive mechanical devices designed to support the vagina. They act as space fillers of the vaginal canal and are an excellent form of noninvasive treatment of POP (**Fig. 5**). Pessaries are the oldest known treatment of POP, dating back more than 2500 years and, until the nineteenth century, it was the only available treatment.[29–31]
    - Pessaries have shown improvement in both POP and urinary symptoms,[32–34] but there remains a paucity of well-designed studies in the literature about their use.
    - In a randomized controlled trial comparing surgery versus pessary use, Abdool and colleagues[35] reported that the only difference between the groups after 1 year was an increase in sexual activity frequency in those who underwent surgery. However, after controlling for age, this difference disappeared. In addition, these results should be interpreted with caution because there was significant loss to follow-up in both groups (32% for pessary and 45% for surgery).

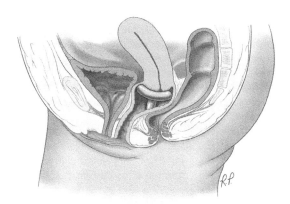

Fig. 5. Vaginal pessary in place supporting the prolapse. (*Reprinted* with permission, Cleveland Clinic Center for Medical Art & Photography © 2015. All Rights Reserved.)

- Many specialists and subspecialists only consider pessaries as a long-term treatment option for patients with contraindications for surgery.[36] However, Kapoor and colleagues[37] showed that two-thirds of patients initially preferred to use a pessary when it was offered as an option. This report highlights the important role of this therapy as a first-line treatment of POP. In addition, pessaries are an excellent option as a bridge to surgery.[36]
- Note that patient age greater than 65 years is one of the characteristics associated with continued long-term use of a pessary.[38] For that reason, this therapy should be considered as a good option in elderly patients as well.
- In terms of patient follow-up, because of the lack of publications on this topic, it is difficult to give guidelines directing patient management during the follow-up period. At present, the recommendation is to return every 3 months to clean the pessary and to check the status of the vaginal mucosa.[39] In cases in which the patient is able to remove the pessary herself, this return visit can be avoided or the increment between visits determined accordingly.

Surgical Treatment Options (if Applicable)

- Surgery is the definitive treatment of POP. In general, the aging population is at a higher risk of perioperative complications than younger patients. However, it is important to consider patient comorbidities and not simply biological age when contemplating surgery because there is no specific age cutoff for anesthesia. Overall, the complications after surgery are low (less than 5%),[40] with cardiovascular effects being the most common. Many elderly women do well, even at ages into the nineties, particularly with transvaginal surgery. In addition, there is no literature to suggest a higher failure rate of POP surgery in elderly patients, regardless of the technique used.[41–44] This information highlights that surgical treatment of POP is feasible and generally safe in elderly patients.
- Therefore, the algorithm regarding surgical technique is very similar to that for the younger population. The only additional technique in non–sexually active elderly patients is the obliterative procedures or colpocleisis.
- Obliterative techniques: in patients who are not sexually active and are not expecting to resume vaginal intercourse, the surgical goals may be slightly different. For this subgroup of patients, the priority is to increase the efficacy and durability of the POP repair.[45] Patients with these characteristics are typically older and, if they have higher surgical risk, a minimally invasive transvaginal extraperitoneal procedure should be considered.[46] A colpocleisis involves closing off most of the vagina thus preventing prolapse. If the patient elects to undergo a colpocleisis, it is essential to give the patient clear information regarding the impossibility of vaginal intercourse in the future and to obtain a careful informed consent. This technique is minimally invasive and is effective, with an overall success rate ranging between 85% and 97%.[47–51]
  - The most commonly used technique in women with a uterus is the Le Fort colpocleisis.[52] Zebede and colleagues[53] reported a large sample size (n = 310) of elderly women (average age, 81 ± 5 years), with a median follow-up of 5.5 months (range, 0.5–87 months) after Le Fort colpocleisis. The subjective and objective cure rates were 92.9% and 98%, respectively. The complication rate was 15%, but the mortality was much lower: 3 of 310 patients (0.9%). The postoperative SUI rate was 9.7%; however, this has previously been reported to be as high as 28%.[47] Smith and colleagues[50] reported a reduction of SUI

when adding a suburethral sling at the time of colpocleisis. One technique that has shown a lower rate of de novo SUI is the Labhardt colpoperineocleisis (5.8% without any concomitant anti-incontinence procedure).[51] The investigators suggest that these differences could be explained by the Labhardt technique involving a bladder neck angle that is not significantly changed compared with the Le Fort procedure.

○ These results highlight that obliterative techniques are a viable and safe option.
- Reconstructive surgeries:
  ○ Regarding the most effective reconstructive surgery in the elderly population, there have been no specific systematic reviews or meta-analyses that focus specifically on this group of patients. Several studies are mentioned earlier that show comparative outcomes in patients older than 65 years compared with younger patients; however, these reports are retrospective and lack well-controlled comparison groups with consistent follow-up.
  ○ The best available evidence regarding the use of reconstructive procedures has been a Cochrane Review that was updated in 2013.[54]
    ■ Sacrocolpopexy: this is an abdominal procedure involving the attachment of the vaginal apex to the sacral anterior longitudinal ligament using a graft, usually of synthetic, nonabsorbable mesh (**Fig. 6**). Nowadays, it is often performed laparoscopically or robotically assisted.[55]
      - Maher and colleagues[54] reported better anatomic outcomes for sacrocolpopexy than for vaginal sacrospinous fixation, but with longer operative and recovery time as well as higher cost. There is no decisive evidence to favor laparoscopic or robotic surgery rather than open abdominal sacrocolpopexy. However, Nygaard and colleagues[56] published the long-term results of the CARE (Colpopexy and Urinary Reduction Efforts) randomized controlled trial for open abdominal sacrocolpopexy, with a disappointing 34% POP recurrence failure rate, mainly in the anterior

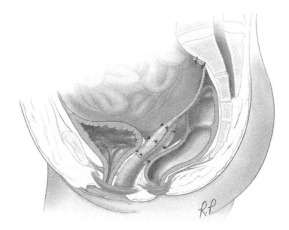

Fig. 6. Sacrocolpopexy: vaginal apex attached to the sacral anterior longitudinal ligament using a mesh. (*Reprinted* with permission, Cleveland Clinic Center for Medical Art & Photography © 2015. All Rights Reserved.)

compartment. Keeping in mind the elderly patient population, the intraoperative risk factors (longer time of an intra-abdominal surgery), the longer recovery time after a transabdominal approach, and the lack of significant differences in outcomes, physicians are likely to pursue nonsurgical treatment or the transvaginal surgical route in this population.

- Transvaginal procedures: in general, these procedures are preferred in older patients based on a much easier recovery, less pain, and lower surgical risk compared with abdominal approaches. These techniques can be classified as native tissue repairs or mesh-augmented procedures.
  - Native tissue repairs:
    - Anterior and posterior compartment defects: for the anterior compartment defect (cystocele) and posterior compartment defects (rectocele), the vaginal mucosa is incised and the bladder or rectum is pushed upwards or downwards, respectively. Then the stronger lateral tissue is plicated in the midline and the vaginal mucosa is closed (**Fig. 7**). For the anterior colporrhaphy, the anatomic recurrence has been reported to be as high as 40% to 60%, but the symptomatic recurrence and the reoperation rate are much lower.[57]
    - Apical defects (uterine prolapse or vault prolapse): several surgical techniques are available. Some of them allow uterine preservation. The most widely used are the sacrospinous ligament fixation and

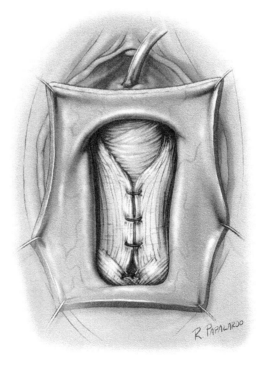

Fig. 7. Anterior colporrhaphy: the stronger anterior lateral tissue is plicated in the midline. (*Reprinted* with permission, Cleveland Clinic Center for Medical Art & Photography © 2015. All Rights Reserved.)

the high uterosacral ligament fixation. In the first procedure, stitches (absorbable or nonabsorbable) are placed through the right sacrospinous ligament through a vaginal incision (**Fig. 8**). These sutures are then tied to the vault or cervix. In the second procedure, bilateral stitches are placed in the uterosacral ligaments and then tied at the vault. For both techniques the reoperation rate for POP recurrence is low.[54]

- Mesh-augmented surgeries: based on the poor anatomic results (mainly for the anterior compartment), new techniques were developed to improve postoperative POP repair results. One such technique was the transvaginal mesh repair. This mesh consisted of a transobturator armed prosthesis to support the anterior vaginal wall (similar to a transobturator tape mesh for incontinence). Even though there is a higher anatomic outcome success rate, there are no significant differences in the subjective outcomes for patients. In addition, there is a much higher complication rate and higher overall reoperation rate compared with native tissue repairs (11% vs 3%).[54]

- Concomitant anti-incontinence procedures: continence surgeries at the time of POP repair are likely to be beneficial. However, in our opinion, prophylactic anti-incontinence surgery may not be beneficial for elderly patients with POP because of the risks of voiding dysfunction. A decision on a concomitant anti-incontinence procedure should be individualized, taking many factors into consideration.

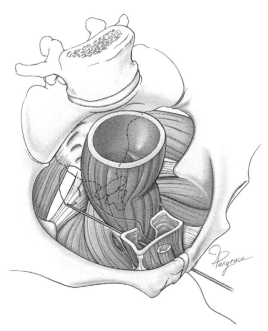

Fig. 8. Sacrospinous ligament fixation: stitches are placed in the right ligament through a vaginal incision. (*Reprinted* with permission, Cleveland Clinic Center for Medical Art & Photography © 2015. All Rights Reserved.)

SUMMARY/DISCUSSION

- POP will continue to be a major health focus in the elderly population over the next few decades. With the older patient population continuing to live longer, it may be expected that patients will be more active and may need to maintain a high QoL standard.
- Although there are no randomized controlled trials for elderly patients with POP, the evaluation, diagnosis, and treatment of these patients should not be very different from those of the general population.
- Although a significant proportion of this population may have POP, many are not bothered by it and only a minority need treatment.
- Specific treatment options in this patient population include pelvic floor therapy, pessaries, and surgery. Many patients do well with a pessary. Surgery is the definitive treatment. In this population, closing off the vagina, colpocleisis, may be a reasonable approach. However, the patient must be appropriately counseled regarding the inability to resume vaginal intercourse after an obliterative procedure.
- This subgroup of patients may be challenging given their increased risk of medical comorbidities. However, physicians should not focus entirely on the biological age to determine patient treatment. Instead, the functional status, sexual status, and desires of the patient must all be taken into account in order to optimize the patient's QoL.

REFERENCES

1. Administration for Community Living, Administration on Aging. Aging statistics. 2014. Available at: http://www.aoa.gov/Aging_Statistics/. Accessed November 25, 2014.
2. Morley GW. Treatment of uterine and vaginal prolapse. Clin Obstet Gynecol 1996; 39(4):959–69.
3. Chen GD. Pelvic floor dysfunction in aging women. Taiwan J Obstet Gynecol 2007;46(4):374–8.
4. Swift SE, Pound T, Dias JK. Case-control study of etiologic factors in the development of severe pelvic organ prolapse. Int Urogynecol J Pelvic Floor Dysfunct 2001;12(3):187–92.
5. Jelovsek JE, Maher C, Barber MD. Pelvic organ prolapse. Lancet 2007; 369(9566):1027–38.
6. Wu JM, Matthews CA, Conover MM, et al. Lifetime risk of stress urinary incontinence or pelvic organ prolapse surgery. Obstet Gynecol 2014;123(6):1201–6.
7. Srikrishna S, Robinson D, Cardozo L, et al. Experiences and expectations of women with urogenital prolapse: a quantitative and qualitative exploration. BJOG 2008;115(11):1362–8.
8. Espuna Pons M, Puig Clota M. Lower urinary tract symptoms in women and impact on quality of life. Results of the application of the King's Health Questionnaire. Actas Urol Esp 2006;30(7):684–91 [in Spanish].
9. Digesu GA, Chaliha C, Salvatore S, et al. The relationship of vaginal prolapse severity to symptoms and quality of life. BJOG 2005;112(7):971–6.
10. Fitzgerald MP, Janz NK, Wren PA, et al. Prolapse severity, symptoms and impact on quality of life among women planning sacrocolpopexy. Int J Gynaecol Obstet 2007;98(1):24–8.
11. Haylen BT, de Ridder D, Freeman RM, et al. An International Urogynecological Association (IUGA)/International Continence Society (ICS) joint report on the terminology for female pelvic floor dysfunction. Neurourol Urodyn 2010;29(1):4–20.

12. Barber MD, Maher C. Epidemiology and outcome assessment of pelvic organ prolapse. Int Urogynecol J 2013;24(11):1783–90.
13. Barber MD. Symptoms and outcome measures of pelvic organ prolapse. Clin Obstet Gynecol 2005;48(3):648–61.
14. Ellerkmann RM, Cundiff GW, Melick CF, et al. Correlation of symptoms with location and severity of pelvic organ prolapse. Am J Obstet Gynecol 2001;185(6): 1332–7 [discussion: 1337–8].
15. Tan JS, Lukacz ES, Menefee SA, et al. Predictive value of prolapse symptoms: a large database study. Int Urogynecol J Pelvic Floor Dysfunct 2005;16(3):203–9 [discussion: 209].
16. Swift SE, Tate SB, Nicholas J. Correlation of symptoms with degree of pelvic organ support in a general population of women: what is pelvic organ prolapse? Am J Obstet Gynecol 2003;189(2):372–7 [discussion: 377–9].
17. Bradley CS, Nygaard IE. Vaginal wall descensus and pelvic floor symptoms in older women. Obstet Gynecol 2005;106(4):759–66.
18. Beverly CM, Walters MD, Weber AM, et al. Prevalence of hydronephrosis in patients undergoing surgery for pelvic organ prolapse. Obstet Gynecol 1997; 90(1):37–41.
19. Dongol A, Joshi KS, K C S. Renal impairment among patients with pelvic organ prolapse in a tertiary care center. Kathmandu Univ Med J (KUMJ) 2013;11(41): 71–4.
20. Bump RC, Mattiasson A, Bo K, et al. The standardization of terminology of female pelvic organ prolapse and pelvic floor dysfunction. Am J Obstet Gynecol 1996; 175(1):10–7.
21. Nager CW, Brubaker L, Litman HJ, et al. A randomized trial of urodynamic testing before stress-incontinence surgery. N Engl J Med 2012;366(21): 1987–97.
22. Bland DR, Earle BB, Vitolins MZ, et al. Use of the pelvic organ prolapse staging system of the International continence Society, American Urogynecologic Society, and Society of gynecologic Surgeons in perimenopausal women. Am J Obstet Gynecol 1999;181(6):1324–7 [discussion: 1327–8].
23. Gilchrist AS, Campbell W, Steele H, et al. Outcomes of observation as therapy for pelvic organ prolapse: a study in the natural history of pelvic organ prolapse. Neurourol Urodyn 2013;32(4):383–6.
24. Bradley CS, Zimmerman MB, Qi Y, et al. Natural history of pelvic organ prolapse in postmenopausal women. Obstet Gynecol 2007;109(4):848–54.
25. Handa VL, Garrett E, Hendrix S, et al. Progression and remission of pelvic organ prolapse: a longitudinal study of menopausal women. Am J Obstet Gynecol 2004;190(1):27–32.
26. Pizarro-Berdichevsky J, Pattillo A, Arellano M, et al. Risk factors for pelvic organ prolapse (POP) progression in a prospective cohort of symptomatic women actively seeking treatment. Int Urogynecol J 2014;25(Suppl 1):S32–3.
27. Stupp L, Resende AP, Oliveira E, et al. Pelvic floor muscle training for treatment of pelvic organ prolapse: an assessor-blinded randomized controlled trial. Int Urogynecol J 2011;22(10):1233–9.
28. McClurg D, Hilton P, Dolan L, et al. Pelvic floor muscle training as an adjunct to prolapse surgery: a randomised feasibility study. Int Urogynecol J 2014;25(7): 883–91.
29. Lamers BH, Broekman BM, Milani AL. Pessary treatment for pelvic organ prolapse and health-related quality of life: a review. Int Urogynecol J 2011;22(6): 637–44.

30. Mutone MF, Terry C, Hale DS, et al. Factors which influence the short-term success of pessary management of pelvic organ prolapse. Am J Obstet Gynecol 2005;193(1):89–94.

31. Powers K, Lazarou G, Wang A, et al. Pessary use in advanced pelvic organ prolapse. Int Urogynecol J Pelvic Floor Dysfunct 2006;17(2):160–4.

32. Clemons JL, Aguilar VC, Tillinghast TA, et al. Patient satisfaction and changes in prolapse and urinary symptoms in women who were fitted successfully with a pessary for pelvic organ prolapse. Am J Obstet Gynecol 2004;190(4):1025–9.

33. Fernando RJ, Thakar R, Sultan AH, et al. Effect of vaginal pessaries on symptoms associated with pelvic organ prolapse. Obstet Gynecol 2006;108(1):93–9.

34. Komesu YM, Rogers RG, Rode MA, et al. Pelvic floor symptom changes in pessary users. Am J Obstet Gynecol 2007;197(6):620.e1–6.

35. Abdool Z, Thakar R, Sultan AH, et al. Prospective evaluation of outcome of vaginal pessaries versus surgery in women with symptomatic pelvic organ prolapse. Int Urogynecol J 2011;22(3):273–8.

36. Bash KL. Review of vaginal pessaries. Obstet Gynecol Surv 2000;55(7):455–60.

37. Kapoor DS, Thakar R, Sultan AH, et al. Conservative versus surgical management of prolapse: what dictates patient choice? Int Urogynecol J Pelvic Floor Dysfunct 2009;20(10):1157–61.

38. Clemons JL, Aguilar VC, Sokol ER, et al. Patient characteristics that are associated with continued pessary use versus surgery after 1 year. Am J Obstet Gynecol 2004;191(1):159–64.

39. Khaja A, Freeman RM. How often should shelf/Gellhorn pessaries be changed? A survey of IUGA urogynaecologists. Int Urogynecol J 2014;25(7):941–6.

40. Menard JP, Mulfinger C, Estrade JP, et al. Pelvic organ prolapse surgery in women aged more than 70 years: a literature review. Gynecol Obstet Fertil 2008;36(1):67–73 [in French].

41. Ghezzi F, Uccella S, Cromi A, et al. Surgical treatment for pelvic floor disorders in women 75 years or older: a single-center experience. Menopause 2011;18(3):314–8.

42. Sung VW, Joo K, Marques F, et al. Patient-reported outcomes after combined surgery for pelvic floor disorders in older compared to younger women. Am J Obstet Gynecol 2009;201(5):534.e1–5.

43. Mohammed N, Raschid Hoda M, Fornara P. Prolapse surgery in octogenarians: are we pushing the limits too far? World J Urol 2013;31(3):623–8.

44. Gabriel B, Rubod C, Cordova LG, et al. Prolapse surgery in women of 80 years and older using the Prolift technique. Int Urogynecol J 2010;21(12):1463–70.

45. FitzGerald MP, Richter HE, Siddique S, et al. Colpocleisis: a review. Int Urogynecol J Pelvic Floor Dysfunct 2006;17(3):261–71.

46. Abbasy S, Kenton K. Obliterative procedures for pelvic organ prolapse. Clin Obstet Gynecol 2010;53(1):86–98.

47. FitzGerald MP, Brubaker L. Colpocleisis and urinary incontinence. Am J Obstet Gynecol 2003;189(5):1241–4.

48. Denehy TR, Choe JY, Gregori CA, et al. Modified Le Fort partial colpocleisis with Kelly urethral plication and posterior colpoperineoplasty in the medically compromised elderly: a comparison with vaginal hysterectomy, anterior colporrhaphy, and posterior colpoperineoplasty. Am J Obstet Gynecol 1995;173(6):1697–701 [discussion: 1701–2].

49. Wheeler TL 2nd, Richter HE, Burgio KL, et al. Regret, satisfaction, and symptom improvement: analysis of the impact of partial colpocleisis for the management of severe pelvic organ prolapse. Am J Obstet Gynecol 2005;193(6):2067–70.

50. Smith AL, Karp DR, Lefevre R, et al. LeFort colpocleisis and stress incontinence: weighing the risk of voiding dysfunction with sling placement. Int Urogynecol J 2011;22(11):1357–62.
51. Pizarro-Berdichevsky J, Galleguillos G, Cuevas R, et al. Labhardt's colpoperineocleisis: subjective results of an alternative treatment for genital prolapse in patients who are not sexually active–2-year follow-up. Int Urogynecol J 2014; 25(3):417–24.
52. Reiffenstuhl G, Platzer W, Knaptein P, et al. Surgical anatomy and technique. Vaginal operations. Baltimore (MD): Williams & Wilkins; 1996. p. 161–80.
53. Zebede S, Smith AL, Plowright LN, et al. Obliterative LeFort colpocleisis in a large group of elderly women. Obstet Gynecol 2013;121(2 Pt 1):279–84.
54. Maher C, Feiner B, Baessler K, et al. Surgical management of pelvic organ prolapse in women. Cochrane Database Syst Rev 2013;(4):CD004014.
55. Visco AG, Advincula AP. Robotic gynecologic surgery. Obstet Gynecol 2008; 112(6):1369–84.
56. Nygaard I, Brubaker L, Zyczynski HM, et al. Long-term outcomes following abdominal sacrocolpopexy for pelvic organ prolapse. JAMA 2013;309(19): 2016–24.
57. Chmielewski L, Walters MD, Weber AM, et al. Reanalysis of a randomized trial of 3 techniques of anterior colporrhaphy using clinically relevant definitions of success. Am J Obstet Gynecol 2011;205(1):69.e1–8.

Underactive Bladder in Older Adults

Yao-Chi Chuang, MD[a], Mauricio Plata, MD[b], Laura E. Lamb, PhD[c],
Michael B. Chancellor, MD[c],*

KEYWORDS

- Underactive bladder • Aging • Overactive bladder • Urinary incontinence

KEY POINTS

- Underactive bladder (UAB) is a major problem that is not well known in the public and health care sectors but is an enormous economic problem that will become more prevalent with the increasing age of populations.
- UAB is a major burden because there are no effective UAB treatments and diagnostic tools.
- Research and education are critical if understanding of UAB is to be advanced; this includes a need for work on the epidemiology, pathophysiology, clinical manifestations, and outcomes of UAB for affected patients and their caregivers.
- There is a critical need for more effective treatment options beyond those currently available. Improved understanding and awareness will in turn lead to changes in health care policy that could have a substantial positive impact on care for patients with UAB.

INTRODUCTION

The average human lifespan has increased globally because of progressive improvements in public health, clinical care, and health technology. Aging is a growth industry in modern society. Individuals born between 1946 and 1964, the last of the so-called baby boomer generation, will reach the age of 65 years in 2030, which will result in 71 million geriatric Americans, constituting 20% of the US population.[1,2] This proportion of older adults will deal with higher rates of chronic conditions affecting the bladder, including lower urinary tract dysfunction, overactive bladder (OAB), urinary incontinence, and underactive bladder (UAB).[3] As the US population continues to grow older, the number of people affected by urinary dysfunction and the associated costs will

[a] Department of Urology, Kaohsiung Chang Gung Memorial Hospital, Chung Shan Medical University Institute of Medicine, Kaohsiung, Taiwan; [b] Department of Urology, Fundación Santa Fe de Bogotá University Hospital, Universidad de los Andes School of Medicine, Bogotá, Colombia; [c] Department of Urology, Aikens Neurourology Research Center, Oakland University William Beaumont School of Medicine, Royal Oak, MI, USA
* Corresponding author.
E-mail address: chancellormb@gmail.com

Clin Geriatr Med 31 (2015) 523–533
http://dx.doi.org/10.1016/j.cger.2015.06.002
0749-0690/15/$ – see front matter © 2015 Elsevier Inc. All rights reserved.

escalate. However, the confounding effects of polypharmacy and multiple comorbidities in the aging population make it hard to determine whether changes are caused by aging alone or related to other conditions.

OAB is a well-known and well-studied condition in urology. However, the opposite syndrome to OAB, UAB, has received scant attention in the scientific community. UAB is used to describe the symptoms of impaired bladder emptying. However, UAB remains under-researched, poorly understood, and underused because of a lack of consensus on terminology, and a lack of standardization of diagnostic criteria. Although detrusor underactivity, defined by the International Continence Society (ICS) as "a contraction of reduced strength and/or duration, resulting in prolonged bladder emptying and/or a failure to achieve complete bladder emptying within a normal time span,"[4] is a term that is urodynamically defined, like its opposite, detrusor overactivity, this definition serves as a foundation to describe the functional abnormality; however, it is hampered by broad subjectivity and lacks strict parameters.

RED FLAGS OF UNDERACTIVE BLADDER

UAB occurs when the bladder loses its ability to contract and fully empty. Part of what makes this condition so vexing is that the symptoms can come and go, and they often mimic those of other diseases, such as prostate enlargement and urinary tract infections, both of which can cause frequent urination (another UAB symptom). With UAB, patients have difficulty telling when their bladders are full. When they do have the urge to urinate, it may be painful, the urine may dribble, or it may not come at all. It may take several minutes to start a stream of urine. They also may feel that there's urine left behind and end up heading to the bathroom again a short time later. When the bladder does not completely empty, urine builds up. This buildup can lead to embarrassing episodes of leakage from overflow incontinence and recurring bladder and kidney infections (**Box 1**).

Box 1
Talk with patients about how to cope with UAB

- Functional steps that may be helpful:

  ○ Double voiding. This technique gives extra time to empty the bladder. After urinating, stay at the toilet for a few additional minutes. After this short break, try to urinate again. If the bladder has not fully emptied, it is often possible to pass more urine.

  ○ Triggered-reflex voiding. This technique involves the use of various stimulation techniques to trigger the brain signals that initiate contractions of the bladder and the flow of urine. The technique may work for anyone with UAB but can be especially useful for a person with a spinal cord injury who still has some reflexes but may not be able to feel whether the bladder is full. Rub the area just above the pubic bone, tug on the pubic hair, or gently squeeze the head of the penis. Try different triggers to see which one works.

- Medications. Men with UAB may get relief from α-blocker drugs used for prostate obstruction. Relaxing the muscle of the bladder neck and proximal urethra helps men to empty the bladder. Bethanechol may be tried but its efficacy is limited.

- Catheterization. With self-catheterization, a catheter is inserted into the urethra to drain urine from the bladder. For people who are unable to do this, an indwelling catheter can be inserted into the urethra by a health care professional to automatically drain urine into a pouch for a set period of time. For people who cannot tolerate an indwelling urethral catheter, a suprapubic catheter may be used.

CAUSES OF UNDERACTIVE BLADDER

When messages between the brain and the bladder are short circuited, the patient's body does not register the normal urge to urinate when the bladder is full. This breakdown in communication may be triggered by a stroke, Parkinson disease, acute urinary tract infection, radiation therapy to the pelvic area, nerve damage after pelvic surgery, or even a herniated disk. In young populations, multiple sclerosis and diabetes are common conditions that can damage sacral spinal cord peripheral nerves that innervate the urinary bladder. As people age, the muscles of the bladder lose some of their elasticity and ability to contract. There is a loss of bladder contractility and voiding efficiency with age. There is also a reduction in muscarinic receptors and acetylcholinesterase-positive nerves in the human bladder as well as a decreased expression of some neuropeptides, such as substance P[4–7] (**Box 2**).

EPIDEMIOLOGY

UAB, like OAB, is a major health issue that shows an age-related increase in prevalence. The clinical symptoms of UAB are indistinguishable from the obstructive lower urinary tract symptoms (LUTS), namely weak stream, intermittency, hesitancy, and straining to void. In patients with OAB with symptoms of frequency and small amounts of voided urine, urgency with or without urge incontinence can be detected with detrusor hyperreflexia and impaired contractility.[5] Therefore, the diagnosis of UAB is difficult from the clinical symptoms only. The epidemiology study regarding detrusor underactivity is based on urodynamic study with variable diagnosis criteria.

Jeong and colleagues[6] examined the prevalence of detrusor underactivity based on bladder contractility index less than 100 for men, and a maximal flow rate (Q_{max}) less than or equal to 12 mL/s combined with a detrusor pressure at Q_{max} less than or equal to 10 cm H_2O for women, in 1179 aged population more than 65 years of age with non-neurogenic voiding dysfunction presenting with urinary tract symptoms. More than 40.2% of men and 13.3% of women had detrusor underactivity, and the numbers increased with age in both groups. In addition, 46.5% of men with detrusor underactivity also had detrusor overactivity or bladder outlet obstruction (BOO) and 72.6% of the women with detrusor underactivity also had detrusor overactivity or stress urinary incontinence.

Box 2
Causes of UAB

- Aging
- Bladder outlet obstruction (BOO)
- Diabetes mellitus (diabetic cystopathy)
- Idiopathic
- Neurologic disorders
  - Injury to the spinal cord, cauda equina, and pelvic plexus
    - Pelvic surgery and fractures, herniated disc, pudendal nerve injury
  - Spinal cord injury, cerebrovascular accidents, multiple sclerosis, Parkinson disease
  - Infectious neurologic problems
    - Acquired immunodeficiency syndrome, neurosyphilis, zoster, herpes simplex, Guillain-Barré syndrome

In men, detrusor underactivity may be caused by BOO or may represent an independent disease process related to aging.[7] Abarbanel and Marcus[8] reported impaired detrusor contractility in 48% of men and 12% of women based on the urodynamic definition of maximal flow rate of less than 10 mL/s, together with a detrusor pressure of less than 30 cm H_2O from 181 patients (82 men and 99 women) aged 70 years or older with LUTS. Two-thirds of men and one-half of women with impaired detrusor contractility also had involuntary contraction. It has been estimated that 10% to 20% of male patients with low flow rate have an element of detrusor underactivity. Detrusor underactivity is present in 9% to 28% of men less than 50 years of age, increasing to 48% in men more than 70 years of age.[7] In older women, detrusor underactivity is also a common condition, with estimated prevalence ranges from 12% to 45%, peaking in the institutionalized population.[7] Thomas and colleagues[9] reported that the natural history of untreated detrusor underactivity in men with a minimum 10-year urodynamic follow-up revealed that detrusor underactivity is not progressive in most nonneurogenic male patients, and detrusor underactivity often does not result in chronic urinary retention. Kuo[10] reported that 33% of men (mean age, 75.3 years) with persistent LUTS after prostatectomy had detrusor underactivity. Also, nearly two-thirds of the incontinent institutionalized elderly population show evidence of detrusor underactivity. UAB rather than obstruction has been found to be the cause of LUTS in 23% to 73% of symptomatic elderly men.[5–8]

THE UNRECOGNIZED PROBLEM

UAB is significant problem that will become more prevalent with an increasingly aged population and the rapid increase in the rate of diabetes that may result in diabetic cystopathy. Lacking effective therapy for UAB, general urologists have hardly noticed the problem. A search on PubMed noted 40-fold fewer publications on UAB than OAB in the medical literature (**Table 1**). A population-based survey by Valente and colleagues[11] highlighted the levels of prevalence and awareness of UAB in the general population. The survey revealed that 23% of the public (54% men; 46% women) reported having a problem emptying the bladder completely, but only 11% had ever heard of UAB.

CONTRIBUTING FACTORS AND PATHOPHYSIOLOGY

Aging and older age have been linked to UAB because of high prevalence in the specific population; however, advanced age is not the only cause of UAB. The presence of UAB in wide range of clinical groups suggests a multifactorial pathogenesis.[7,8,12] Risk factors related to the pathophysiologic processes of UAB include diabetes mellitus,

Table 1 Peer-reviewed published research on PubMed in September 2014	
Terms	Peer Review Publications
Urinary incontinence	34,623
Aging bladder	1134
Detrusor overactivity	1876
OAB	4632
Detrusor underactivity	170
UAB	114

BOO, neurologic problems involving the lumbosacral nerve roots, and pelvic surgery that causes the damage of the pelvic nerve plexus. In aged women, a profound lack of estrogen could also potentially contribute to UAB by favoring the development of degenerative or biochemical changes involving key components of the contractility of detrusor muscle, or its innervations.[5,8,13] Furthermore, it is also common for older people with polypharmacy, which may include medications such as calcium channels blockers, neuroleptics, and alpha-receptor agonists, to develop UAB.

Putative mechanisms of UAB include neural, nonneural, and aging factors:

- Neural: surgical injuries, trauma, or diseases affecting the central or peripheral nervous systems, which cause defects in either afferent innervation or in its integrative control at spinal and supraspinal centers, and leads to poor efferent outflow and impaired voiding efficiency.
- Nonneural: diseases affecting the bladder, including urothelium and detrusor muscle. Changes in neurotransmitter release from the urothelium as well as in the sensitivity and coupling of the suburothelial interstitial cell-afferent network lead to loss of bladder volume sensitivity and impaired voiding efficiency. The disability of the detrusor to contract efficiently, or decreased excitability, imply a defect in the muscle.
- Aging: progressive decrease in neural and/or nonneural functions related to degeneration, random cellular damage, and genetic aging programs. Caveolae are vesicles involved in bladder muscle cell signaling, the numbers of which increase with bladder maturation but decrease with aging.[14,15] Muscarinic and purinergic receptors are molecules involved in bladder contraction and are known to cluster in caveolae. The dense-band pattern with caveolar depletion has been described as the ultrastructural pattern associated with normative aging bladder and this change is increased in older adults with detrusor underactivity.[14]

PROGRESSION OF OVERACTIVE BLADDER TO UNDERACTIVE BLADDER

Chancellor has hypothesized that UAB and OAB may not be separate disease entities.[16] Instead, chronic untreated or treatment-refractory OAB, caused by neurologic diseases such as diabetes, BOO, or aging, may progress to detrusor hyperreflexia with impaired contractility and eventually UAB.[16] The progression of OAB to UAB hypothesis suggests that early education, behavioral modification, and medical treatment may alter and/or prevent progression to UAB.

CLINICAL EVALUATION

The physical examination may reveal a distended bladder and large amount of postmicturition residual urine in patients with UAB. It is common that loss of neurologic control is one of the major causes of UAB in aged adults. Neurologic injury might be caused by occult or overt pelvic or sacral injury and should have a careful physical examination. Assessment of bulbocavernosus reflex, perianal sensation, and anal sphincter tone is used to detect the integrity of the sacral dermatomes. Parasympathetic denervation causes UAB, whereas sympathetic damage produces loss of function of the bladder neck and urethra and leads to urinary incontinence.[17] The clinical symptoms of UAB include straining to urinate, diminished and interrupted urinary stream, sensation of incomplete emptying, and may also include incontinence.

Sensory loss or anesthesia in the perineum or perianal area is associated with S2 to S4 dermatomes, which is a useful predictive clinical index in patients with lumbar disc prolapse or lumbar canal stenosis. It has been reported that the bulbocavernosus reflex was absent or significantly diminished in 84% of cases with cauda equina injury, whereas the perineal sensation and muscle stretch reflexes were compromised in 77% of cases.[18] A complete injury of the pelvic plexus disrupts the nerve supply to the bladder and the urethra, but most injuries are incomplete. If sensation is lost, the drive of micturition is lost and the resultant symptoms are usually urinary retention and overflow incontinence.[19]

EVALUATION OF UNDERACTIVE BLADDER

- Urinalysis: rule out infection and diabetes
- Residual urine volume measurement: via ultrasonography bladder scan or catheterization for measurement of residual urine
- Uroflow: noninvasive test to evaluate for diminished flow rate that may indicate impaired contractility, BOO, or both
- Urodynamics: catheter-based test that can measure bladder sensation and contractility power

UNDERACTIVE BLADDER QUESTIONNAIRE

UAB, especially UAB with chronic urinary retention, has a negative impact on the patients' quality of life, interfering with daily activities, and increasing the threat of recurrent urinary tract infection. Previous epidemiologic studies have shown that detrusor underactivity is highly prevalent in the aged population based on urodynamic definition. However, a popular symptom score for UAB is still lacking. Clinicians are working toward development of a validated UAB symptom score (UAB questionnaire [UAB-Q]) (**Table 2**) by using a self-reported questionnaire to quantify UAB symptoms. If total UAB-Q score is 3 or greater, the patient may have UAB and may need to talk with a

Table 2
UAB-Q

(1) In the past week, how often did you have the urge to urinate but could not urinate?	Three or more times □	Two times □	One time □	None of the time □
(2) In the past week, on a typical night, how often did you wake up in the night to urinate?	Three or more times □	Two times □	One time □	None of the time □
(3) In the past week, during the day, how often did you have to urinate again just after you urinated?	All of the time □	Most of the time □	Some of the time □	None of the time □
(4) In the past week, how often have you had to strain/push to empty your bladder?	All of the time □	Most of the time □	Some of the time □	None of the time □
(5) In the past week, during the day, how strong was the feeling that you did not empty your bladder after you urinated?	Extremely strong □	Moderately strong □	A little strong □	Not at all strong □
Score	3	2	1	0

Directions: please check the box that best describes your bladder symptoms or the impact of your bladder symptoms.
Adapted from Underactive Bladder Foundation. Available at: http://www.underactivebladder.org/index.php/bladder-health-survey; with permission. Accessed September 29, 2014.

health care professional. For more information, visit http://www.underactivebladder.org/.

UAB-Q may be a useful tool for research and clinical practice if the posttreatment reduction in the UAB-Q is consistent with the global impression of patients of the therapeutic efficacy. Correlation with the urodynamic parameters needs to be assessed and additional studies of the UAB-Q as a symptom assessment tool are needed.

THERAPEUTIC DIRECTIONS

LUTS associated with OAB or BOO caused by urethral dysfunction or benign prostate hyperplasia have traditionally been treated with antimuscarinic agents or alpha-adrenergic blockers. However, the treatment of UAB symptoms focused on increasing detrusor smooth muscle strength by using muscarinic receptor agonists, such as bethanechol, to stimulate detrusor muscarinic receptors fails to prove the therapeutic effects for UAB.[20] The causes of detrusor underactivity are variable and the degree to which UAB attributes to detrusor underactivity is not known.[12] Therefore, the proposed causes of UAB, and detrusor underactivity, must be reconsidered. There is an emergent need to define specific phenotypes of UAB through pathophysiologic categorizations of the underlying causes of UAB to provide new, effective, and safe therapies for UAB (**Box 3**).

CHOLINESTERASE INHIBITORS

Tanaka and colleagues[21] reported that a total of 14 poor voiders after transurethral resection of the prostate who were 50 years old or older with weak detrusor

---

Box 3
Treatment options for UAB

Bladder

Afferent: improve sensation

- Sacral neuromodulation

Efferent/myogenic: increase contractility

- Cholinergic agonist and cholinesterase inhibitor
- Brindley neuromodulation
- Latissimus dorsi flap and bladder reduction surgeries
- Stem cell regenerative therapy

Urethra

Reduce outlet resistance

- Alpha-adrenergic blocker
- Botulinum toxin
- Bladder neck and prostate surgery
- Phosphodiesterase inhibitor
- Skeletal muscle relaxant, including baclofen and benzodiazepines
- Urethrolysis and sphincterotomy

Combination

Combine agents to both stimulate bladder emptying and induce urethral relaxation

contractility as shown by Schäfer diagram received 4 weeks of daily treatment with 15 mg of oral distigmine. Detrusor contractility according to Schäfer diagram had a tendency to improve and maximum flow rate improved significantly from 8.9 mL/s to a mean of more than 12 mL/s after oral distigmine treatment. Bougas and colleagues[22] reported on 27 patients with UAB treated with distigmine (choline esterase inhibitor) 5 mg 3 times a day with resultant improvements in voided volumes and decreased postvoid residuals. In addition, pressure/flow measurements improved, but not significantly, in this study.

PROSTAGLANDIN E2 AND PROSTAGLANDIN RECEPTORS

Prostaglandin E2 (PGE2) can increase detrusor contraction, relax urethra, and enhance sensory function by stimulating capsaicin sensitive afferent nerves.[23–25] The effects of PGE2 are produced through 4 types of prostaglandin receptors (EP1–EP4), each mediating separate actions. EP1 and EP3 are stimulatory receptors, mediating smooth muscle contraction by an increase of phosphoinositol turnover and calcium mobilization, or a decrease of adenylate cyclase and cyclic AMP levels, respectively.[24,25] EP2 receptors are known to mediate bladder and urethral relaxation. In a test of an additive approach, bethanechol 50 mg 4 times daily and intravesical PGE2 treatment (1.5 mg in 20 mL of 0.9% saline, once weekly) together for 6 weeks showed limited therapeutic effect compared with placebo in a study of 17 male and 2 female patients with detrusor underactivity.[26] However, it would be interesting to test agents with these receptor agonists in patients with UAB.

SACRAL NEUROMODULATION

A subset of patients with UAB symptoms have idiopathic retention, for which sacral neuromodulation (Interstim, Medtronic) is the only regulatory approved therapy. The control of guarding and voiding reflexes is located in close proximity in the S2 to S4 levels of the human spinal cord in response to different clinical scenarios.[27] It has been shown that it is possible to modulate these reflexes via sacral nerve stimulation (SNS) and restore voluntary micturition. Fowler syndrome is thought to be caused by poorly relaxing sphincter–induced poor bladder sensation and detrusor underactivity.[28] The study of functional MRI in women with retention associated with Fowler syndrome has shown diminished brain activations in relevant visceral receptive areas. SNS can normalize brain responses, improve bladder sensations, and restore voiding function in nonobstructive urinary retention.[29] However, the positive responses to SNS in patients with idiopathic retention may be limited to those with nonneurogenic urethral overactivity/sphincteric dyssynergia and the sensory suppression in Fowler syndrome.[28]

STEM CELL THERAPY FOR UNDERACTIVE BLADDER

Cell therapy is intended to improve creation of detrusor force by directly augmenting both the existing muscle mass and contractility. Degeneration or loss of detrusor smooth muscle is regarded as one of contributors to UAB associated with aging.[14] In addition, oxidative stress associated with benign prostatic obstruction, a common condition in aged men, results in neurodegeneration within the bladder wall. Skeletal muscle–derived stem cells injected into the bladder wall show evidence of smooth muscle differentiation and induced innervation, with urodynamic evidence of enhanced detrusor contraction.[30] Autologous muscle–derived stem cells injected into the failing bladder may improve bladder emptying in some patients with UAB

(Chancellor, personal communication). The first US Food and Drug Administration–approved clinical trial of this technology started in 2014 at Beaumont Health System in Michigan (Chancellor, personal communication, 2015).

EDUCATION AND NEXT STEP

With the significant global inadequacies regarding understanding and perception of UAB,[31] the First International Congress of Urologic Research and Education on Underactive Bladder (CURE-UAB) brought together diverse stakeholders to identify major scientific challenge areas and initiate a call to action among the medical community. The meeting, held in February 2014 in Washington DC, was supported by the Aikens Center at Beaumont Health Systems, the National Institutes of Health, and the Underactive Bladder Foundation. The proceeds of the First International CURE-UAB, including video of all the lectures, are available at (www.underactivebladder.org).[32] The next International Congress on Underactive Bladder will be held on December 3 to 4, 2015, in Denver, Colorado. Meeting publications are included in a special supplemental issue of the *International Journal of Urology and Nephrology* (http://dx.doi.org/10.1007/s11255-014-0789-8).

SUMMARY

UAB is a major problem that is not well known in the public and health care sectors but is an enormous economic problem that will become more prevalent with increasing aging populations. UAB is a major burden because there are no effective UAB treatments and diagnostic tools. Research and education are critical if understanding of UAB is to be advanced. This requirement includes a need for work on the epidemiology, pathophysiology, clinical manifestations, and outcomes of UAB for affected patients and their caregivers. There is a critical need for more effective treatment options beyond those currently available. Improved understanding and awareness will in turn lead to changes in health care policy that could have a substantial positive impact on care for patients with UAB.

REFERENCES

1. Centers for Disease Control and Prevention. Life expectancy. United States, 2010. Available at: http://www.cdc.gov/nchs/fastats/life-expectancy.htm. Accessed May 7, 2014.
2. Werner CA. The older population: 2010. 2010 census briefs. Washington, DC: US Census Bureau; 2011. Available at: http://www.census.gov/prod/cen2010/briefs/c2010br-09.pdf/. Accessed May 7, 2014.
3. DuBeau CE. The aging lower urinary tract. J Urol 2006;175:S11–5.
4. Abrams P, Cardozo L, Fall M, et al, Standardisation Sub-committee of the International Continence Society. The standardisation of terminology of lower urinary tract function: report from the Standardisation Sub-committee of the International Continence Society. Neurourol Urodyn 2002;21(2):167–78.
5. Resnick NM, Yalla SV. Detrusor hyperactivity with impaired contractile function. An unrecognized but common cause of incontinence in elderly patients. JAMA 1987;257:3076–81.
6. Jeong SJ, Kim HJ, Lee YJ, et al. Prevalence and clinical features of detrusor underactivity among elderly with lower urinary tract symptoms: a comparison between men and women. Korean J Urol 2012;53(5):342–8.

7. Osman NI, Chapple CR, Abrams P, et al. Detrusor underactivity and the underactive bladder: a new clinical entity? A review of current terminology, definitions, epidemiology, aetiology, and diagnosis. Eur Urol 2014;65(2):389–98.
8. Abarbanel J, Marcus EL. Impaired detrusor contractility in community-dwelling elderly presenting with lower urinary tract symptoms. Urology 2007;69:436–40.
9. Thomas AW, Cannon A, Bartlett E, et al. The natural history of lower urinary tract dysfunction in men: minimum 10-year urodynamic follow-up of untreated detrusor underactivity. BJU Int 2005;96:1295–300.
10. Kuo HHC. Analysis of the pathophysiology of lower urinary tract symptoms in patient after prostatectomy. Urol Int 2002;68:99–104.
11. Valente S, DuBeau C, Chancellor DD, et al. Epidemiology and demographics of the underactive bladder: a cross-sectional survey. Int Urol Nephrol 2014;46: S7–10.
12. Smith PP. Aging and the underactive detrusor: a failure of activity or activation. Neurourol Urodyn 2010;29:408–12.
13. Sanchez-Ortiz RF, Wang Z, Menon C, et al. Estrogen modulates the expression of myosin heavy chain in detrusor smooth muscle. Am J Physiol Cell Physiol 2001; 280(3):C433–40.
14. Elbadawi A, Yalla SV, Resnick NM. Structural basis of geriatric voiding dysfunction. II. Aging detrusor: normal versus impaired contractility. J Urol 1993;150(5 Pt 1):1657–67.
15. Dixon JS, Gosling JA. Ultrastructure of smooth muscle cells in the urinary system. In: Motta PM, editor. Ultrastructure of smooth muscle. Boston (MA): Kluwer; 1990. p. 153–69.
16. Chancellor MB. The overactive bladder progression to underactive bladder hypothesis. Int Urol Nephrol 2014;46:S23–7.
17. de Groat WC. Anatomy and physiology of the lower urinary tract. Urol Clin North Am 1993;20(3):383–401.
18. Pavlakis AJ. Cauda equina and pelvic plexus injury. In: Krane RJ, Siroky MB, editors. Clinical Neuro-urology. Boston (MA): Little Brown; 1991. p. 333–4.
19. Neal DE, Boguc PRI, Williams RE. Histological appearances of the nerves of the bladder in patients with denervation of the bladder after excision of the rectum. Br J Urol 1982;54:658–66.
20. Andersson KE. Detrusor underactivity/underactive bladder: new research initiatives needed. J Urol 2010;184:1829–30.
21. Tanaka Y, Masumori N, Itoh N, et al. Symptomatic and urodynamic improvement by oral distigmine bromide in poor voiders after transurethral resection of the prostate. Urology 2001;57:270–4.
22. Bougas DA, Mitsogiannis IC, Mitropoulos DN, et al. Clinical efficacy of distigmine bromide in the treatment of patients with underactive detrusor. Int Urol Nephrol 2004;36(4):507–12.
23. Andersson KE, Wein AJ. Pharmacology of the lower urinary tract: basis for current and future treatments of urinary incontinence. Pharmacol Rev 2004;56: 581–631.
24. Coleman RA, Smith WL, Narumiya S. International Union of Pharmacology classification of prostanoid receptors: properties, distribution, and structure of the receptors and their subtypes. Pharmacol Rev 1994;46:205–29.
25. Sugimoto Y, Narumiya S. Prostaglandin E receptors. J Biol Chem 2007;282: 11613–7.
26. Hindley RG, Brierly RD, Thomas PJ. Prostaglandin E2 and bethanechol in combination for treating detrusor underactivity. BJU Int 2004;93(1):89–92.

27. Chancellor MB, Chartier-Kastler EJ. Principles of sacral nerve stimulation (SNS) for the treatment of bladder and urethral sphincter dysfunctions. Neuromodulation 2000;3:16–26.
28. De Ridder D, Ost D, Bruyninckx F. The presence of Fowler's syndrome predicts successful long-term outcome of sacral nerve stimulation in women with urinary retention. Eur Urol 2007;51(1):229–33 [discussion: 233–4].
29. Kavia R, Dasgupta R, Critchley H, et al. A functional magnetic resonance imaging study of the effect of sacral neuromodulation on brain responses in women with Fowler's syndrome. BJU Int 2010;105(3):366–72.
30. Huard J, Yokoyama T, Pruchnic R, et al. Muscle-derived cell-mediated ex vivo gene therapy for urological dysfunction. Gene Ther 2002;9(23):1617–26.
31. Chancellor MB, Kaufman J. Case for pharmacotherapy development for underactive bladder. Urology 2008;72(5):966–7.
32. Underactive Bladder Foundation. Available at: www.underactivebladder.org. Accessed September 29, 2014.

Translational Research and Functional Changes in Voiding Function in Older Adults

CrossMark

Florenta Aura Kullmann, PhD[a], Lori Ann Birder, PhD[b,c],
Karl-Erik Andersson, MD, PhD[d,e],*

KEYWORDS

- Urinary bladder • Voiding dysfunctions • Ischemia • LUTS • Overactive bladder
- Underactive detrusor • Urinary incontinence • Animal models

KEY POINTS

- Lower urinary tract symptoms (LUTS) significantly increase with age and include a prevalence of overactive bladder symptoms and even impaired bladder contractility.
- The pathophysiology of LUTS in older adults is multifactorial and includes comorbid medical illness, neurologic and psychiatric conditions, medications, functional impairments, and environmental factors.
- Many age-related changes in bladder function have an origin that is myogenic, neurogenic, and/or ischemic.
- Many of the structural and functional changes observed in animal models of aging seem to be similar to those described in humans.
- Although several factors have been identified as playing a potential role in these age-related symptoms, the influence in any patient group is unknown.

Disclosure: None.
This work was supported by the following grants: RO1 DK57284 and R37 DK54824 to L.A. Birder, P30 DK079307 Pittsburgh Center for Kidney Research - O'Brien Pilot to F.A. Kullmann, and a grant from Samuel and Emma Winters Foundation to F.A. Kullmann.
[a] Renal-Electrolyte Division, Medicine Department, University of Pittsburgh School of Medicine, 3500 Terrace Street, A1220 Scaife Hall, Pittsburgh, PA 15261, USA; [b] Renal-Electrolyte Division, Medicine Department, University of Pittsburgh School of Medicine, 3500 Terrace Street, A1207 Scaife Hall, Pittsburgh, PA 15261, USA; [c] Pharmacology and Chemical Biology, University of Pittsburgh School of Medicine, 200 Lothrop Street, Pittsburgh, PA 15213, USA; [d] Department of Urology, Institute for Regenerative Medicine, Wake Forest Baptist Medical Center, Wake Forest University School of Medicine, Medical Center Boulevard, Winston Salem, NC 27157, USA; [e] AIAS, Aarhus Institute of Advanced Studies, Aarhus University, Høegh-Guldbergs Gade 6B, Building 1632, Aarhus C 8000, Denmark
* Corresponding author. AIAS, Aarhus Institute of Advanced Studies, Aarhus University, Høegh-Guldbergs Gade 6B, Building 1632, Aarhus C 8000, Denmark.
E-mail address: kea@aias.au.dk

Clin Geriatr Med 31 (2015) 535–548
http://dx.doi.org/10.1016/j.cger.2015.06.001
0749-0690/15/$ – see front matter © 2015 Elsevier Inc. All rights reserved.

geriatric.theclinics.com

INTRODUCTION

Aging-related bladder dysfunction and associated lower urinary tract symptoms (LUTS) represent an increasing problem in developed countries because of increased life expectancy. LUTS are generally divided into storage (irritative), voiding (obstructive), and postmicturition components. Storage symptoms include urgency, frequency, nocturia, and urgency incontinence (ie, the overactive bladder [OAB] syndrome). Voiding symptoms comprise reduced force of stream, hesitancy, inability to empty the bladder, and straining. Postmicturition symptoms include feeling of incomplete emptying and postmicturition dribble.[1,2] However, none of these symptoms is disease specific or has a high correlation with a specific urodynamic pattern. Most of these symptoms have been suggested to be age dependent, and are attributed to various factors, including reduced bladder capacity, changes in bladder sensation, and, on urodynamic investigation, detrusor overactivity (DO). However, the pathophysiology behind the dysfunctions is sometimes difficult to establish because what can be attributed to normal aging cannot be separated from what is caused by comorbidities. LUTS is an increasing problem: an estimated 45% of the 2008 worldwide population (4.3 billion) was affected by at least one LUTS, reducing the quality of life. By 2018, an estimated 2.3 billion individuals will be affected by at least one LUTS (18.4% increase).[3]

FUNCTIONAL AGING-RELATED VOIDING CHANGES

Functional changes in the urinary tract occur with both normal aging and in elderly individuals with different types of diseases. The pathophysiology of LUTS in older adults is multifactorial and includes comorbid medical illness, neurologic and psychiatric conditions, medications, functional impairments, and environmental factors.[4,5]

The Overactive Bladder

The OAB symptom complex comprises urinary urgency, with or without urgency incontinence, usually with frequency and nocturia in the absence of other disorders.[6] Several articles have discussed different aspects of OAB in older adults[5,7–10] and it has been well established that the syndrome increases with age, and that aging alone can be considered a major risk factor for developing these symptoms.

The OAB syndrome as defined by the International Continence Society refers to idiopathic OAB.[6] Because the same symptoms can occur with known comorbidities probably involved in the pathophysiology of the symptoms, such as Parkinson disease, multiple sclerosis, spinal injuries, Alzheimer disease, and diabetes cystopathy, epidemiologic studies focusing on idiopathic OAB underestimate the true prevalence of the symptom complex. Because aging can be considered a major risk factor for developing the symptoms, current population forecasts predicting a worldwide increase in the proportion of people aged more than 65 years, with the greatest increase being in those aged more than 80 years,[11] also predict an increase in patients with OAB symptoms. According to Irwin and colleagues[3] (2011) an estimated 455 million individuals worldwide experienced OAB in 2008, with numbers of affected individuals anticipated to increase to 500 million by 2013 (10.0% increase) and to 546 million by 2018 (20.1% increase). It can be expected that the health care burden associated with OAB and other LUTS will increase and that the occurrence of OAB in the aging population will have important quality-of-life and economic consequences.[4,12–15]

Urinary incontinence, in addition to urgency, may be one of the most relevant symptoms, given that other comorbidities may also limit the ability to remain dry.[16] The impact on the quality of life in this population is vast; incontinence remains a risk factor for nursing home placement[17–19] and links with other conditions, including an increased risk of falls and fractures,[20] sleep disorders, and depression.[21–23] The factor of age is in itself likely to exacerbate the problem because elderly men with LUTS report a poorer quality of life than younger men with the same condition.[24]

Detrusor Underactivity

Uroflow studies have shown an age-dependent decrease in maximum flow rate (Q_{max}),[25,26] which was confirmed and shown to be similar in both sexes,[27,28] but was not demonstrable in symptomatic elderly men with nonobstructive voiding dysfunction.[29] Difficulties to empty the bladder (detrusor underactivity [DU]) may have many underlying causes and has been the subject of recent interest.[30–34] Some of the most frequently discussed causes are impaired detrusor contractility and decreased bladder/urethral sensation.[35,36] Urodynamic assessment in older patients of both sexes without overt neurologic disease showed higher residual volumes and lower detrusor shortening velocities, but no changes in isometric detrusor function.[37] In a series of patients in whom the bladder capacity at first void was taken as measure of bladder sensation, this parameter showed a progressive increase with age, suggesting an age-dependent decrease in bladder sensation,[35,36] a finding confirmed by several other investigators.[28,38] In a clinical study of patients referred for LUTS or urinary incontinence, Madersbacher and colleagues[27] (1998) found an increase in postvoid residual, along with a decrease of flow rates, voided volumes, and bladder capacity associated with increasing age. These findings were similar in both genders. Pfisterer and colleagues[28] (2006) assessed a group of 85 female volunteers aged between 20 and 90 years using bladder diary, uroflowmetry, and detailed videourodynamics. Bladder capacity did not change with age, but was smaller in women with DO on urodynamics. Urine production and urine frequency did not differ significantly with age. Bladder sensation, detrusor contraction strength, maximal flow rate, and maximum urethral closure pressure were all negatively associated with age. It was concluded that there is a normal functional decline with aging in otherwise asymptomatic women. This study thus suggested a progressive decrease in detrusor contraction strength, which was in line with the findings of van Mastrigt[39] (1992), who showed a statistically significant age-related decrease of the detrusor contractility parameter, W_{max} (maximum Watt factor), in both sexes. Other investigators were unable to show any correlations between bladder contractility and age in symptomatic elderly men with nonobstructive bladder dysfunction,[29] or between maximum detrusor pressure and detrusor pressure at peak flow rate and age in patients of both sexes with LUTS.[27] Direct study of detrusor contractility in vitro did not show any correlation between contractile force and age.[40]

Normal age-related changes in the bladder and lower urinary tract (LUT) should be clearly differentiated from pathologic alterations seen with conditions such as OAB or LUTS. DO and the related condition, detrusor hyperactivity with impaired contractile function,[41] can also present with advancing age and should be diagnosed adequately in elderly individuals. The currently available data from animal and human studies show that aging affects the LUT function through ultrastructural and physiologic alterations. The reported age-related changes in animals do not always correspond with what is found in humans, and should be interpreted with caution. Overall, in humans, bladder sensation and contractility seem to decrease with advancing age as a possible consequence of neuronal loss and remodeling of the bladder and urethra.

ANIMAL MODELS OF AGING-RELATED BLADDER DYSFUNCTION
In Vivo Studies of Bladder Function

Animal models allow detailed investigation of structural and functional aspects of the micturition pathways and changes occurring with aging. In addition, the genetically modified mouse models allow further understanding and targeting of specific genes. The influence of aging on bladder structure and/or function was studied in vivo and/ or in vitro, mostly in rodents of different strains and/or gender. These rodents include C57Bl6 mice (male, female, 22–25 months old),[42–44] the senescent-accelerated prone mice (senescent-accelerated prone mice [SAMP8]; male, female, 36–38 weeks old),[45] Fisher 344 rats (male, 22–24 months old),[46,47] Fischer/Brown Norway rats (male, 28–30 months old),[48] Wistar rats (male or female, 22–37 months old),[49–51] Fisher 344 rats (female, 24 months old),[52] Sprague-Dawley (SD) rats (male, 18–24 months old).[53,54] Other species included dogs[55,56] and guinea pigs.[57–61] As pointed out previously, the relation between aging per se and external influences on the detrusor from diseases in the nervous system, in the vascular supply, and in the LUT smooth muscles is poorly understood in humans.[62–64] In animals kept under constant laboratory conditions, theoretically the impact of external influences can be reduced, which should enable the effect of age only on bladder function to be studied. However, this does not seem to provide consistent results, in part because of differences between species, genders, or strains. A small number of studies have used in vivo methods, such as the use of metabolic cages or cystometry, for characterization of age-related changes.[42,45–49] Metabolic cage data obtained from aged mice and SAMP8[42,45] showed a significant increase in the number of urine spots, suggesting an increase in the frequency of voiding. Similarly, the frequency of voiding was increased in aging rats as well as in rats with chronic bladder ischemia (also a risk factor in aging).[46,47,65] Cystometry studies yielded variable results. Smith and colleagues,[44] using a pressure/flow multichannel urethane-anesthetized mouse cystometry model, tested the hypothesis that in vivo detrusor performance does not degrade with aging. Aging was associated with an impaired ability to respond to the challenge of continuous bladder filling with cyclic voiding. However, among responsive animals, voiding detrusor contraction strength did not degrade with aging in this murine model and indirect measures suggested that bladder volume sensitivity was diminished. These findings seem to be in agreement with findings in humans showing that maximal detrusor pressure did not correlate with age,[66] and that no age-related changes in maximum detrusor pressure ($p_{det.Qmax}$) could be shown in men and women with LUTS.[27] In contrast, Pfisterer and colleagues[28] (2006) found that maximum urethral closure pressure, detrusor contraction strength, and urine flow rate declined significantly with age, and so did bladder sensation. Other reports indicate increase in voiding pressure threshold in aged rodents,[52,53] suggesting possible disturbances in the afferent system that can include decreased afferent excitability, impaired communication between urothelium and afferent nerves, and/or other mechanisms. Baseline intravesical pressure was also increased,[48,53] suggesting changes in the smooth muscle/bladder wall that may affect storage function. Micturition pressure (reflects contractility of the smooth muscle as well as function of the efferent system) was variable,[44,48,53] suggesting changes in more than one component of the system.

In Vitro Studies of Bladder Function

To further understand the in vivo data, several studies have performed various types of in vitro experiments. The overriding goals were to investigate individual components of the micturition pathway, including bladder nerves (afferent, efferent), the urothelium and lamina propria, as well as the smooth muscle.

Afferent nerves

Although scarce, studies using aged mice revealed augmented afferent nerve firing during bladder filling and increased afferent discharge in response to low threshold volumes only (male mice[42]). These results suggest that afferent activity during the filling phase may be enhanced and this may be an underlying mechanism for symptoms of urgency and frequency reported in older adults. Studies in rats indicated that the conduction velocity of myelinated and unmyelinated fibers did not seem to change with age; however, there was a reduction in the number of small-diameter (predominantly unmyelinated) fibers.[50] These changes, if occurring in humans, may account for alterations in bladder sensations in older adults.

Urothelium/lamina propria

Histologic evaluation indicated several structural changes in the urothelium and lamina propria. These changes include urothelial thinning (male Fischer/Brown Norway rats),[48] granular appearance of umbrella cell layer, discoidal vesicles, electron-dense bodies, and vacuoles in the umbrella layer, often containing what appears to be cellular debris in all layers and increased cellularity (number of different cell types, many around blood vessels) in lamina propria in female mice.[67] Other studies have shown increased reactive oxygen species in cultured urothelial cells from male mice,[68] decreased total antioxidant capacity and significantly increased levels of lipid peroxides (malondialdehyde [MDA]) and inducible nitric oxide synthase (iNOS) (markers of oxidative stress), and ultrastructural alterations in mitochondria with accumulation of lipofuscin.[69] Furthermore, alterations in the collagen content have been reported, although results are not consistent. For example, changes include a generalized increase in collagen content in male Fischer/Brown Norway rats[48] versus an increase only in the bladder neck in male SD rats[53] compared with decreases in the smooth muscle and lamina propria areas in female Wistar/Rij rats.[49] In contrast, few functional studies of aging urothelium have been performed. For example, aging mice have been associated with increased ATP release and a corresponding decrease in acetylcholine. Urothelial cells were also more sensitive to purinergic agonists and $P2X_3$ receptors expression was increased.[42] These changes may contribute to bladder overactivity and hypersensitivity.

Efferent transmission and smooth muscle

The efferent transmission is mostly cholinergic in humans and cholinergic and purinergic in rodents. In aged bladder tissue from humans and rats, a decrease in the atropine-sensitive component of the efferent transmission has been reported.[48,53,70] This decrease correlates with structural changes reporting a reduction ($\sim$40%) in the number of AChE-positive neurons in the intramural plexus in guinea pigs.[60] These alterations may affect the strength of the contraction and may contribute to changes in voiding function (underactive bladder).

A number of structural and functional changes have been reported in the smooth muscle. Several studies investigated the ability of smooth muscle to handle changes in intracellular calcium. Although responses to strong depolarization using KCl were shown to be variable,[42,43,48,49,51,53] muscle strips from aged rodents were more susceptible to calcium channel antagonists and to reduced extracellular calcium.[54] Also, aged dissociated smooth muscle cells show differences in mobilization of intracellular calcium.[43] Altogether, impaired ability of the smooth muscle to handle changes in levels of intracellular calcium coupled with decreased muscle mass and increased collagen content[48] may represent underlying mechanisms for changes in bladder contraction strength with age.

Bladder storage and voiding phases involve several main transmitters (norepinephrine, Ach, and ATP) and their associated smooth muscle receptors (beta-adrenergic, muscarinic, and purinergic receptors). During storage, norepinephrine released from the sympathetic nerves relaxes the smooth muscle via beta-adrenergic receptors (β-ARs), particularly β_3-ARs in humans.[71,72] Studies on the effect of aging on bladder β-ARs have yielded inconsistent results.[5] In the bladder of male SD rats and female Wistar/Rij, the receptor density did not seem to change significantly.[49,53] Latifpour and colleagues[73] (1990) reported that the number of β-ARs increased with age in rabbit bladder dome and base. In contrast, a study using male Fischer 344 rats reported a decrease in β-ARs in aged rats.[74] A similar decrease was also reported for human bladder.[75] Functionally, weaker smooth muscle response (relaxation) to noradrenaline, isoproterenol, or the β3-AR agonist BRL37344 have been reported in bladder from male Wistar rats.[51] Even if changes in β-AR function in older adults cannot be excluded, there is no evidence that the clinical response to β3-AR agonist treatment (mirabegron) is reduced in the geriatric population.[76]

Voiding is achieved via release of ACh in human (and ACh and ATP in rodents) from the parasympathetic nerves to contract the bladder, concomitant with NO release in the urethra to relax the urethra smooth muscle. In the detrusor, muscarinic receptors (particularly M3) mediate the bladder contraction. Aging-dependent changes in muscarinic receptors have yielded contradictory results, in part because of species and strain differences. In male Fischer 344 rats[77] and male mice,[42] muscarinic receptor–mediated detrusor contraction was increased. In contrast, in male SD rats,[53,78,79] male Fisher/Brown Norway,[48] and male mice,[43] muscarinic receptor–mediated detrusor contraction was decreased, whereas in male Wistar[80] and female Wistar/Rij rats[49] there was no change. Even if there may be aging-dependent changes in muscarinic receptor function in humans, this does not seem to affect the clinical response to antimuscarinic drugs.[81–83]

In summary, although several reports indicated structural and functional changes in the aged bladder, in vitro data do not always match the in vivo observations. The potential translational value may be increased if both in vivo and in vitro parameters could be studied in the same animal.

RISK FACTORS
Gender Differences

Irwin and colleagues[3] (2011) estimated the prevalence of OAB worldwide as being greater in women versus men in 2008 (11.6% vs 9.7%, respectively). The difference was expected to be maintained in 2013 (11.7% vs 9.8%) and 2018 (11.9% vs 10.0%). Some of the gender differences in bladder function and control can be attributed to gross anatomic differences, but there is evidence that other factors can contribute.[18,84,85] For example, there are significant gender differences in coping strategies, with better coping mechanisms shown among elderly women.[86] This finding may be related to differences in health care–seeking behavior and receiving treatment. Older men seek professional help for their incontinence more often compared with women. However, women are more often treated.[87,88] The risk of incontinence in older individuals with restricted mobility may be greater in women than in men, depending on the greater physical effort required by women in preparing for micturition. Urinary incontinence has been shown to be associated with a higher mortality, but only among elderly men.[89] Urinary incontinence has a greater negative impact on sexuality in elderly men compared with elderly women.[90,91] However, in older women with incontinence a main reason for not being sexually active was lack of a partner. Although urinary incontinence was the main reason for not having sex in only 5%, about 25% of the sexually active women reported a negative influence of urine loss on their sex lives.[91]

Atherosclerosis and Oxidative Stress

Aging is associated with an impairment of blood vessel function and changes may occur in the vasculature on the molecular, cellular, structural, and functional levels.[92–94] Vascular aging is characterized by endothelial dysfunction[95,96] and starts in young adults with slow and progressive vascular remodeling, and early signs of declining endothelial function may manifest before the fourth decade of life.[97] Endothelial dysfunction leads to oxidative stress, and increased levels of proinflammatory cytokines,[94,98] which represents an independent risk factor for development of atherosclerosis and hypertension. Recent evidence from epidemiologic, clinical, and animal basic research suggests that aging-associated changes in the pelvic vasculature, resulting in atherosclerosis and vascular dysfunction, may be important factors in the generation of LUTS.

Benign prostatic hyperplasia (BPH)/bladder outlet obstruction (BOO) is a common condition in elderly men and BOO can be associated with reduced bladder blood flow. Berger and colleagues (2006) found that in patients with BPH/BOO with severe vascular damage (diabetes mellitus type 2), LUT perfusion and International Prostate Symptom Score (IPSS) were significantly worse compared with patients with BPH/BOO without diabetes and healthy controls.

Chronic bladder ischemia can occur independently of BOO in older adults. The vascular supply to the human genitourinary tract, including the bladder, prostate, uterus, urethra, and penis, is primarily derived from the iliac arteries. The abdominal aorta and its branches, especially the bifurcation of the iliac arteries, are particularly vulnerable to atherosclerotic lesions.[99] Atherosclerotic obstructive changes distal to the aortic bifurcation have consequences for the distal vasculature and LUT blood flow. Epidemiologic studies have investigated the association between LUTS and vascular risk factors for atherosclerosis, such as hypertension, hyperlipidemia, diabetes mellitus, and nicotine use,[100,101] and Ponholzer and colleagues[100] (2006) suggested a potential role of atherosclerosis in the development of LUTS in both sexes. Takahashi and colleagues[102] (2012) also indicated the association between severity of atherosclerosis and male LUTS. Pinggera and colleagues[103] (2006), using transrectal color Doppler ultrasonography, showed that elderly patients with LUTS had a significant decrease in bladder blood flow compared with asymptomatic young individuals. They also found a negative correlation between decreased LUT perfusion and IPSS in these elderly patients. This finding implies that coexisting vascular disease–related chronic ischemia may be more detrimental to bladder dysfunction than BPH/BOO alone. Histologic studies have shown fibrosis formation or denervation in the bladder samples from elderly male and female patients without BOO.[104–106] These observations were supported by the study of Kershen and colleagues[107] (2002), which showed that decreased bladder blood flow and decreased bladder wall compliance correlated strongly, suggesting structural changes in the bladder wall induced by ischemia. Moreover, pelvic arterial insufficiency, such as caused by atherosclerosis, is also strongly associated with erectile dysfunction (ED).[108,109] The close association between LUTS and ED has been documented in elderly men.[110–112] Thus, these clinical studies may suggest aging-associated alteration of pelvic vasculature as a common cause in the development of both conditions.[113,114]

Evidence from clinical and basic research suggests that atherosclerosis in both genders can induce a reduction of bladder blood flow, leading to chronic ischemia. Chronic bladder ischemia and repeated ischemia/reperfusion during a micturition cycle may produce oxidative stress, leading to denervation of the bladder and the expression of tissue-damaging molecules in the bladder wall.[65,115,116] Masuda and colleagues[117] (2008) suggested that oxidative stress mediates bladder hyperactivity through sensitization of afferent pathway in the bladder of rats. Studies in animal models suggest that the extent of bladder dysfunction in chronic ischemia depends on the degree and duration of ischemia.[118–120] This process seems to be responsible for the development of DO progressing to DU and the inability to empty the bladder.[120] When bladder ischemia becomes severe and prolonged, progression of denervation and damage to detrusor muscle with fibrosis formation may cause DU and voiding symptoms.

SUMMARY

In view of the complex control of the LUT, underlying symptoms of the aging bladder include incontinence, overactivity, and/or the inability to empty. The underlying mechanisms that may contribute to these symptoms are not known but are likely to be controlled by multiple genetic, epigenetic, and environmental factors. Future translational studies should be designed to unravel pathologic processes in the aging bladder and to develop new modalities targeting these pathologic processes for the treatment of age-related bladder control problems.

REFERENCES

1. Andersson KE. Storage and voiding symptoms: pathophysiologic aspects. Urology 2003;62:3–10.
2. Andersson KE. LUTS treatment: future treatment options. Neurourol Urodyn 2007;26:934–47.
3. Irwin DE, Kopp ZS, Agatep B, et al. Worldwide prevalence estimates of lower urinary tract symptoms, overactive bladder, urinary incontinence and bladder outlet obstruction. BJU Int 2011;108:1132–8.
4. Coyne KS, Wein A, Nicholson S, et al. Comorbidities and personal burden of urgency urinary incontinence: a systematic review. Int J Clin Pract 2013;67: 1015–33.
5. Yoshida M. Perspectives on overactive bladder in the elderly population. World J Urol 2009;27:729–37.
6. Abrams P, Cardozo L, Fall M, et al. The standardisation of terminology of lower urinary tract function: report from the Standardisation Sub-Committee of the International Continence Society. Neurourol Urodyn 2002;21:167–78.
7. Kraus SR, Bavendam T, Brake T, et al. Vulnerable elderly patients and overactive bladder syndrome. Drugs Aging 2010;27:697–713.
8. Griebling TL. Overactive bladder in elderly men: epidemiology, evaluation, clinical effects, and management. Curr Urol Rep 2013;14:418–25.
9. Natalin R, Lorenzetti F, Dambros M. Management of OAB in those over age 65. Curr Urol Rep 2013;14:379–85.
10. Gibson W, Wagg A. New horizons: urinary incontinence in older people. Age Ageing 2014;43:157–63.
11. United Nations, Department of Economic and Social Affairs, Population Division. World population prospects: the 2012 revision, highlights and advance tables. 2013. Available at: http://esa.un.org/unpd/wpp/Documentation/pdf/WPP2012_HIGHLIGHTS.pdf.
12. Abrams P, Kelleher CJ, Kerr LA, et al. Overactive bladder significantly affects quality of life. Am J Manag Care 2000;6:S580–90.
13. Coyne KS, Payne C, Bhattacharyya SK, et al. The impact of urinary urgency and frequency on health-related quality of life in overactive bladder: results from a national community survey. Value Health 2004;7:455–63.
14. Currie CJ, McEwan P, Poole CD, et al. The impact of the overactive bladder on health-related utility and quality of life. BJU Int 2006;97:1267–72.

15. Tang DH, Colayco DC, Khalaf KM, et al. Impact of urinary incontinence on healthcare resource utilization, health-related quality of life and productivity in patients with overactive bladder. BJU Int 2014;113:484–91.
16. Wagg A, Cohen M. Medical therapy for the overactive bladder in the elderly. Age Ageing 2002;31:241–6.
17. Thom DH, Haan MN, Van Den Eeden SK. Medically recognized urinary incontinence and risks of hospitalization, nursing home admission and mortality. Age Ageing 1997;26:367–74.
18. Nuotio M, Tammela TL, Luukkaala T, et al. Predictors of institutionalization in an older population during a 13-year period: the effect of urge incontinence. J Gerontol A Biol Sci Med Sci 2003;58:756–62.
19. DuBeau CE, Kuchel GA, Johnson T 2nd, et al. Incontinence in the frail elderly: report from the 4th International Consultation on Incontinence. Neurourol Urodyn 2010;29:165–78.
20. Wagner TH, Hu TW, Bentkover J, et al. Health-related consequences of overactive bladder. Am J Manag Care 2002;8:S598–607.
21. Brown JS, McGhan WF, Chokroverty S. Comorbidities associated with overactive bladder. Am J Manag Care 2000;6:S574–9.
22. Wong SY, Hong A, Leung J, et al. Lower urinary tract symptoms and depressive symptoms in elderly men. J Affect Disord 2006;96:83–8.
23. Nuotio M, Tammela TL, Luukkaala T, et al. Association of urgency symptoms with self-rated health, mood and functioning in an older population. Aging Clin Exp Res 2007;19:465–71.
24. Engstrom G, Henningsohn L, Walker-Engstrom ML, et al. Impact on quality of life of different lower urinary tract symptoms in men measured by means of the SF-36 questionnaire. Scand J Urol Nephrol 2006;40:485–94.
25. Jorgensen JB, Jensen KM, Mogensen P. Age-related variation in urinary flow variables and flow curve patterns in elderly males. Br J Urol 1992;69:265–71.
26. Jorgensen JB, Jensen KM, Mogensen P. Longitudinal observations on normal and abnormal voiding in men over the age of 50 years. Br J Urol 1993;72:413–20.
27. Madersbacher S, Pycha A, Schatzl G, et al. The aging lower urinary tract: a comparative urodynamic study of men and women. Urology 1998;51:206–12.
28. Pfisterer MH, Griffiths DJ, Schaefer W, et al. The effect of age on lower urinary tract function: a study in women. J Am Geriatr Soc 2006;54:405–12.
29. Ameda K, Sullivan MP, Bae RJ, et al. Urodynamic characterization of nonobstructive voiding dysfunction in symptomatic elderly men. J Urol 1999;162:142–6.
30. van Koeveringe GA, Vahabi B, Andersson KE, et al. Detrusor underactivity: a plea for new approaches to a common bladder dysfunction. Neurourol Urodyn 2011;30:723–8.
31. Miyazato M, Yoshimura N, Chancellor MB. The other bladder syndrome: underactive bladder. Rev Urol 2013;15:11–22.
32. Drake MJ, Williams J, Bijos DA. Voiding dysfunction due to detrusor underactivity: an overview. Nat Rev Urol 2014;11:454–64.
33. Osman NI, Chapple CR, Abrams P, et al. Detrusor underactivity and the underactive bladder: a new clinical entity? A review of current terminology, definitions, epidemiology, aetiology, and diagnosis. Eur Urol 2014;65:389–98.
34. Osman NI, Chapple CR. Contemporary concepts in the aetiopathogenesis of detrusor underactivity. Nat Rev Urol 2014;11(11):639–48.
35. Smith PP. Aging and the underactive detrusor: a failure of activity or activation? Neurourol Urodyn 2010;29:408–12.

36. Smith PP, Chalmers DJ, Feinn RS. Does defective volume sensation contribute to detrusor underactivity? Neurourol Urodyn 2014. [Epub ahead of print].

37. Malone-Lee J, Wahedna I. Characterisation of detrusor contractile function in relation to old age. Br J Urol 1993;72:873–80.

38. Kenton K, Lowenstein L, Simmons J, et al. Aging and overactive bladder may be associated with loss of urethral sensation in women. Neurourol Urodyn 2007;26: 981–4.

39. Van Mastrigt R. Age dependency of urinary bladder contractility. Neurourol Urodyn 1992;11:315–7.

40. Fry CH, Bayliss M, Young JS, et al. Influence of age and bladder dysfunction on the contractile properties of isolated human detrusor smooth muscle. BJU Int 2011;108:E91–6.

41. Resnick NM, Yalla SV. Detrusor hyperactivity with impaired contractile function. An unrecognized but common cause of incontinence in elderly patients. JAMA 1987;257:3076–81.

42. Daly DM, Nocchi L, Liaskos M, et al. Age-related changes in afferent pathways and urothelial function in the male mouse bladder. J Physiol 2014; 592:537–49.

43. Gomez-Pinilla PJ, Pozo MJ, Camello PJ. Aging differentially modifies agonist-evoked mouse detrusor contraction and calcium signals. Age 2011;33:81–8.

44. Smith PP, DeAngelis A, Kuchel GA. Detrusor expulsive strength is preserved, but responsiveness to bladder filling and urinary sensitivity is diminished in the aging mouse. Am J Physiol Regul Integr Comp Physiol 2012;302: R577–86.

45. Triguero D, Lafuente-Sanchis A, Garcia-Pascual A. Changes in nerve-mediated contractility of the lower urinary tract in a mouse model of premature ageing. Br J Pharmacol 2014;171:1687–705.

46. Chun AL, Wallace LJ, Gerald MC, et al. Effect of age on in vivo urinary bladder function in the rat. J Urol 1988;139:625–7.

47. Chun AL, Wallace LJ, Gerald MC, et al. Effects of age on urinary bladder function in the male rat. J Urol 1989;141:170–3.

48. Zhao W, Aboushwareb T, Turner C, et al. Impaired bladder function in aging male rats. J Urol 2010;184:378–85.

49. Lluel P, Palea S, Barras M, et al. Functional and morphological modifications of the urinary bladder in aging female rats. Am J Physiol Regul Integr Comp Physiol 2000;278:R964–72.

50. Nakayama H, Noda K, Hotta H, et al. Effects of aging on numbers, sizes and conduction velocities of myelinated and unmyelinated fibers of the pelvic nerve in rats. J Auton Nerv Syst 1998;69:148–55.

51. Frazier EP, Schneider T, Michel MC. Effects of gender, age and hypertension on beta-adrenergic receptor function in rat urinary bladder. Naunyn Schmiedebergs Arch Pharmacol 2006;373:300–9.

52. Kohan AD, Danziger M, Vaughan ED Jr, et al. Effect of aging on bladder function and the response to outlet obstruction in female rats. Urol Res 2000;28: 33–7.

53. Lluel P, Deplanne V, Heudes D, et al. Age-related changes in urethrovesical coordination in male rats: relationship with bladder instability? Am J Physiol Regul Integr Comp Physiol 2003;284:R1287–95.

54. Yu HJ, Wein AJ, Levin RM. Age-related differential susceptibility to calcium channel blocker and low calcium medium in rat detrusor muscle: response to field stimulation. Neurourol Urodyn 1996;15:563–76.

55. Takahashi S, Moriyama N, Yamazaki R, et al. Urodynamic analysis of age-related changes of alpha 1-adrenoceptor responsiveness in female beagle dogs. J Urol 1996;156:1485–8.
56. Suzuki Y, Moriyama N, Okaya Y, et al. Age-related change of the role of alpha1l-adrenoceptor in canine urethral smooth muscle. Gen Pharmacol 1999;33:347–54.
57. Gomez-Pinilla PJ, Gomez MF, Sward K, et al. Melatonin restores impaired contractility in aged guinea pig urinary bladder. J Pineal Res 2008;44:416–25.
58. Gomez-Pinilla PJ, Pozo MJ, Baba A, et al. Ca2+ extrusion in aged smooth muscle cells. Biochem Pharmacol 2007;74:860–9.
59. Gomez-Pinilla PJ, Pozo MJ, Camello PJ. Aging impairs neurogenic contraction in guinea pig urinary bladder: role of oxidative stress and melatonin. Am J Physiol Regul Integr Comp Physiol 2007;293:R793–803.
60. Mizuno MS, Pompeu E, Castelucci P, et al. Age-related changes in urinary bladder intramural neurons. Int J Dev Neurosci 2007;25:141–8.
61. Wheeler MA, Pontari M, Dokita S, et al. Age-dependent changes in particulate and soluble guanylyl cyclase activities in urinary tract smooth muscle. Mol Cell Biochem 1997;169:115–24.
62. Elbadawi A, Yalla SV, Resnick NM. Structural basis of geriatric voiding dysfunction. II. Aging detrusor: normal versus impaired contractility. J Urol 1993;150: 1657–67.
63. Hald T, Horn T. The human urinary bladder in ageing. Br J Urol 1998;82(Suppl 1):59–64.
64. Nordling J. The aging bladder–a significant but underestimated role in the development of lower urinary tract symptoms. Exp Gerontol 2002;37:991–9.
65. Nomiya M, Yamaguchi O, Andersson KE, et al. The effect of atherosclerosis-induced chronic bladder ischemia on bladder function in the rat. Neurourol Urodyn 2012;31:195–200.
66. Karram MM, Partoll L, Bilotta V, et al. Factors affecting detrusor contraction strength during voiding in women. Obstet Gynecol 1997;90:723–6.
67. Phillips JI, Davies I. The comparative morphology of the bladder and urethra in young and old female c57bl/icrfat mice. Exp Gerontol 1980;15:551–62.
68. Nocchi L, Daly DM, Chapple C, et al. Induction of oxidative stress causes functional alterations in mouse urothelium via a trpm8-mediated mechanism: implications for aging. Aging Cell 2014;13:540–50.
69. Perse M, Injac R, Erman A. Oxidative status and lipofuscin accumulation in urothelial cells of bladder in aging mice. PLoS One 2013;8:e59638.
70. Yoshida M, Homma Y, Inadome A, et al. Age-related changes in cholinergic and purinergic neurotransmission in human isolated bladder smooth muscles. Exp Gerontol 2001;36:99–109.
71. de Groat WC. Integrative control of the lower urinary tract: preclinical perspective. Br J Pharmacol 2006;147(Suppl 2):S25–40.
72. Michel MC. Beta-adrenergic receptor subtypes in the urinary tract. Handb Exp Pharmacol 2011;(202):307–18.
73. Latifpour J, Kondo S, O'Hollaren B, et al. Autonomic receptors in urinary tract: sex and age differences. J Pharmacol Exp Ther 1990;253:661–7.
74. Nishimoto T, Latifpour J, Wheeler MA, et al. Age-dependent alterations in beta-adrenergic responsiveness of rat detrusor smooth muscle. J Urol 1995;153: 1701–5.
75. Li G, Zheng XH, Li K, et al. Age-dependent alternations in beta-adrenoceptor function in human detrusor and possible mechanism. Zhonghua wai ke za zhi 2003;41:526–9 [in Chinese].

76. Wagg A, Cardozo L, Nitti VW, et al. The efficacy and tolerability of the beta3-adrenoceptor agonist mirabegron for the treatment of symptoms of overactive bladder in older patients. Age Ageing 2014;43:666–75.

77. Kolta MG, Wallace LJ, Gerald MC. Age-related changes in sensitivity of rat urinary bladder to autonomic agents. Mech Ageing Dev 1984;27:183–8.

78. Hegde SS, Mandel DA, Wilford MR, et al. Evidence for purinergic neurotransmission in the urinary bladder of pithed rats. Eur J Pharmacol 1998;349:75–82.

79. Yu HI, Wein AJ, Levin RM. Contractile responses and calcium mobilization induced by muscarinic agonists in the rat urinary bladder: effects of age. Gen Pharmacol 1997;28:623–8.

80. Schneider T, Hein P, Michel-Reher MB, et al. Effects of ageing on muscarinic receptor subtypes and function in rat urinary bladder. Naunyn Schmiedebergs Arch Pharmacol 2005;372:71–8.

81. Dubeau CE, Kraus SR, Griebling TL, et al. Effect of fesoterodine in vulnerable elderly subjects with urgency incontinence: a double-blind, placebo controlled trial. J Urol 2014;191:395–404.

82. DuBeau CE, Morrow JD, Kraus SR, et al. Efficacy and tolerability of fesoterodine versus tolterodine in older and younger subjects with overactive bladder: a post hoc, pooled analysis from two placebo-controlled trials. Neurourol Urodyn 2012; 31:1258–65.

83. Wagg AS. Antimuscarinic treatment in overactive bladder: special considerations in elderly patients. Drugs Aging 2012;29:539–48.

84. Wilson MM. Urinary incontinence: bridging the gender gap. J Gerontol A Biol Sci Med Sci 2003;58:752–5.

85. Norton P, Brubaker L. Urinary incontinence in women. Lancet 2006;367:57–67.

86. Talbot LA, Cox M. Differences in coping strategies among community-residing older adults with functional urinary continence, dysfunctional urinary continence and actual urinary incontinence. Ostomy Wound Manage 1995;41: 30–2, 34–7.

87. Teunissen D, Lagro-Janssen T. Urinary incontinence in community dwelling elderly: are there sex differences in help-seeking behaviour? Scand J Prim Health Care 2004;22:209–16.

88. Li Y, Cai X, Glance LG, et al. Gender differences in healthcare-seeking behavior for urinary incontinence and the impact of socioeconomic status: a study of the Medicare managed care population. Med Care 2007;45:1116–22.

89. Herzog AR, Diokno AC, Brown MB, et al. Urinary incontinence as a risk factor for mortality. J Am Geriatr Soc 1994;42:264–8.

90. Temml C, Haidinger G, Schmidbauer J, et al. Urinary incontinence in both sexes: prevalence rates and impact on quality of life and sexual life. Neurourol Urodyn 2000;19:259–71.

91. Visser E, de Bock GH, Berger MY, et al. Impact of urinary incontinence on sexual functioning in community-dwelling older women. J Sex Med 2014;11:1757–65.

92. Ungvari Z, Kaley G, de Cabo R, et al. Mechanisms of vascular aging: new perspectives. J Gerontol A Biol Sci Med Sci 2010;65:1028–41.

93. Oakley R, Tharakan B. Vascular hyperpermeability and aging. Aging Dis 2014;5: 114–25.

94. Rubio-Ruiz ME, Perez-Torres I, Soto ME, et al. Aging in blood vessels. Medicinal agents for systemic arterial hypertension in the elderly. Ageing Res Rev 2014; 18C:132–47.

95. El Assar M, Angulo J, Vallejo S, et al. Mechanisms involved in the aging-induced vascular dysfunction. Front Physiol 2012;3:132.

96. Bachschmid MM, Schildknecht S, Matsui R, et al. Vascular aging: chronic oxidative stress and impairment of redox signaling-consequences for vascular homeostasis and disease. Ann Med 2013;45:17–36.

97. Kotsis V, Stabouli S, Karafillis I, et al. Early vascular aging and the role of central blood pressure. J Hypertens 2011;29:1847–53.

98. El Assar M, Angulo J, Rodriguez-Manas L. Oxidative stress and vascular inflammation in aging. Free Radic Biol Med 2013;65:380–401.

99. Tarcan T, Azadzoi KM, Siroky MB, et al. Age-related erectile and voiding dysfunction: the role of arterial insufficiency. Br J Urol 1998;82(Suppl 1):26–33.

100. Ponholzer A, Temml C, Wehrberger C, et al. The association between vascular risk factors and lower urinary tract symptoms in both sexes. Eur Urol 2006;50: 581–6.

101. Kim S, Jeong JY, Choi YJ, et al. Association between lower urinary tract symptoms and vascular risk factors in aging men: the Hallym Aging Study. Korean J Urol 2010;51:477–82.

102. Takahashi N, Shishido K, Sato Y, et al. The association between severity of atherosclerosis and lower urinary tract function in male patients with lower urinary tract symptoms. LUTS 2012;4:9–13.

103. Pinggera GM, Mitterberger M, Steiner E, et al. Association of lower urinary tract symptoms and chronic ischaemia of the lower urinary tract in elderly women and men: assessment using colour Doppler ultrasonography. BJU Int 2008;102: 470–4.

104. Lepor H, Sunaryadi I, Hartanto V, et al. Quantitative morphometry of the adult human bladder. J Urol 1992;148:414–7.

105. Holm NR, Horn T, Hald T. Detrusor in ageing and obstruction. Scand J Urol Nephrol 1995;29:45–9.

106. Mills IW, Greenland JE, McMurray G, et al. Studies of the pathophysiology of idiopathic detrusor instability: the physiological properties of the detrusor smooth muscle and its pattern of innervation. J Urol 2000;163:646–51.

107. Kershen RT, Azadzoi KM, Siroky MB. Blood flow, pressure and compliance in the male human bladder. J Urol 2002;168:121–5.

108. Kostis JB, Jackson G, Rosen R, et al. Sexual dysfunction and cardiac risk (The Second Princeton Consensus Conference). Am J Cardiol 2005;96:85M–93M.

109. Montorsi P, Ravagnani PM, Galli S, et al. Association between erectile dysfunction and coronary artery disease: matching the right target with the right test in the right patient. Eur Urol 2006;50:721–31.

110. Braun MH, Sommer F, Haupt G, et al. Lower urinary tract symptoms and erectile dysfunction: co-morbidity or typical "aging male" symptoms? Results of the "Cologne Male Survey". Eur Urol 2003;44:588–94.

111. Kohler TS, McVary KT. The relationship between erectile dysfunction and lower urinary tract symptoms and the role of phosphodiesterase type 5 inhibitors. Eur Urol 2009;55:38–48.

112. Ponholzer A, Temml C, Obermayr R, et al. Association between lower urinary tract symptoms and erectile dysfunction. Urology 2004;64:772–6.

113. Coyne KS, Kaplan SA, Chapple CR, et al. Risk factors and comorbid conditions associated with lower urinary tract symptoms: EpiLUTS. BJU Int 2009;103(Suppl 3):24–32.

114. McVary K. Lower urinary tract symptoms and sexual dysfunction: epidemiology and pathophysiology. BJU Int 2006;97(Suppl 2):23–8 [discussion: 44–5].

115. Azadzoi KM. Effect of chronic ischemia on bladder structure and function. Adv Exp Med Biol 2003;539:271–80.

116. Azadzoi KM, Chen BG, Radisavljevic ZM, et al. Molecular reactions and ultra-structural damage in the chronically ischemic bladder. J Urol 2011;186: 2115–22.
117. Masuda H, Kihara K, Saito K, et al. Reactive oxygen species mediate detrusor overactivity via sensitization of afferent pathway in the bladder of anaesthetized rats. BJU Int 2008;101:775–80.
118. Azadzoi KM, Tarcan T, Kozlowski R, et al. Overactivity and structural changes in the chronically ischemic bladder. J Urol 1999;162:1768–78.
119. Azadzoi KM, Tarcan T, Siroky MB, et al. Atherosclerosis-induced chronic ischemia causes bladder fibrosis and non-compliance in the rabbit. J Urol 1999;161:1626–35.
120. Nomiya M, Yamaguchi O, Akaihata H, et al. Progressive vascular damage may lead to bladder underactivity in rats. J Urol 2014;191:1462–9.

Functional Brain Imaging and the Neural Basis for Voiding Dysfunction in Older Adults

Phillip P. Smith, MD[a],*, George A. Kuchel, MD[b],
Derek Griffiths, PhD[c]

KEYWORDS

• Urinary incontinence • Aging • Elderly • Frailty • Bladder • Lower urinary tract

KEY POINTS

• Brain abnormalities may contribute to the increased prevalence of urinary dysfunction such as overactive bladder and urge incontinence in older individuals.

• Functional brain imaging suggests that 3 independent neural circuits (frontal, midcingulate, and subcortical) control voiding by suppressing the voiding reflex in the brainstem periaqueductal gray.

• Damage to the connecting pathways subserving these circuits (white matter hyperintensities) increases with age and is associated both with severity of urge incontinence and changes in brain function.

• The pathway between the medial frontal cortex (circuit 1) and the periaqueductal gray seems particularly sensitive to the effects of white matter hyperintensities.

• These types of neurologic deficits may also contribute to declines in the ability of many older adults to sense, process, and execute appropriate decisions if there is urgency, thus rendering them more vulnerable to becoming incontinent.

• All of these considerations suggest that multicomponent therapies targeting these structural and functional neural abnormalities may be more effective than any single treatment focused on the bladder.

Funding Sources: D. Griffiths, none at present.
Conflicts of Interest: D. Griffiths is a consultant with Laborie Medical and Johnson & Johnson.
[a] Urology Division, Department of Surgery, UConn Center on Aging, University of Connecticut Health Center, 263 Farmington Avenue, Farmington, CT 06030, USA; [b] Division of Geriatrics, UConn Center on Aging, University of Connecticut Health Center, 263 Farmington Avenue, Farmington, CT 06030, USA; [c] Geriatric Medicine, University of Pittsburgh, 3471 Fifth Avenue, Suite 500, Pittsburgh, PA 15213, USA
* Corresponding author.
E-mail address: ppsmith@uchc.edu

INTRODUCTION

Disorders related to urinary control become increasingly prevalent and troublesome with age.[1–4] Symptoms of urgency, frequency, nocturia, and incontinence increase with age, even in the absence of an obvious genitourinary cause.[5] In contrast, many older adults with noticeable urodynamic abnormalities manage to remain dry and/or symptom free.[5] Unlike younger adults, the cause of incontinence in older adults becomes increasingly multifactorial, with nongenitourinary factors assuming important roles as both predisposing and precipitating risk factors. Thus this clinical problem assumes the mantle of a geriatric syndrome in elderly patients.[6] An association of storage, voiding, and incontinence symptoms with conditions increasingly common in older adults, including diabetes, hypertension, depression, and constipation,[7] further influences clinical presentation and outcomes, compounding the impact of urinary symptoms on life quality in older adults.

The standard approach to voiding symptoms and incontinence generally links symptoms to measurable function at the level of urodynamic studies, and function directly to the bladder and urethra; this is the bladder-centric model. This model is formalized by the terms overactive bladder and underactive bladder as descriptions of common storage and voiding symptom complexes, which are close to the terms describing urodynamic observations of detrusor performance during filling and voiding: detrusor overactivity and detrusor underactivity. The standard parsing of urinary incontinence symptoms into stress versus urge suggests a simplistic causal dichotomy of sphincteric insufficiency (urodynamic stress incontinence) or detrusor misbehavior (detrusor overactivity incontinence). Such bladder-focused associations have proved to be therapeutically useful in younger populations, thus reinforcing their apparent value. It has long been recognized that lower urinary tract symptoms are poorly predictive of observed (urodynamic) function.[8] Nevertheless, the presumption that incontinence, overactive bladder, and underactive bladder symptoms have something to do with the capabilities of the detrusor smooth muscle and urethral sphincteric mechanism has persisted.

Any presumed linkage of symptoms to dysfunction therefore hinges on an understanding of the impact of aging on lower urinary tract function and, by extension, structure and organ physiology. In contrast with a universal functional decline, aging is better characterized as a downward broadening of the spectrum of function; median levels of functionality trend downwards, the distribution widens, with many individuals retaining high levels of cognitive, visceral, and somatic performance.[9] Furthermore, at times, it can be difficult to disentangle the impact of aging per se from disease-induced changes. A growing body of knowledge suggests that aging and chronic diseases for which advanced age is a major risk factor may share common biological pathways.[10,11] These concerns are reflected in the sometimes contradictory reports regarding the impact of aging on lower urinary tract function. A consistent finding is a loss of sensitivity. The Pittsburgh group reported on urodynamics performed in a small number of healthy and asymptomatic women.[12] The threshold volume for strong desire to void increased, and urethral closure pressures and detrusor pressures at maximum flow decreased with increasing age and achievement of menopausal status. Animal models provide supportive evidence for a loss of system sensitivity to bladder volume.[13–15] Ultrastructural studies have shown evidence of depleted caveolae and slightly widened muscle intercellular spaces (so-called dense band pattern) in otherwise asymptomatic patients who did not strain to void or have a large postvoid residual volume.[16] Similar changes have been observed in an animal model.[17] Moreover, given the known role of caveolae in calcium signaling, the deletion of the caveolin gene results in impaired bladder muscle contractility.[18] Although caveolar depletion has been suggested as a contributor to impaired detrusor contractility[19] (and therefore by extension to underactive bladder and detrusor underactivity in the traditional paradigm), neither animal nor human studies in healthy asymptomatic individuals have conclusively shown a loss of voiding efficiency or detrusor strength during voiding; most in vitro and in vivo animal models suggest that voiding strength is preserved with aging despite loss of calcium sensitivity, resistance to oxidative damage, and diminished mitochondrial efficiency.[15,20–31]

Further complicating the association of aging and dysfunction is the assumption of normal function traditionally derived from younger healthy populations. For example, asymptomatic detrusor overactivity is observed in older adults,[32] and may not be truly pathologic, especially in geriatric patients. The prevalence of asymptomatic detrusor underactivity is not known, although postvoid residual volumes in asymptomatic individuals might increase with advancing age.[33] Furthermore, the natural history of objective dysfunction, without or with treatment of symptoms, is often not known. With few exceptions, once the patient's symptoms have sufficiently resolved, it is not standard practice to repeat costly and invasive urodynamic evaluation. Therefore, any linkages between symptom relief and dysfunction resolution are generally unknown.

In addition, available corrective therapies based on a bladder-centric therapeutic model are frequently suboptimal (eg, antimuscarinics, neuromodulatory techniques, and surgeries for sphincteric incontinence) or nonexistent (eg, detrusor underactivity, detrusor hyperactivity with impaired contractility). Occasionally, compensatory or palliative treatment with diapers or catheters is the only management option,[34] condemning the increasing population of elders to a much reduced quality of life. After more than a century of drug development, this fact must serve as notice that urinary symptoms are multifactorial and not inherent to the bladder.

Thus evidence at several levels suggests that a bladder-centric paradigm is an incomplete approach to urinary symptoms in older adults. Lower urinary tract symptoms are common, not dependent on or well-correlated with objective function, and the available evidence suggests minimal consistent age impact on inherent lower tract structure or function. Moreover, the nervous system assumes an increasingly important role in ensuring the maintenance of normal homeostasis in the context of lower genitourinary tract function, However, these 3 increasingly problematic themes (symptoms, function, treatment) are firmly linked by control and perceptual brain processes. The lower urinary tract is under constant brain control, in response to a steady stream of afferent data derived from bladder wall tension.[35] Beyond the standard teaching of autonomic control over bladder filling and emptying, the importance of real-time dynamic brain control is shown by evidence that aging is associated with increased volume-derived afferent stimulation[21,30] despite direct and indirect evidence of diminished system sensitivity to volume. Furthermore, indirect evidence suggests an age-associated increase in brain forward control over bladder-filling characteristics,[36] thus implicating a brain-bladder interaction in functional urinary changes of aging. The past 2 decades in particular have seen the development of methodologies allowing more direct evaluation and interrogation of brain processes responsible for urinary control and perceptions. Functional and structural brain imaging have become the main methods of studying brain control of voiding and urine storage in humans, in both health and disease.

BRAIN IMAGING OF BLADDER CONTROL

Until a few decades ago, knowledge about the brain structures involved in bladder control was derived mainly from animal experiments. In humans, studies of the outcome of trauma, stroke, or tumors suggested that the frontal lobes were important for bladder control[37–43] because, if they were damaged, urinary incontinence (ie, inability to voluntarily control voiding) resulted (**Fig. 1**). Building on these foundations, modern brain imaging techniques have permitted development of new understandings of urinary control in intact animals and humans. These techniques are rooted in the idea that oxygen use, and therefore blood flow, is increased in active brain areas and decreased in less active areas. This concept was first proposed more than a century ago.[43] Regional blood flow changes can be measured by single-photon emission computed tomography (SPECT) or PET but functional MRI (fMRI), perhaps the current standard imaging technique, depends on magnetic differences between deoxyhemoglobin and oxyhemoglobin and uses a blood oxygen level dependent (BOLD) signal to create functional images of activations/deactivations[44] (for a historical review see ref.[42]).

The first functional brain imaging study in the urinary field was made 20 years ago, using SPECT to show brain regions that were underperfused (and therefore presumably underactive) at rest.[45,46] Despite poor spatial resolution, the study showed, in a group of older men and women (mean age, 79 years), that a particularly severe form of incontinence (urge urinary incontinence [UUI] with reduced bladder-filling sensation) was associated with reduced perfusion of the frontal lobes. A further

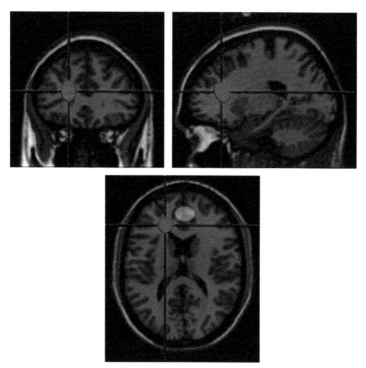

Fig. 1. Sagittal (*top right*), coronal (*top left*) and axial (*bottom*) brain sections showing frontal regions where stroke or trauma caused temporary (*blue-green ellipse*) or permanent (*red ellipse*) lower urinary tract dysfunction, especially incontinence. (*Data from* Andrew J, Nathan PW. Lesions on the anterior frontal lobes and disturbances of micturition and defaecation. Brain 1964;87:233–62; and *From* Fowler CJ, Griffiths DJ. A decade of functional brain imaging applied to bladder control. Neurourol Urodyn 2010;29(1):52; with permission.)

association between incontinence and impaired cognition confirmed that a brain factor contributed to severe geriatric incontinence,[47] presumably reflecting a white or gray matter defect in a region critical to both bladder control and aspects of cognition.

The modern era of brain imaging of bladder control began in 1997 when Blok and colleagues[48] published their landmark PET studies of filling and voiding in normal men and women.[48,49] With its good spatial resolution, PET confirmed that brainstem regions important for voiding in cats[50–52] and prominent in a working model of cerebral control (the periaqueductal gray [PAG] and the pontine micturition center [PMC]) were active during human micturition (**Fig. 2**). There was activity also in the hypothalamus and the right inferior frontal gyrus (lateral prefrontal cortex [lPFC] in **Fig. 3**). During unsuccessful attempts to micturate, increased activity was found in a different brainstem nucleus that was thought to control the motor neurons of the pelvic floor.[52] These results were supported by PET observations made by other investigators during micturition[53] and withholding of urine.[54]

Since then, functional brain imaging has transformed the knowledge of bladder control. PET and SPECT have been largely superseded by fMRI, yielding functional images with improved spatial and temporal resolution. Most studies have used healthy adults, although a few have examined brain-bladder relationships in specific conditions such as postprostatectomy incontinence,[55] normal pressure hydrocephalus,[56] and incomplete spinal cord injury.[57]

In 2001, an influential PET study[58] of normal men was published. During storage, brain activity related to increasing bladder volume was seen in the PAG, the midline pons, the midcingulate cortex (dorsal anterior cingulate cortex [dACC]), and bilaterally in the frontal lobes (**Fig. 4**). Increased brain activity associated with decreased urge to void was seen in a different portion of the cingulate cortex, in the premotor cortex, and in the hypothalamus. These findings confirmed the important role of the PAG in sensation during urine storage.

A working model of brain-bladder control emerged, helping to visualize the brain regions involved and their interconnections. According to the model, the bladder and urethra are governed by a spinobulbospinal voiding reflex that acts as a switch between 2 phases: storage of urine and voiding. Afferent data derived from bladder volume status impinges on the midbrain PAG. When it reaches a critical level the reflex is triggered: the PMC is activated, the urethral sphincter relaxes, and the bladder contracts, resulting in bladder emptying. Normally this reflex is under the control of

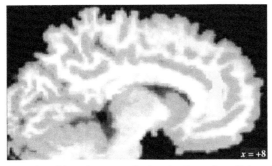

Fig. 2. PET scan during micturition shows marked activation of medial prefrontal cortex and, just visible on the lower boundary, activation of a small region thought to be the PMC, indicating that the voiding reflex has fired. (*From* Blok BF, Willemsen AT, Holstege G. A PET study on brain control of micturition in humans. Brain 1997;120(Pt 1):119; with permission.)

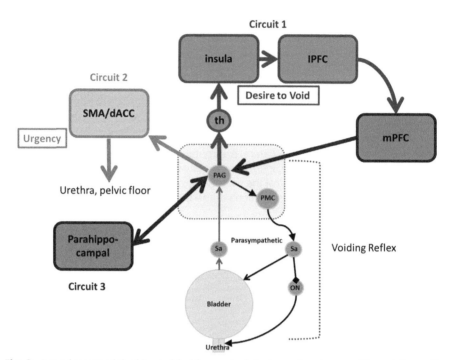

Fig. 3. A working model of brain-bladder control during urine storage. The voiding reflex is shown in green. Three forebrain circuits generate sensation and control voiding by suppressing the voiding reflex at the PAG. dACC, dorsal anterior cingulate cortex (midcingulate cortex); lPFC, lateral prefrontal cortex; mPFC, medial prefrontal cortex; ON, Onuf nucleus; Sa, sacral cord; SMA, supplementary motor area; th, thalamus. (*From* de Groat WC, Griffiths D, Yoshimura N. Neural control of the lower urinary tract. Compr Physiol 2015;5(1):327–96; with permission.)

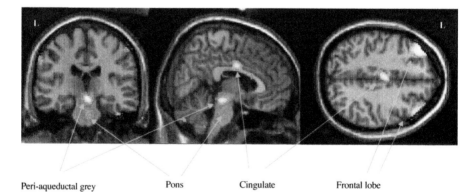

Fig. 4. PET study of normal men, showing regions activated with increasing bladder volume. (*From* Athwal BS, Berkley KJ, Hussain I, et al. Brain responses to changes in bladder volume and urge to void in healthy men. Brain 2001;124(2):373; with permission.)

forebrain circuits that generate bladder sensation (desire to void) and suppress void-ing (mainly at the PAG) unless it would be safe, socially acceptable, and consciously desired. Failure of this forebrain mechanism allows voiding to be triggered involun-tarily; the hallmark of incontinence.

FUNCTIONAL MRI STUDIES IN HEALTHY SUBJECTS

With the widespread adoption in the twenty-first century of fMRI, brain imaging with good spatial resolution and the ability to follow rapid changes ($\sim$1 second) became possible. Most investigators studied healthy young adults, using various protocols (paradigms) to elicit changes in brain activity that could be followed by fMRI. In these studies the brain regions of the working model (see **Fig. 3**) appeared repeatedly, although little was learned about the effect of aging on bladder control.

One group[59] performed fMRI during alternating periods of rest and pelvic muscle contraction, both with empty and with full bladder. Activation maps intended to show the brain areas involved in inhibition of the voiding reflex were calculated by subtracting the empty from the full bladder condition. The supplementary motor area (SMA) (see dACC/SMA in **Fig. 3**), bilateral putamen, right parietal cortex, right limbic system (called parahippocampal complex in **Fig. 3**), and right cerebellum were all activated.

Another group[60,61] identified brain mechanisms active during intentional modula-tion of the desire to void (but without allowing urine to pass). Significant brain activity was found in the insula and nearby opercula, in the SMA, the cingulate motor area (dACC), and the right prefrontal cortex (**Fig. 5**). Trends toward activation were detected in the thalamus, PAG, and ventral pons. Suppression of the urge to void significantly activated the left superior frontal lobe (lPFC in **Fig. 3**). Modulation of the desire to void also changed the effective connectivity of the brain regions

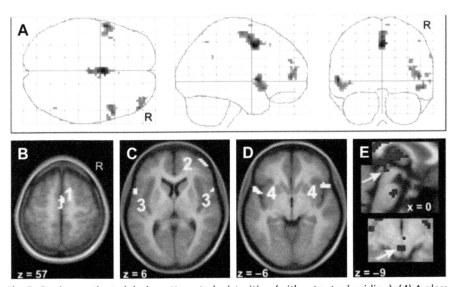

Fig. 5. Regions activated during attempted micturition (without actual voiding). (A) A glass-brain view. (B–D) Axial brain sections. 1, SMA; 2, right lateral prefrontal cortex; 3 and 4, operculum and insula. Yellow arrow in (E) shows PAG. (From Griffiths DJ, McCracken PN, Harrison GM, et al. Cerebral aetiology of urinary urge incontinence in elderly people. Age Ageing 1994;23(3):246–50; with permission.)

involved.[61] During voluntary pelvic floor muscle contractions,[62] the SMA was strongly activated, with peak activity in the posterior portion (near dACC), suggesting that this region is specifically involved in pelvic floor muscle control. Correspondingly, in healthy men and women,[63,64] relaxation and contraction of pelvic floor muscles induced strong activation patterns in the frontal cortex (lPFC), sensorimotor cortex (possibly the SMA), cerebellum, and basal ganglia, with well-localized activations in the PMC and the PAG.

The Pittsburgh group studied mechanisms of continence, incontinence, and therapy in a series of studies of older women with UUI,[65] and in healthy women for comparison, using a repeated infusion/withdrawal paradigm to stimulate repetitive brain activity. In a small group of healthy older women carefully selected for no symptoms or bladder-diary variables suggestive of UUI, and no detrusor overactivity under any circumstances,[66] there was evidence, at small bladder volumes, of activation of the PAG and the parahippocampal cortex (**Fig. 6** left) (these are parts of circuit 3) and also a trend to activation of the insula, suggesting that this subcortical circuit monitors bladder events that occur near the level of conscious awareness, with little or no activation of the prefrontal cortex, dACC, or SMA. In contrast, at large bladder volumes with strong sensation of desire to void,[65] there was activation of the insula, particularly on the right, extending into the right inferior frontal gyrus (see **Fig. 6** right). There was also a trend to activation of the dACC/SMA and a region in the hypothalamus.

Based on these findings, there seem to be 3 interacting circuits that provide sensory recognition, contextualization, decision making, and motor preparations:

- Circuit 1, frontal, involving the medial prefrontal cortex (mPFC); contextualization of bladder sensory information with preconscious and conscious control over bladder filling and voiding; the seat of the void/no void decision.
- Circuit 2, midcingulate, involving the dACC and adjacent SMA; registration of bladder sensory information and preparation of motor responses.

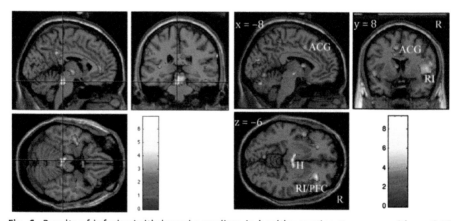

Fig. 6. Results of infusion/withdrawal paradigm in healthy continent women with no OAB or detrusor overactivity. (*Left*) At small bladder volumes, regions activated include PAG and a bilateral parahippocampal region (*bottom left*). (*Right*) At large bladder volumes, there is activation of right insula (RI) extending into right lateral prefrontal cortex (PFC). ACG, anterior cingulate gyrus; dACC/SMA, dorsal ACG/supplemental motor area; H, hypothalamus. (*From* Griffiths D, Tadic SD, Schaefer W, et al. Cerebral control of the bladder in normal and urge-incontinent women. Neuroimage 2007;37(1):4; with permission.)

- Circuit 3, subcortical, involving regions such as the hippocampal complex; corresponding with the limbic system, pattern/environmental recognition, and relating urinary status to emotional state.

In addition the insula is thought to act as the autonomic sensory cortex[67] and therefore is involved in bladder sensation and/or appreciation of bladder fullness.

CONNECTIVITY

Discussion of separate but interacting control circuits emphasizes the important but understudied role of connectivity in the operation of the working model. White matter pathways can be located or tracked directly using a special form of MRI: detrusor tensor imaging. However, most published connectivity studies rely on correlation analyses applied to the regional activations, known as functional or effective connectivity, which do not necessarily imply an anatomic connection.

One such study[68] suggested that in continent older women many regions of the working model were effectively connected with right insula and dACC/SMA, including frontotemporal and sensorimotor cortex, midbrain, and pontine regions. Among urge-incontinent individuals, the effective connectivity was shifted to a parietotemporal complex. A follow-up study[69] in healthy women confirmed connectivity of insula and dACC with putamen and right PMC (**Fig. 7**).

Another study of healthy adults[61] found that the dACC had stronger connectivity with the PAG and medial motor areas during simulated micturition (ie, without voiding) than at baseline, possibly reflecting monitoring of urethral sphincter contractions. The insula, conversely, showed decreased connectivity during simulated micturition. Thus intentional modulation of the desire to void changed the effective connectivity of supraspinal regions involved in bladder control.

EFFECT OF AGING ON BRAIN ACTIVATION AND CONNECTIVITY

Only a few studies have explicitly addressed the brain activity changes associated with aging. Griffiths and colleagues[69] showed that, in healthy adult women, there was strong activation of the right insula as well as the thalamus (see **Fig. 7**). This activation (and that of dACC/SMA and surrounding areas) decreased with age (**Figs. 8**, left and **9**). Because the insula is the seat of visceral awareness and dACC/SMA also is concerned with bladder sensation, the observation of diminishing activation in these regions is consistent with the age-associated decrease of bladder-filling sensation found on urodynamics in normal women (discussed earlier).[70] However, among subjects with UUI, insular activation increased with age (see **Fig. 8** right).[65] Presumably an age-associated abnormality in bladder afferents or their handling in the brain allows easier triggering of the voiding reflex, resulting in incontinence. This abnormality may be the white matter anomaly in mPFC or its connecting pathways.

Among older women with proven UUI, scanned with full bladder, there were strong cortical activations in dACC/SMA and the insula was activated (**Fig. 10**). There was a trend to deactivation near the mPFC[65] and also in parahippocampal areas. This pattern of activation and deactivation (see also **Fig. 5**) seems to be characteristic of urgency: a sensation, not usually felt by normal individuals, of a sudden and compelling desire to void that is difficult to defer.[71] Deactivation implies that activity in that region becomes weaker during bladder filling, a finding consistent with increased attention to bladder events,[72] resulting in stronger conscious control of the bladder, exerted via the return pathway from mPFC to PAG in the working model (see **Fig. 3**).

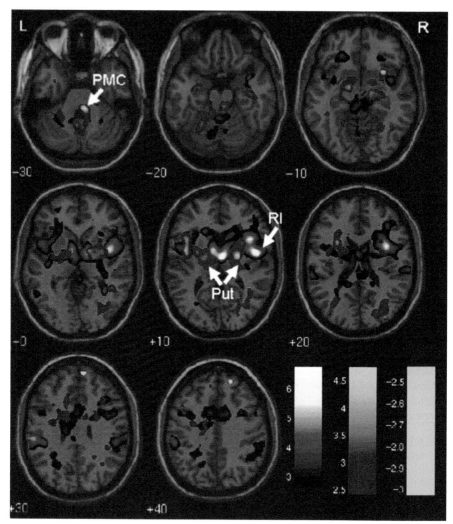

Fig. 7. Among continent women of mixed ages, blue regions show effective connectivity with RI and dACC (dACC/SMA). Red/yellow regions are activated by rapid bladder filling. PMC, right pontine micturition center; Put, bilateral putamen; RI, right insula. (*From* Griffiths DJ, Tadic SD, Schaefer W, et al. Cerebral control of the lower urinary tract: how age-related changes might predispose to urge incontinence. Neuroimage 2009;47(3):982; with permission.)

To better understand this, behavior subgroup analyses were performed. All these women had UUI with detrusor overactivity (DO) on regular urodynamics, but not all showed DO while in the scanner. Those without DO in scanner behaved differently than those with DO, even though none of the scans were made during DO: during urgency the DO group showed significantly stronger dACC/SMA activation than the no-DO group, suggesting that increased activity in this region is not a cause of incontinence but represents a compensatory reaction of circuit 2 (sphincter contraction together with urgency) to a failure occurring elsewhere.

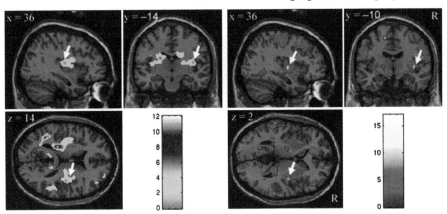

Fig. 8. (*Left*) Normal female patients at small bladder volume, showing regions (*blue*) where activation by rapid bladder filling decreases with age. (*Right*) Incontinent patients, showing regions where activation increases with age. White arrows indicate that activation of right posterior insula increases with age in normal controls but decreases with age in urge-incontinent patients. (*From* Griffiths D, Tadic SD, Schaefer W, et al. Cerebral control of the bladder in normal and urge-incontinent women. Neuroimage 2007;37(1):5; with permission.)

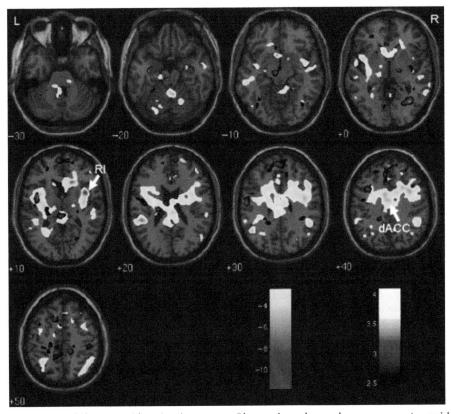

Fig. 9. Normal changes with aging in women. Blue regions show where response to rapid bladder filling has diminished with age, including RI and dACC. Red/yellow regions show where connectivity has changed with age, including mPRC (*middle row*). (*From* Griffiths DJ, Tadic SD, Schaefer W, et al. Cerebral control of the lower urinary tract: how age-related changes might predispose to urge incontinence. Neuroimage 2009;47(3):983; with permission.)

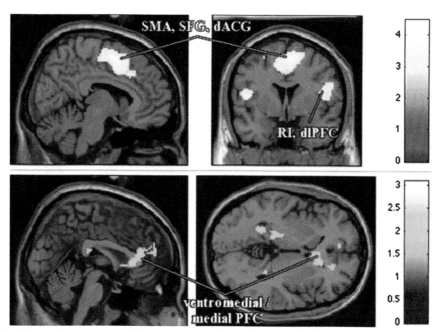

Fig. 10. In older women with proven urge incontinence, with large bladder volume, the infusion/withdrawal paradigm generates activation of dACC/SMA and insula (*yellow regions, upper row*); it leads to deactivation of the mPRC and some other regions (*blue*). dACG, dorsal anterior cingulate gyrus; dlPFC, dorsolateral PFC; SFG, superior frontal gyrus. (*From* Tadic SD, Griffiths D, Schaefer W, et al. Brain activity underlying impaired continence control in older women with overactive bladder. Neurourol Urodyn 2012;31(5):657; with permission.)

Connectivity too depends on age. In normal women there is an age-associated change in the effective connectivity of the mPRC (circuit 1) with the insula and dACC/SMA (circuit 2; see **Fig. 9**). This change supports the view that abnormality of the connecting pathways of the mPFC, perhaps caused by white matter hyperintensities (WMHs), contributes to the development of UUI in older people.

Structural imaging of cerebral WMHs (white matter damage) has helped to explain the meaning of fMRI findings vis-à-vis activation/deactivation patterns in older women with UUI: there was greater WMH burden in the DO group than in the no-DO group, especially in a prominent white matter tract known as the right anterior thalamic radiation (ATR). As shown in **Fig. 11**, the ATR connects the prefrontal cortex with the thalamus and brainstem.[73] It seems to connect many of the regions deactivated by bladder filling, including the parahippocampal complex (bright blue areas, top left; circuit 3) and the mPRC (blue region at top of the figures are the frontal brain; circuit 1).

Thus WMH burden in the ATR may cause the mPFC or its connecting pathways to function abnormally, disabling circuit 1. This causal role of white matter damage was supported by a study[73] in which similar regional activations and deactivations became more prominent with increasing WMH burden. Because WMH become more common with age, this type of incontinence (UUI with WMH as a cause or contributing factor) is likely to be characteristic of old age. Further study of the relation between incontinence and WMH has been performed by the Connecticut group.[74] The critical upshot

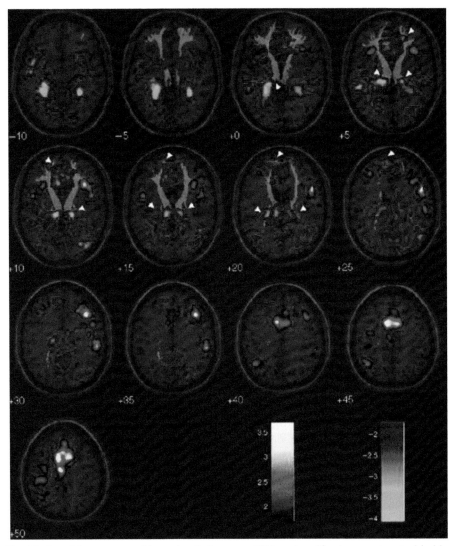

Fig. 11. For older women with moderate to severe UUI, regional brain responses to bladder filling (*blue areas* indicate deactivation) superimposed on a white matter tract (ATR; shown in *light gray*). White pointers show some of the regions where the tract appears to project to deactivated areas. (*From* Tadic SD, Griffiths D, Murrin A, et al. Brain activity during bladder filling is related to white matter structural changes in older women with urinary incontinence. Neuroimage 2010;51(4):1300; with permission.)

of this work has been the recognition of the primary association of WMH disease burden in relevant brain areas with symptom severity rather than symptom occurrence. Prefrontal cortex, ACC, and insula participate in the attentional biasing required for the conscious recognition and preparation for action in response to visceral input.[72] Disruption of this monitoring system by WMH (as suggested by the imaging) may delay or remove bladder volume recognition, replacing typical sensations of the filling bladder with atypical and potentially overwhelming sensations (typifying urgency). By impeding motor area preparation, sphincteric and mobility responses may be slowed or absent, further contributing to symptom severity. This finding directly suggests the importance of perceptual and integrative processes in the generation of symptoms.

SUMMARY

Brain processes are critical to the control of bladder filling and emptying, adaptive integration with other visceral and somatic processes, and to the perceptions of these functions. Several complementary imaging techniques have provided static and real-time information contributing to a greatly enhanced understanding of visceral control. Emerging evidence suggests that the increased prevalence of lower urinary tract symptoms with aging, especially overactive bladder symptoms and incontinence, is more likely to relate to disordered brain processes than end-organ changes. Key questions remain, including delineating the impact of aging versus brain changes caused by coexistent disease, the specific brain processes responsible for homeostatic control over the aging lower urinary tract in the context of the overall aging organism, and how these functional and perceptual integrative processes might be therapeutically manipulated.

REFERENCES

1. Resnick NM. Urinary incontinence. Lancet 1995;346:94–9.
2. Naughton MJ, Wyman JF. Quality of life in geriatric patients with lower urinary tract dysfunction. Am J Med Sci 1997;314(4):219–27.
3. Nuotio M, Jylha M, Luukkaala T, et al. Urgency, urge incontinence and voiding symptoms in men and women aged 70 years and over. BJU Int 2002;89(4):350–5.
4. Smith PP. Aging and the underactive detrusor: a failure of activity or activation? Neurourol Urodyn 2010;29(3):408–12.
5. Araki I, Zakoji H, Komuro M, et al. Lower urinary tract symptoms in men and women without underlying disease causing micturition disorder: a cross-sectional study assessing the natural history of bladder function. J Urol 2003; 170(5):1901–4.
6. Inouye SK, Studenski S, Tinetti ME, et al. Geriatric syndromes: clinical, research, and policy implications of a core geriatric concept. J Am Geriatr Soc 2007;55(5): 780–91.
7. Coyne KS, Sexton CC, Irwin DE, et al. The impact of overactive bladder, incontinence and other lower urinary tract symptoms on quality of life, work productivity, sexuality and emotional well-being in men and women: results from the EPIC study. BJU Int 2008;101(11):1388–95.
8. Bates CP, Whiteside CG, Turner-Warwick R. Synchronous cine-pressure-flow-cysto-urethrography with special reference to stress and urge incontinence. Br J Urol 1970;42(6):714–23.
9. Kuchel GA. Aging and homeostatic regulation. In: Halter JB, Ouslander JG, Tinetti ME, et al, editors. Hazzard's principles of geriatric medicine and gerontology. 6th edition. New York: McGraw-Hill; 2010. p. 621–9.
10. Burch JB, Augustine AD, Frieden LA, et al. Advances in geroscience: impact on healthspan and chronic disease. J Gerontol A Biol Sci Med Sci 2014;69(Suppl 1): S1–3.
11. Kennedy BK, Berger SL, Brunet A, et al. Geroscience: linking aging to chronic disease. Cell 2014;159(4):709–13.

12. Pfisterer MH, Griffiths DJ, Rosenberg L, et al. Parameters of bladder function in pre-, peri-, and postmenopausal continent women without detrusor overactivity. Neurourol Urodyn 2007;26(3):356–61.

13. Rodrigues AA Jr, Suaid HJ, Tucci S Jr, et al. Long term evaluation of functional and morphological bladder alterations on alloxan-induced diabetes and aging: experimental study in rats. Acta Cir Bras 2008;23:53–8.

14. Hotta H, Morrison JF, Sato A, et al. The effects of aging on the rat bladder and its innervation. Jpn J Physiol 1995;45(5):823–36.

15. Chai TC, Andersson KE, Tuttle JB, et al. Altered neural control of micturition in the aged F344 rat. Urol Res 2000;28(5):348–54.

16. Elbadawi A, Yalla SV, Resnick NM. Structural basis of geriatric voiding dysfunction. II. Aging detrusor: normal versus impaired contractility. J Urol 1993;150(5 Pt 2):1657–67.

17. Lowalekar SK, Cristofaro V, Radisavljevic ZM, et al. Loss of bladder smooth muscle caveolae in the aging bladder. Neurourol Urodyn 2012;31(4):586–92.

18. Sadegh MK, Ekman M, Rippe C, et al. Biomechanical properties and innervation of the female caveolin-1-deficient detrusor. Br J Pharmacol 2010;162(5):1156–70.

19. Lai HH, Boone TB, Yang G, et al. Loss of caveolin-1 expression is associated with disruption of muscarinic cholinergic activities in the urinary bladder. Neurochem Int 2004;45(8):1185–93.

20. Chun AL, Wallace LJ, Gerald MC, et al. Effect of age on in vivo urinary bladder function in the rat. J Urol 1988;139(3):625–7.

21. Daly DM, Nocchi L, Liaskos M, et al. Age-related changes in afferent pathways and urothelial function in the male mouse bladder. J Physiol 2014;592(Pt 3):537–49.

22. Lluel P, Palea S, Barras M, et al. Functional and morphological modifications of the urinary bladder in aging female rats. Am J Physiol Regul Integr Comp Physiol 2000;278(4):R964–72.

23. Munro DD, Wendt IR. Contractile and metabolic properties of longitudinal smooth muscle from rat urinary bladder and the effects of aging. J Urol 1993;150(2 Pt 1):529–36.

24. Ordway GA, Kolta MG, Gerald MC, et al. Age-related change in alpha-adrenergic responsiveness of the urinary bladder of the rat is regionally specific. Neuropharmacology 1986;25(12):1335–40.

25. Pagala MK, Tetsoti L, Nagpal D, et al. Aging effects on contractility of longitudinal and circular detrusor and trigone of rat bladder. J Urol 2001;166(2):721–7.

26. Saito M, Gotoh M, Kato K, et al. Influence of aging on the rat urinary bladder function. Urol Int 1991;47(Suppl 1):39–42.

27. Saito M, Kondo A, Gotoh M, et al. Age-related changes in the rat detrusor muscle: the contractile response to inorganic ions. J Urol 1991;146(3):891–4.

28. Saito M, Kondo A, Gotoh M, et al. Age-related changes in the response of the rat urinary bladder to neurotransmitters. Neurourol Urodyn 1993;12(2):191–200.

29. Saito M, Ohmura M, Kondo A. Effect of ageing on blood flow to the bladder and bladder function. Urol Int 1999;62(2):93–8.

30. Smith PP, DeAngelis A, Kuchel GA. Detrusor expulsive strength is preserved, but responsiveness to bladder filling and urinary sensitivity is diminished in the aging mouse. Am J Physiol Regul Integr Comp Physiol 2012;302(5):R577–86.

31. Tugay M, Yildiz F, Utkan T, et al. Age-related smooth muscle reactivity changes in the rat bladder: an in vitro study. Pharmacol Res 2003;48(4):329–34.

32. Branch LG, Walker LA, Wetle TT, et al. Urinary incontinence knowledge among community-dwelling people 65 years of age and older. J Am Geriatr Soc 1994;42(12):1257–62.

33. Gehrich A, Stany MP, Fischer JR, et al. Establishing a mean postvoid volume in asymptomatic perimenopausal and postmenopausal women. Obstet Gynecol 2007;110(4):827–32.
34. Hartmann KE, McPheeters ML, Biller DH, et al. Treatment of overactive bladder in women. Evid Rep Technol Assess (Full Rep) 2009;(187):1–120, v.
35. le Feber J, van Asselt E, van Mastrigt R. Afferent bladder nerve activity in the rat: a mechanism for starting and stopping voiding contractions. Urol Res 2004;32(6): 395–405.
36. Smith PP, DeAngelis A, Simon R. Evidence of increased centrally enhanced bladder compliance with ageing in a mouse model. BJU Int 2015;115(2):322–9.
37. Andrew J, Nathan PW. Lesions on the anterior frontal lobes and disturbances of micturition and defaecation. Brain 1964;87:233–62.
38. Maurice-Williams RS. Micturition symptoms in frontal tumours. J Neurol Neurosurg Psychiatry 1974;37(4):431–6.
39. Griffiths DJ, Fowler CJ. The micturition switch and its forebrain influences. Acta Physiol (Oxf) 2013;207(1):93–109.
40. Ueki K. Disturbances of micturition observed in some patients with brain tumour. Neurol Med Chir 1960;2:25.
41. Sakakibara R, Hattori T, Yasuda K, et al. Micturitional disturbance after acute hemispheric stroke: analysis of the lesion site by CT and MRI. J Neurol Sci 1996;137:47–56.
42. Thulborn KR. My starting point: the discovery of an NMR method for measuring blood oxygenation using the transverse relaxation time of blood water. Neuroimage 2012;62(2):589–93.
43. Roy CS, Sherrington CS. On the regulation of the blood-supply of the brain. J Physiol 1890;11(1–2):85–158, 17.
44. Ogawa S, Lee TM, Kay AR, et al. Brain magnetic resonance imaging with contrast dependent on blood oxygenation. Proc Natl Acad Sci U S A 1990;87(24): 9868–72.
45. Griffiths DJ, McCracken PN, Harrison GM, et al. Cerebral aetiology of urinary urge incontinence in elderly people. Age Ageing 1994;23(3):246–50.
46. Griffiths DJ, McCracken PN, Harrison GM, et al. Urinary incontinence in the elderly: the brain factor. Scand J Urol Nephrol 1994;28(Suppl. 157):83–8.
47. Griffiths D. Clinical studies of cerebral and urinary tract function in elderly people with urinary incontinence. Behav Brain Res 1998;92(2):151–5.
48. Blok BF, Willemsen AT, Holstege G. A PET study on brain control of micturition in humans. Brain 1997;120(Pt 1):111–21.
49. Blok BF, Sturms LM, Holstege G. Brain activation during micturition in women. Brain 1998;121(Pt 11):2033–42.
50. Barrington FJ. The component reflexes of micturition in the cat. Parts I and II. Brain 1931;54(2):177–8.
51. Barrington FJ. The component reflexes of micturition in the cat. Part III. Brain 1941;64(2):239–43.
52. Holstege G, Griffiths D, de Wall H, et al. Anatomical and physiological observations on supraspinal control of bladder and urethral sphincter muscles in the cat. J Comp Neurol 1986;250(4):449–61.
53. Nour S, Svarer C, Kristensen JK, et al. Cerebral activation during micturition in normal men. Brain 2000;123(Pt 4):781–9.
54. Matsuura S, Kakizaki H, Mitsui T, et al. Human brain region response to distention or cold stimulation of the bladder: a positron emission tomography study. J Urol 2002;168(5):2035–9.

55. Seseke S, Baudewig J, Ringert RH, et al. Monitoring brain activation changes in the early postoperative period after radical prostatectomy using fMRI. Neuroimage 2013;78:1–6.
56. Sakakibara R, Uchida Y, Ishii K, et al. Correlation of right frontal hypoperfusion and urinary dysfunction in iNPH: a SPECT study. Neurourol Urodyn 2012;31(1):50–5.
57. Zempleni MZ, Michels L, Mehnert U, et al. Cortical substrate of bladder control in SCI and the effect of peripheral pudendal stimulation. Neuroimage 2010;49(4): 2983–94.
58. Athwal BS, Berkley KJ, Hussain I, et al. Brain responses to changes in bladder volume and urge to void in healthy men. Brain 2001;124(Pt 2):369–77.
59. Zhang H, Reitz A, Kollias S, et al. An fMRI study of the role of suprapontine brain structures in the voluntary voiding control induced by pelvic floor contraction. Neuroimage 2005;24(1):174–80.
60. Kuhtz-Buschbeck JP, van der Horst C, Pott C, et al. Cortical representation of the urge to void: a functional magnetic resonance imaging study. J Urol 2005;174(4 Pt 1):1477–81.
61. Kuhtz-Buschbeck JP, Gilster R, van der Horst C, et al. Control of bladder sensations: an fMRI study of brain activity and effective connectivity. Neuroimage 2009; 47(1):18–27.
62. Kuhtz-Buschbeck JP, van der Horst C, Wolff S, et al. Activation of the supplementary motor area (SMA) during voluntary pelvic floor muscle contractions–an fMRI study. Neuroimage 2007;35(2):449–57.
63. Seseke S, Baudewig J, Kallenberg K, et al. Gender differences in voluntary micturition control: an fMRI study. Neuroimage 2008;43(2):183–91.
64. Seseke S, Baudewig J, Kallenberg K, et al. Voluntary pelvic floor muscle control–an fMRI study. Neuroimage 2006;31(4):1399–407.
65. Griffiths D, Tadic SD, Schaefer W, et al. Cerebral control of the bladder in normal and urge-incontinent women. Neuroimage 2007;37(1):1–7.
66. Tadic SD, Tannenbaum C, Resnick NM, et al. Brain responses to bladder filling in older women without urgency incontinence. Neurourol Urodyn 2013;32(5):435–40.
67. Craig AD. Interoception: the sense of the physiological condition of the body. Curr Opin Neurobiol 2003;13(4):500–5.
68. Tadic SD, Griffiths D, Schaefer W, et al. Abnormal connections in the supraspinal bladder control network in women with urge urinary incontinence. Neuroimage 2008;39(4):1647–53.
69. Griffiths DJ, Tadic SD, Schaefer W, et al. Cerebral control of the lower urinary tract: how age-related changes might predispose to urge incontinence. Neuroimage 2009;47(3):981–6.
70. Pfisterer MH, Griffiths DJ, Rosenberg L, et al. The impact of detrusor overactivity on bladder function in younger and older women. J Urol 2006;175(5):1777–83.
71. Abrams P, Cardozo L, Fall M, et al. The standardisation of terminology of lower urinary tract function: report from the Standardisation Sub-committee of the International Continence Society. Neurourol Urodyn 2002;21(2):167–78.
72. Raichle ME, Snyder AZ. A default mode of brain function: a brief history of an evolving idea. Neuroimage 2007;37(4):1083–90 [discussion: 1097–9].
73. Tadic SD, Griffiths D, Murrin A, et al. Brain activity during bladder filling is related to white matter structural changes in older women with urinary incontinence. Neuroimage 2010;51(4):1294–302.
74. Kuchel GA, Moscufo N, Guttmann CR, et al. Localization of brain white matter hyperintensities and urinary incontinence in community-dwelling older adults. J Gerontol A Biol Sci Med Sci 2009;64(8):902–9.

The Role of Urodynamics in Elderly Patients

Joseph E. Yared, MD, E. Ann Gormley, MD*

KEYWORDS

- Urodynamics • Elderly • Stress incontinence • Urgency • Parkinson • Stroke

KEY POINTS

- Urodynamic testing (UDS) is the study of the storage and voiding functions of the bladder and its outlet. UDS is used to determine if lower urinary tract symptoms (LUTS) is due to a dysfunction of the bladder, the outlet or both. UDS should only be performed when there is a particular question to be answered and when that answer might lead to a different management strategy.
- UDS attempts to reproduce the patient's symptoms. The patient should be prepared for the test and should be positioned comfortably and safely.
- UDS includes measurement of post void residual, a cystometrogram, a pressure-flow study, and electromyography of the pelvic floor.
- UDS may be used to diagnose bladder storage or voiding dysfunctions, but its greatest utility is to confirm the presence of a particular problem before operating.

INTRODUCTION

Urodynamic testing (UDS) is the study of the storage and voiding functions of the bladder and its outlet. According to a United Nations report on aging, those who are older than 60 will be 21.1% of the world's population by 2050 and the probability of a 65-year-old in more developed regions today living to 85 years or older continues to increase.[1] In the elderly population, lower urinary tract symptoms (LUTS) consisting of increased urgency, frequency, and nocturia and increased symptoms of both urgency and stress incontinence are common.[2] The population older than 65 years is a heterogenous group in terms of frailty, those who present with impairment in their physical activity, mobility, balance, strength, cognition and have coexistent chronic medical conditions and need for assistance with activities of daily living and those who are not frail. Separation of those older than 65 into frail and nonfrail groups is beyond the scope of this article. The existence of LUTS in any patient does not warrant the use of UDS to establish a diagnosis. In fact, level I evidence is lacking for the exact

Section of Urology, Department of Surgery, 1 Medical Center Drive, Lebanon, NH 03756, USA
* Corresponding author.
E-mail address: Elizabeth.Ann.Gormley@hitchcock.org

Clin Geriatr Med 31 (2015) 567–579
http://dx.doi.org/10.1016/j.cger.2015.06.003   geriatric.theclinics.com

indication of UDS.[3] LUTS should be initially investigated with a thorough history, physical examination, voiding diary, urinalysis, and urine culture. A pad weight test may be helpful in some incontinent patients. In female patients during the physical examination, the health of the vaginal mucosa is assessed, urethral hypermobility is noted, a stress test is performed and pelvic organ prolapse is graded. Before performing other tests and before treatment the impact of the patient's symptoms on their quality of life is assessed.

UDS is used to determine whether LUTS is owing to a dysfunction of the bladder, the outlet, or both. UDS should only be performed when there is a particular question to be answered and when that answer might lead to a different management strategy. It is also reasonable to perform UDS before considering an operative procedure, particularly in elderly patients who may not be ideal surgical candidates.

UDS should be performed with an attempt to reproduce the patient's symptoms to present an accurate clinical picture of the patient's condition. The clinician and the staff in the UDS suite must alleviate any anxiety the patient might have by preparing the patient for the test by explaining the procedure, telling patients what to expect throughout the test and explaining the purpose of the test and how it may impact treatment.

POSITIONING

Usually, the patient is placed in a seated or standing position on a special table that can accommodate fluoroscopy equipment, including a C-arm.[4] Ideally, patients should not be placed supine during filling because this may minimize overactive bladder symptoms.[5] During the voiding phase of UDS, patients should be positioned in whatever position they normally use to void. When positioning the patient for UDS, the clinician should keep in mind that older patients might have limited mobility, impaired balance, and reduced strength, and may require assistance in positioning. Patients should be positioned so that they are comfortable and feel safe without fear or risk of falling.

URODYNAMIC TESTING

UDS is composed of different components that do not necessarily need to be used together. The clinician should use their judgment to pick the most appropriate parts of the study to answer the question that they are trying to address and to establish a diagnosis. It is reasonable to start with minimally invasive studies first and then decide whether more invasive testing is warranted.

The International Continence Society has guidelines in place for good UDS technique.[6] The bladder is catheterized to ensure that the patient's bladder is empty and to obtain a postvoid volume. A dual-lumen catheter is used in the bladder to measure pressures and to allow for filling. A single-lumen catheter is inserted in the rectum to record intraabdominal pressure. In females, this can be placed in the vagina. Electromyography (EMG) electrodes are then attached to the perineal skin to record sphincter activity. Once the catheters are placed and the patient positioned, the transducers are zeroed. UDS comprise the following tests.

Postvoid Residual

The postvoid residual (PVR) is the amount of urine left in the bladder after voiding. This can be assessed noninvasively with an ultrasound/bladder scanner (**Fig. 1**) or via straight catheterization. A high PVR could be indicative of dysfunctional bladder emptying, obstruction, or both. In patients with ascites, straight catheterization is

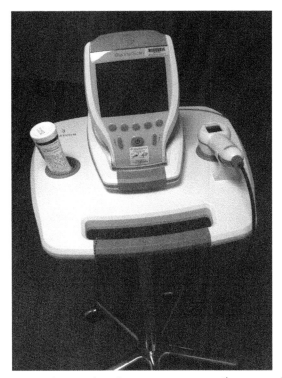

Fig. 1. A bladder scanner is a noninvasive way to measure the post void residual urine. (Verathon Inc, Bothell, WA.)

preferred because the bladder scanner could inaccurately measure intraabdominal fluid as intravesical fluid.[3,7]

Uroflowmetry

Uroflowmetry is a noninvasive method that measures the rate of urine flow over time.[3] Most uroflometry machines use a gravimetric meter to calculate the hydrostatic pressure caused by the accumulated urine.[7] A normal result is a bell shaped curve and a flat curve with a rate of less than 12 mL/s is suggestive of obstruction (**Fig. 2**). Uroflowmetry alone is not diagnostic and a decision to undertake an operative intervention should not be based solely on a uroflowmetry result.

Multichannel Urodynamics

Multichannel urodynamics is a multicomponent evaluation that includes the following tests.

Cystometry

Cystometry (CMG) is the measurement of change in bladder pressure during filling and voiding. Detrusor pressure (P_{det}) is calculated by subtracting abdominal pressure (P_{abd}) measured by the rectal catheter from vesical pressure (P_{ves}) measured by the catheter in the bladder (**Fig. 3**). CMG allows for evaluation of involuntary detrusor contractions, compliance, sensation, and bladder capacity during filling. The bladder is usually filled with water, saline, or contrast over different rates while the pressures

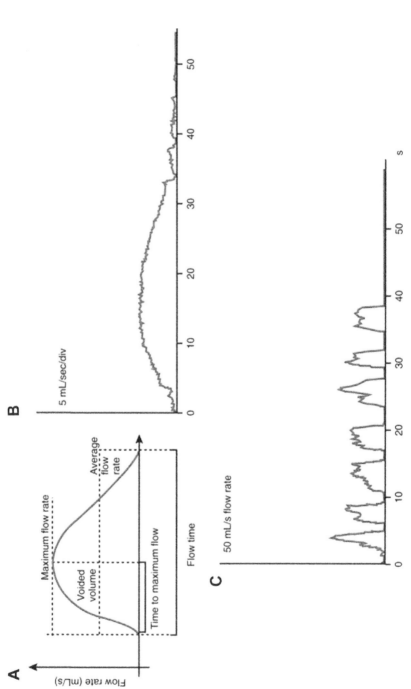

Fig. 2. Examples of uroflow curves. (*A*) Normal bell-shaped flow curve of flow rate versus time. (*B*) A flattened pattern is usually indicative of obstruction. (*C*) An interrupted or straining pattern can be seen with impaired bladder contractility, obstruction, or voiding with or by abdominal straining. (*From* [*A*] Wein AJ, English WS, Whitemore KE. Office urodynamics. Urol Clin North Am 1988;15:609, with permission; and [*B, C*] Boone TB, Kim YH. Uroflowmetry. In: Nitti VW, editor. Practical urodynamics. Philadelphia: WB Saunders; 1998. p. 31; with permission.)

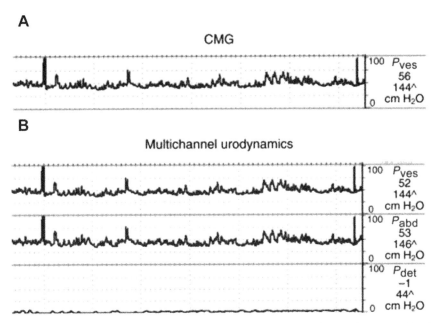

Fig. 3. (*A*) Single-channel cystometry (CMG) where only the total vesical pressure (P_{ves}) is measured. Note the multiple spikes and rises in pressure. Without having simultaneous monitoring of intra-abdominal pressure, it is impossible to determine if these pressure spikes are owing to an increase in detrusor or abdominal pressure. (*B*) This same tracing with intraabdominal pressure (P_{abd}) monitoring added (multichannel urodynamic testing). This allows for the determination of (subtracted) detrusor pressure (P_{det}). Now it can be clearly seen that changes in P_{ves} were owing to the changes in P_{abd} (eg, movement, coughing). The P_{det} curve is noted to be flat and without any increases in pressure. (*From* Nitti VW. Cystometry and abdominal pressure monitoring. In: Nitti VW, editor. Practical urodynamics. Philadelphia: WB Saunders; 1998. p. 44; with permission.)

are being measured. Fill rates usually start at 50 to 70 mL/minute and can be decreased or increased, depending on bladder capacity and patient comfort.

Before performing a CMG, patients are instructed that they will be asked to report on sensation throughout the test. Sensation is measured as a first sensation of bladder filling, first desire to void, and strong desire to void.[3,7]

Electromyography
EMG uses patch or needle electrodes to measure the electric potentials that generate the contraction of pelvic floor muscles. This measurement is continuous and is contrasted to detrusor contractions to assess if the respective contractions are synergistic or dyssenergistic. EMG is extremely useful in the evaluation of neurologic disorders.[3,7]

Pressure Flow Studies

Pressure flow studies (PFS) measure urine flow and detrusor pressure at the same time. Unlike uroflowmetry, PFS is an invasive study. PFS is the most appropriate study for the evaluation of bladder contractility and outlet obstruction. There exist multiple nomograms in which pressure and flow are plotted against each other and are used in clinical practice to establish and quantitate the diagnosis of obstruction.[3,7,8] These are discussed elsewhere in this article.

Videourodynamics

Videourodynamics combines multichannel UDS and fluoroscopy of the genitourinary tract and is used when both anatomy and function are needed to establish a diagnosis.[9] The bladder is filled with x-ray contrast and a C-arm fluoroscopy machine is used to take radiographic images during filling and voiding. This modality is important in patients with neurologic disease, history of anatomic anomalies, and in the evaluation of bladder neck obstruction, detrusor external sphincter dyssynergia, vesicoureteral reflux, incontinence, fistulas and outlet obstruction in women (**Fig. 4**).[4,10]

Although newer fluoroscopy units are designed to use less radiation than older units, appropriate shielding should be used and the number of images taken should be minimized for the protection of both the patient and the operator.[4]

Abdominal Leak Point Pressure and Valsalva Leak Point Pressure

Abdominal leak point pressure (ALPP) and Valsalva leak point pressure (VLPP) are interchangeable terms that define the lowest pressure generated by the abdomen in the absence of detrusor contraction that causes leakage of urine. ALPP/VLPP is used in the evaluation of stress incontinence. It is measured by asking the patient to perform a standard set of maneuvers, typically a Valsalva maneuver and a cough, at incremental bladder volumes.

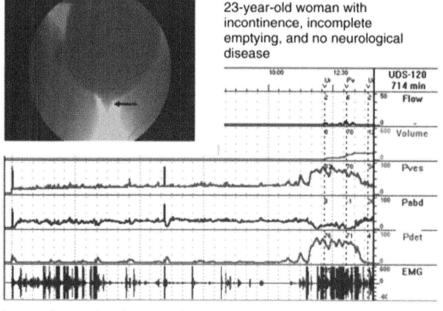

Fig. 4. Dysfunctional voiding—a urodynamics study of a 23-year-old woman with urgency incontinence, incomplete emptying, and no neurologic disease. Just before voiding there is an involuntary detrusor contraction. With voiding there is increased EMG activity. The fluoroscopic picture taken during voiding shows a characteristic "spinning top urethra" with the level of obstruction at the external sphincter. The high-pressure–low-flow voiding is also characteristic of obstruction. (*From* Nitti VW. Urodynamic and video-urodynamic evaluation of the lower urinary tract. In: Wein AJ, Kavoussi LR, Novick AC, et al., editors. Campbell-Walsh urology. 10th edition. Philadelphia: Elsevier Saunders, 2012; with permission.)

Detrusor Leak Point Pressure

Detrusor leak point pressure is the lowest detrusor pressure capable of causing urine leakage. It is used as a surrogate to assess risk for the upper urinary tract. Detrusor leak point pressure of 40 cm H_2O and greater is generally considered a risk for upper tract deterioration.[4] A phasic rise in detrusor pressure during filling that is involuntary is termed detrusor overactivity and may or may not result in urine leakage. Some individuals who do not have symptoms of bladder overactivity will have detrusor overactivity during filling.

Urethral Pressure Profile

Urethral pressure profile uses a transducer catheter to measure the pressure at different points in the urethra after the bladder is filled and while the catheter is slowly being removed. The difference between this pressure and the intravesical pressure is the maximum urethral closure pressure. The urethral pressure profile and maximum urethral closure pressure have been used in the diagnosis of stress urinary incontinence (SUI).

LOWER URINARY TRACT SYMPTOMS THAT ARE COMMON IN THE GERIATRIC POPULATION

Stress Urinary Incontinence in Females

Urinary incontinence is defined as the involuntary loss of urine while SUI is defined as the involuntary loss of urine during effort.[11] Urinary incontinence was estimated to be responsible for 1.1 million office visits in the United States in 2000.[12]

In the patient who describes SUI, if the sign of SUI can be observed during physical examination, the necessity of UDS to diagnose SUI is questionable. Placing a sling immediately for women with pure SUI has been shown to be more cost effective than basing the decision on UDS.[13] In the geriatric population, patients often present with symptoms of mixed incontinence, SUI, and urgency urinary incontinence, or the patient may have a difficult time describing exactly what she is doing when she is incontinent. In these situations, UDS may help to better define the type of incontinence. In the patient who describes severe incontinence, the diagnosis of intrinsic sphincter deficiency should be entertained. Advanced age and menopausal status correlate with intrinsic sphincter deficiency.[14] Although the exact definition of intrinsic sphincter deficiency is controversial, the only way to make the diagnosis is to perform UDS. UDS are also recommended when a diagnosis cannot be established with a history and physical examination and when patients have recurrent SUI after prior surgical treatment.[3,13]

Urodynamic SUI is observed during filling CMG. To establish the diagnosis, loss of urine during UDS must be accompanied with an increase in abdominal pressure and no change in detrusor pressure. If SUI cannot be demonstrated in a patient with subjective symptoms, the study should be repeated after the catheter is removed.[3,7]

In women with significant prolapse, if urodynamic SUI is not demonstrated the prolapse should be reduced and testing repeated to determine ALPP/VLPP. Urodynamic SUI that only occurs with prolapse reduction is termed occult SUI. UDS in the patient with SUI should include urethral evaluation, usually with the measurement of VLPP. A urethral pressure profile and measurement of maximum urethral closure pressure is performed by some practitioners to assess urethral function. Poor urethral function, previously described as a VLPP lower than 60 cm H_2O, is associated with poorer outcomes of surgical procedures, such as suspensions.[15] UDS, when performed for SUI should also include measurement of voiding efficacy with a PVR measurement and a pressure flow study if the PVR is high or if there is concern about voiding dysfunction. Patients with high PVR and impaired emptying may benefit preoperatively from conservative management, like more frequent self-catheterization, and they should be warned that they are more likely to go into retention postoperatively.[3]

Overactive Bladder, Urgency Urinary Incontinence, and Mixed Urinary Incontinence

Overactive bladder (OAB) is a symptom complex that includes frequency and urinary urgency with or without incontinence.[3] When it is not accompanied by incontinence, it is known as OAB–dry and when it is, it is known as OAB–wet or UUI. UUI is the most common urinary incontinence in older people.[16] Whereas OAB is a symptom, detrusor overactivity is a urodynamic finding characterized by involuntary contractions during the filling phase of CMG.[3] OAB may exist with or without detrusor overactivity and not all patients with detrusor overactivity complain of OAB.

Behavioral treatment is the first line treatment for OAB and pharmacologic treatment is the second line. UDS should be performed only when patients are refractory to conservative management and when invasive treatments, like botulinum toxin injections and sacral stimulation, are being considered. One of the reasons to perform UDS in this setting is to ensure that the patient does not also have SUI. PFS should be considered to rule out bladder outlet obstruction in patients with urgency incontinence, particularly in patients at risk for obstruction including those with refractory OAB after a bladder outlet procedure.[3]

Nocturia

Nocturia is defined as having to wake up at night 1 or more times to void. In people older than 60, the prevalence in the Danish population was 77%. Nocturnal polyuria is defined as having more than 33% of the 24-hour urine output at night. Both conditions can be a manifestation of systemic diseases that might be outside the scope of a urologist.[17] UDS evaluation of nocturia is limited. In the patient with nocturia and a high PVR, a PFS can be used to rule out obstruction, provided that the patient is a candidate for surgery to relieve outlet obstruction. Patients with nocturia in conjunction with daytime frequency and urgency likely have OAB and, as noted, should only undergo UDS when more invasive treatments are being considered.

Neurogenic Bladder

Neurogenic bladder is a broad term that describes bladder dysfunction that is owing to an underlying neurologic etiology. The most common causes of neurogenic bladder seen by the urologist are owing to spinal cord injury, multiple sclerosis, Parkinson disease, cerebrovascular accident (CVA), traumatic brain injury, myelomeningocele, diabetes, peripheral nerve injury, and back or spine disease.[3] The neurologic conditions common in the older population are discussed in more detail elsewhere in this article.

None of these conditions necessarily correlate with any 1 pattern of LUTS, making UDS indispensable to establish the correct urologic diagnosis and start treatment with the following goals: preventing upper tract damage, maintaining continence, and ensuring complete emptying. Most of the components of the UDS examination have some utility in testing the neurogenic bladder.

When neurogenic bladder is suspected, UDS should include measuring a PVR. This should be done at the time of diagnosis, and may be done on a regular basis during subsequent visits to track changes in bladder function.[3] The finding of increased PVR is usually a trigger for change in the management of the neurogenic bladder because it has been associated with the risk of infections and sepsis, bladder stones, and worsening kidney function.[3]

CMG is also recommended during initial evaluation of the neurogenic bladder. It is useful when there is suspicion of renal impairment as one of the tenets of managing neurogenic bladder is to maintain low intravesical pressures. It is also the best test to assess for detrusor dysfunction.[3] Videourodynamics can be combined with CMG to investigate anatomic abnormalities like reflux and hydronephrosis. Last, PFS can be very valuable to distinguish bladder contraction problems from urethral obstruction.[18]

Benign Prostatic Hyperplasia

As mentioned, LUTS is common in the older population.[2] The main cause of these symptoms in males is BPH caused by bladder outlet obstruction.[19] The American Urological Association symptom score is a validated standard scoring system[20] and is probably an adequate evaluation, along with history and physical examination, of the patient who is not interested in an invasive treatment.

Patients with UDS-proven obstruction have more successful outcomes after bladder outlet surgeries like transurethral resection of the prostate.[19] PFS remains the gold standard for diagnosing bladder outlet obstruction. There are 3 nomograms used in clinical practice: Abrams-Griffith, urethra resistance factor, and Schafer. The 3 use the same classification of obstructed, equivocal, and nonobstructed. More recently, Griffiths and colleagues[21] described a less invasive method using a penile cuff to establish a modified nomogram predicting bladder outlet obstruction with a 68% positive predictive value and 78% negative predictive value.

SPECIAL CIRCUMSTANCES IN ELDERLY PATIENTS
Parkinson Disease

Parkinson disease is the second most common neurodegenerative disease after Alzheimer disease, it is uncommon before the age of 40, and its incidence increases with age. It is currently thought to affect more than 1 million Americans and it is more prevalent in men than women. PD is due to the loss of the dopaminergic neurons in the substantia nigra of the basal ganglia. Although therapy can decrease the symptoms, the disease is still associated with a significant degree of morbidity and mortality.[22]

Urinary symptoms are very common in PD and can appear at any stage of the disease.[23] The most common urinary symptoms in PD are related to bladder storage and consist mostly of OAB symptoms; urgency, frequency and nocturia. The most common UDS finding on CMG is detrusor overactivity. This is thought to be owing to the loss of the inhibitory effect of the basal ganglia D1 neurons on the micturition reflex. Treating the symptoms of OAB in someone with PD can be problematic, because anticholinergic medications can increase confusion in this population.[23] Detrusor underactivity is only present in a small number of patients[24] and can be used to differentiate PD from Shy–Drager disease, where detrusor underactivity is a common finding.[25] Patients with Shy–Drager disease will also generally have an open bladder neck seen during filling on a videourodynamic study. Shy–Drager disease is among the few neurologic diseases where UDS can actually help to make the diagnosis. In the patient with PD in whom a transurethral resection of the prostate is being considered, UDS is important to ensure that the patient is obstructed and also to rule out Shy–Drager disease, because the open bladder neck may cause postoperative incontinence. Detrusor–sphincter dyssynergia on EMG studies is uncommon in PD but could be indicative of the disease. It is likely that this dyssynergia is not real, but related to sphincter bradykinesia. A high PVR is the only finding that correlates with the severity of the symptoms in PD.[26]

Stroke and Cerebrovascular Accidents

CVA, both ischemic and hemorrhagic, is a major cause of disability and death worldwide and its incidence steadily increases with advancing age. In the west, 80% of strokes are ischemic and the rest are hemorrhagic. Mortality in the first month after a CVA can be as high as 78%.[27]

The symptoms seen after a stroke can be separated into acute and delayed symptoms. In the acute phase, it has been reported that 47% of patients are in retention and 29% remained in it after 1 month of the event. In the delayed phase, the prevalence of incontinence is anywhere between 37% and 79%.[28] In a prospective study that obtained UDS on 106 patients at a mean of 22 days after stroke, the most common finding on CMG was detrusor overactivity in both continent and incontinent patients. Just like in the case of PD, this is thought to be owing to the dysfunction of the suprapontine nervous system. Detrusor underactivity was only found in 6% of the patients; however, it was distributed equally between continent and incontinent patients. There was no correlation between incontinence and the laterality of the lesion and incontinent patients had worse functional status and prognosis. Although incontinence decreased with time, age greater than 75 years was an independent factor in failure to regain continence.[29,30]

It is thought that sphincter function and sensation are intact in patients with CVA. This makes incontinence extremely challenging to explain and brings up different theories about the etiology, like incontinence being owing to poor cognitive function, mobility, the severity of the stroke, and other risk factors, rather than the disruption of particular neural pathways.[29]

Bladder management should be undertaken by the urologist with the goal of reestablishing continence in post CVA patients to prevent skin breakdowns and improve their quality of life. In patients with detrusor overactivity, this can be done with the use of behavioral therapy like timed voiding, anticholinergic medications, and botulinum toxin injections. Patients with underactive detrusor should be managed with clean intermittent catheterization with the goal of minimizing PVR and preventing upper tract damage.

Many stroke patients can be evaluated with a careful history, a physical examination, and an assessment of PVR. Although an argument can be made that UDS is necessary to completely diagnose the bladder dysfunction that may accompany a CVA, a counterargument can be made for not doing UDS if the results of the test are not going to impact management. In patients with detrusor overactivity after a CVA, bladder pressures are rarely high enough or sustained so that the risk of upper tract damage is low. Before obtaining UDS in the patient who has had a CVA, the clinician should also take into account the patient's physical and cognitive abilities to allow them to undergo the test.

Dementia

Dementia is the loss of cognitive ability; it is extremely common in the elderly population with an incidence around 1% to 2% per year.[31] Dementia is poorly understood and is associated with multiple conditions like vascular disease, Alzheimer disease, Lewy body disease, and others. Alzheimer disease is responsible for more than 50% of dementia cases. Urinary incontinence is very common in this population and the most common UDS finding is detrusor overactivity. The assessment of these patients presents many challenges like the inability to use validated questionnaires and the inability to ask about symptoms during UDS. A recent study by Lee and colleagues[32] performed UDS on 144 patients with Alzheimer disease and incontinence and confirmed the finding of detrusor overactivity in 57.6% of the patients. Detrusor overactivity was found to correlate with the severity of the dementia. Another study performed UDS on Alzheimer disease patients taking donepezil and found that it did not adversely affect lower urinary tract function.[18]

Spinal Stenosis/Disk Herniation

Neurodegenerative disease of the spine is a common cause of pain and disability in the geriatric population. In patients older than 65 years of age, lumbar spinal stenosis is the most common reason for spine surgery. It is mostly owing to age-related, degenerative changes of the discs and facet joints. Patients are usually comfortable with sitting and uncomfortable with standing.[33]

Urologic symptoms of stenosis are similar to these of disc herniation and are related to the level and the degree of the compression. The most common discs to herniate are at the lumbar level and herniation does not necessarily cause symptoms. When the herniation or the stenosis compress the nerve roots at the lumbar level, this is known as cauda equina syndrome. The incidence of cauda equina syndrome in the United States is estimated to be around 0.12%, which is less of that of lumbar disc herniation estimated at 0.15%.[34] In a series of 122 patients with lumbar disc herniation and associated neurologic symptoms, 32 had the finding of detrusor areflexia on UDS.[35] In patients with cauda equina syndrome and neurogenic bladder, Kim and colleagues[36] found detrusor underactivity or acontractility in 60.7% of the patients and detrusor overactivity in 32.8% of the patients. This study confirms the previous findings of Podnar and colleagues,[37] who presented a series of 65 patients in 2006, which showed detrusor underactivity or acontractility in 59% of men and 85% of women. It also showed that women were more frequently incontinent than men and that there was no correlation between LUTS and urodynamic findings, stressing again on the importance of UDS to diagnose bladder dysfunction in neurogenic bladder cases.

SUMMARY

UDS can be a very useful diagnostic tool in the elderly population. Although it is considered to be safe and has minimal morbidity, it is costly and invasive. Although its use is controversial in some instances, it is of great benefit in other instances, such as before embarking on invasive therapy. Like any other test, care should be taken to only use it when the results will change the management of the disease and when its benefits outweigh any harm.

REFERENCES

1. World population ageing 2013. Geneva: United Nations, Department of Economic and Social Affairs, Population Division (2013). 2013. Available at: http://www.un.org/en/development/desa/population/publications/pdf/ageing/World PopulationAgeing2013.pdf.
2. Pfisterer MH, Griffiths DJ, Schaefer W, et al. The effect of age on lower urinary tract function: a study in women. J Am Geriatr Soc 2006;54(3):405.
3. Winters JC, Dmochowski RR, Goldman HB, et al. Urodynamic studies in adults: AUA/SUFU guideline. J Urol 2012;188(6 Suppl):2464–72.
4. Marks BK, Goldman HB. Videourodynamics: indications and technique. Urol Clin North Am 2014;41(3):383–91, vii–viii.
5. Al-Hayek S, Belal M, Abrams P. Does the patient's position influence the detection of detrusor overactivity? Neurourol Urodyn 2008;27:279–86.

6. Gammie A, Clarkson B, Constantinou C, et al. International Continence Society guidelines on urodynamic equipment performance. Neurourol Urodyn 2014; 33(4):370–9.

7. MacLachlan LS, Rovner ES. Good urodynamic practice: keys to performing a quality UDS study. Urol Clin North Am 2014;41(3):363–73, vii.

8. Onyishi SE, Twiss CO. Pressure flow studies in men and women. Urol Clin North Am 2014;41(3):453.

9. McGuire EJ, Cespedes RD, O'Connell HE. Leak-point pressures. Urol Clin North Am 1996;23(2):253.

10. Nitti VW, Tu LM, Gitlin J. Diagnosing bladder outlet obstruction in women. J Urol 1999;161(5):1535.

11. Haylen BT, de Ridder D, Freeman RM, et al. An International Urogynecological Association (IUGA)/International Continence Society (ICS) joint report on the terminology for female pelvic floor dysfunction. Neurourol Urodyn 2010;29(1): 4–20.

12. Hu TW, Wagner TH, Bentkover JD, et al. Costs of urinary incontinence and over-active bladder in the United States: a comparative study. Urology 2004;63(3): 461–5.

13. Campeau L. Urodynamics in stress incontinence: when are they necessary and how do we use them? Urol Clin North Am 2014;41(3):393–8, viii.

14. Pajoncini C, Costantini E, Guercini F, et al. Clinical and urodynamic features of intrinsic sphincter deficiency. Neurourol Urodyn 2003;22(4):264–8.

15. Nitti VW, Combs AJ. Correlation of Valsalva leak point pressure with subjective degree of stress urinary incontinence in women. J Urol 1996;155(1):281–5.

16. Wagg AS, Cardozo L, Chapple C, et al. Overactive bladder syndrome in older people. BJU Int 2007;99(3):502–9. Available at: http://onlinelibrary.wiley.com/doi/10.1111/j.1464-410X.2006.06677.x/epdf. Accessed September 22, 2014.

17. Gulur DM, Mevcha AM, Drake MJ. Nocturia as a manifestation of systemic disease. BJU Int 2011;107(5):702–13.

18. Sakakibara R, Fowler CJ, Hattori T, et al. Pressure-flow study as an evaluating method of neurogenic urethral relaxation failure. J Auton Nerv Syst 2000; 80(1–2):85–8.

19. Min DS, Cho HJ, Kang JY, et al. Effect of transurethral resection of the prostate based on the degree of obstruction seen in urodynamic study. Korean J Urol 2013;54(12):840–5.

20. Barry MJ, Fowler FJ Jr, O'Leary MP, et al. The American Urological Association symptom Index for benign prostatic hyperplasia. The Measurement Committee of the American Urological Association. J Urol 1992;148(5):1549–57 [discussion: 1564].

21. Griffiths CJ, Harding C, Blake C, et al. A nomogram to classify men with lower urinary tract symptoms using urine flow and noninvasive measurement of bladder pressure. J Urol 2005;174(4 Pt 1):1323–6 [discussion: 1326]; [author reply: 1326].

22. Nutt JG, Wooten GF. Clinical practice. Diagnosis and initial management of Parkinson's disease. N Engl J Med 2005;353(10):1021–7.

23. Jost WH. Urological problems in Parkinson's disease: clinical aspects. J Neural Transm 2013;120(4):587–91.

24. Ragab MM, Mohammed ES. Idiopathic Parkinson's disease patients at the urologic clinic. Neurourol Urodyn 2011;30(7):1258–61.

25. Kim M, Jung JH, Park J, et al. Impaired detrusor contractility is the pathognomonic urodynamic finding of multiple system atrophy compared to idiopathic Parkinson's disease. Parkinsonism Relat Disord 2015;21(3):205–10.

26. Araki I, Kitahara M, Oida T, et al. Voiding dysfunction and Parkinson's disease: urodynamic abnormalities and urinary symptoms. J Urol 2000;164(5):1640–3.

27. van der Worp HB, van Gijn J. Acute ischemic stroke. N Engl J Med 2007;357(6): 572–9.

28. Yum KS, Na SJ, Lee KY, et al. Pattern of voiding dysfunction after acute brainstem infarction. Eur Neurol 2013;70(5–6):291–6.

29. Linsenmeyer TA. Post-CVA voiding dysfunctions: clinical insights and literature review. NeuroRehabilitation 2012;30(1):1–7.

30. Pizzi A, Falsini C, Martini M, et al. Urinary incontinence after ischemic stroke: clinical and urodynamic studies. Neurourol Urodyn 2014;33(4):420–5.

31. Petersen RC. Mild cognitive impairment. N Engl J Med 2011;364(23):2227–34.

32. Lee SH, Cho ST, Na HR, et al. Urinary incontinence in patients with Alzheimer's disease: relationship between symptom status and urodynamic diagnoses. Int J Urol 2014;21(7):683–7.

33. Katz JN, Harris MB. Lumbar spinal stenosis. N Engl J Med 2008;358(8):818–25.

34. Podnar S. Epidemiology of cauda equina and conus medullaris lesions. Muscle Nerve 2007;35(4):529–31.

35. Bartolin Z, Savic I, Persec Z. Relationship between clinical data and urodynamic findings in patients with lumbar intervertebral disk protrusion. Urol Res 2002; 30(4):219–22.

36. Kim SY, Kwon HC, Hyun JK. Detrusor overactivity in patients with cauda equina syndrome. Spine (Phila Pa 1976) 2014;39(16):E955–61.

37. Podnar S, Trsinar B, Vodusek DB. Bladder dysfunction in patients with cauda equina lesions. Neurourol Urodyn 2006;25(1):23–31.

Associations Between Urinary Symptoms and Sexual Health in Older Adults

Cara Tannenbaum, MD, MSc

KEYWORDS

- Sexual dysfunction • Incontinence • Overactive bladder • Treatment
- Older men and women

KEY POINTS

- There is evidence that urinary and sexual symptoms coexist in older men and women.
- Although the relationship may be causal, sexual dysfunction involves a complex interplay of partner factors, relationship factors, individual factors, mental health disorders, life stressors, medical comorbidity, and medication intake.
- Men with overactive bladder and urgency incontinence are less likely to report being sexually active, as are men with erectile dysfunction and stress incontinence after prostatectomy.
- Data on the relationship between sexual dysfunction and urinary symptoms in older women are scarce, and may be mediated by overall poor health and function. In contrast with young and midlife women, little is known about coital incontinence in older women and its response to surgical intervention.
- Surgical and nonsurgical interventions for lower urinary tract symptoms may be effective for treating sexual dysfunction, suggesting the need for inquiry during clinical encounters and future research.

SEXUAL HEALTH AMONG OLDER ADULTS

Sexual activity declines with age, but many older adults remain sexually active well into the ninth decade.[1] In a large population-based survey of sexual activity among older adults in the United States, 67% of men and 40% of women aged 65 to 74 years reported sexual activity with a partner in the previous 12 months.[1] Among men and women aged 75 to 85 years, 39% and 17% respectively reported sexual activity.[1] Most engaged in coital intercourse. Oral sex was performed by nearly half of men and women aged 65 to 74 years, and by up to one-third of those aged 75 years and older.

Disclosure: The author has no financial conflicts of interest to disclose.
Division of Geriatric Medicine, Université de Montréal, 4565 Queen Mary Road, Montreal, Quebec H3W1W5, Canada
E-mail address: cara.tannenbaum@umontreal.ca

Clin Geriatr Med 31 (2015) 581–590
http://dx.doi.org/10.1016/j.cger.2015.06.007
0749-0690/15/$ – see front matter © 2015 Elsevier Inc. All rights reserved.
geriatric.theclinics.com

PREVALENCE OF SEXUAL DYSFUNCTION

Sexual problems increase with age and are common. Almost 50% of sexually active older men and women complain of 1 or more sexual problems.[1] Sexual dysfunction, as defined by the *Diagnostic and Statistical Manual of Mental Disorders, Fifth Edition* (DSM-5), refers to a clinically significant disturbance in a person's ability to respond sexually or to experience sexual pleasure.[2] Common sexual dysfunctions in older age and their definitions are listed in **Box 1**. The prevalence of different sexual problems by age group among older men and women is described in **Table 1**.[1] Higher rates of medication-induced/substance-induced sexual dysfunction likely exist among the geriatric population with polypharmacy, but the exact prevalence and incidence remain unknown. **Box 2** describes examples of medications and substances that can cause or contribute to sexual dysfunction.[2–6]

THE MULTIFACTORIAL NATURE OF SEXUAL DYSFUNCTION

Sexual dysfunction involves a complex interplay of physiologic, psychological, and social factors. Partner factors, relationship factors, individual factors, concomitant mental health disorders, life stressors, medical comorbidity, and cultural or religious influences can all play a role in sexual dysfunction.[1,2] **Table 2** lists all elements of assessment that are required in a thorough examination of sexual dysfunction.

OVERALL HEALTH STATUS AND SEXUAL DYSFUNCTION

Older men and women who rate their health as being poor are less likely to be sexually active.[1] Furthermore, among those with poor health who remain sexually active, there is a higher occurrence of sexual problems.[1] Older women who report poor overall health are nearly 3 times more likely to report diminished sexual pleasure; in men, mental health problems have a negative impact.[7] Chronic medical conditions, depression, polypharmacy, cognitive decline, and functional impairment contribute to a lack of libido and many of the other sexual problems listed in **Table 2**.

Box 1
DSM-5 definitions of common sexual dysfunctions in older age

Erectile dysfunction: the repeated failure to obtain or maintain erections during partnered sexual activities.

Delayed ejaculation: marked delay in or inability to achieve ejaculation.

Female orgasmic disorder: difficulty experiencing orgasm and/or markedly reduced intensity of orgasmic sensations.

Sexual interest/arousal disorder: lack of, or significantly reduced, sexual interest/arousal.

Genitopelvic pain/penetration disorder: difficulty having intercourse, genitopelvic pain, fear of pain or vaginal penetration, and/or tension of the pelvic floor muscles.

Medication or substance-induced sexual dysfunction: a disturbance in sexual function that has a temporal relationship with medication/substance initiation, dose increase, or medication/substance discontinuation.

Adapted from Diagnostic and statistical manual of mental disorders, 5th edition. DSM-5. Arlington (VA): American Psychiatric Association; 2013.

Table 1
Prevalence of sexual problems by age group in older men and women

Type of Sexual Dysfunction	Percentage of People Aged 65–74 y Who Are Sexually Active (95% Confidence Intervals)	Percentage of People Aged 75–85 y Who Are Sexually Active (95% Confidence Intervals)
Men		
Erectile dysfunction	44.6 (38.7–52.4)	43.5 (34.5–52.4)
Lack of interest in sex	28.5 (22.8–34.3)	24.2 (16.5–32.0)
Delayed ejaculation	22.7 (17.5–27.9)	33.2 (25.0–41.5)
Sex not pleasurable	7.0 (3.7–10.4)	5.1 (1.2–9.0)
Anxiety about performance	28.9 (22.9–34.9)	29.3 (19.8–38.9)
Women		
Female orgasmic disorder	32.8 (24.9–40.6)	38.2 (23.7–52.8)
Lack of interest in sex	38.4 (29.5–47.4)	49.3 (36.8–61.9)
Difficulty with lubrication	43.2 (34.8–51.5)	43.6 (27.0–60.2)
Pain during intercourse	18.6 (10.8–26.3)	11.8 (4.3–19.4)
Sex not pleasurable	22.0 (15.0–29.0)	24.9 (14.8–35.0)
Anxiety about performance	12.5 (6.1–18.9)	9.9 (1.7–18.2)

Adapted from Lindau ST, Schumm LP, Laumann EO, et al. A study of sexuality and health among older adults in the United States. N Engl J Med 2007;357:762–74.

INTERRELATIONSHIP BETWEEN URINARY DISORDERS AND SEXUAL DYSFUNCTION

There is evidence that urinary and sexual symptoms are often comorbid in older men and women.[8–10] However, because poor health and functional impairment are associated with both sexual problems and urinary disorders, especially urinary incontinence in older adults, it is often difficult to establish whether there is a direct effect of storage or voiding dysfunction on sexual activity, or whether the association is caused by shared common risk factors and correlates.[11–13] A direct relationship may be represented by a case in which coital incontinence (ie, loss of urine during coital sexual activity) in women leads to subsequent avoidance or fear of sexual activity. An indirect relationship likely occurs in older men with postprostatectomy urinary incontinence who also experience erectile dysfunction, both as a result of non–nerve sparing prostate resection.[14] Similarly, the association between urinary incontinence and lack of sexual function in older community-dwelling women loses significance when physical health is accounted for in the analysis.[11] Recognizing that correlation does not imply causation in these cases is critical in order to provide older men and women with a realistic notion of how treatment of urinary symptoms can be expected to improve sexual function.[15]

ASSOCIATION BETWEEN LOWER URINARY TRACT SYMPTOMS AND SEXUAL DYSFUNCTION IN MEN
Data from Epidemiologic Studies

To date, the Multinational Survey of the Aging Male (MSAM-7) is the largest nationally representative survey of lower urinary tract symptoms (LUTS) and their association with sexual dysfunction, conducted among 12,815 men aged 50 to 60 years, 60 to 70 years, and 70 to 80 years across the United States and 6 European countries.[16]

Box 2
Examples of medications and substances that can induce sexual dysfunction

Antidepressants: approximately 25% to 80% of individuals of all ages taking selective serotonergic reuptake inhibitors (SSRIs) and tricyclic antidepressants report sexual side effects. The most common side effect with SSRIs is difficulty achieving orgasm in women and a delay in or inability to ejaculate in men. Problems with desire and erection are less frequent.

Antipsychotics: nearly 50% of users report problems with sexual desire, erection, lubrication, ejaculation, and orgasm with typical and atypical agents.

Sedative-hypnotic medication: there may be a higher prevalence of erectile and orgasmic problems associated with the use of benzodiazepines. Over-the-counter antihistamines may diminish sexual arousal.

Opioids: increased rates of sexual dysfunction have been reported with high-dose opioid drugs for pain, and with methadone.

Alcohol: alcohol abuse is related to higher rates of erectile problems.

Stimulants: approximately 60% to 70% of heroine users report sexual problems. Cocaine users are also at increased risk.

Hormonal agents: erectile dysfunction occurs in 5% to 9% of men using 5-alpha reductase inhibitors to treat benign prostatic hypertrophy.

Antihypertensive agents: centrally acting sympatholytic drugs and β-blockers may have a greater impact on sexual function than other classes.

Indication bias: many psychiatric and medical disorders are associated with disturbances of sexual function, making it difficult to distinguish a medication-induced or substance-induced sexual problem from a manifestation of the underlying condition for which the drug was prescribed. The temporal onset and resolution of symptoms with respect to the initiation, discontinuation, or reintroduction of a medicinal substance is the best way to establish causality.

Adapted from Diagnostic and statistical manual of mental disorders, 5th edition. DSM-5. Arlington (VA): American Psychiatric Association; 2013.

Table 2
Factors that play a role in sexual health and dysfunction

Factor	Examples
Partner issues	Availability of a healthy partner, partner illness, or partner's sexual problems
Relationship issues	Lack of intimacy, poor communication, partner violence, discrepancies in desire for sexual activity
Individual issues	Poor body image, history of sexual or emotional abuse
Psychiatric comorbidity	Depression, anxiety, dementia
Life stressors	Bereavement; illness among friends, family, or children; financial worries
Medical conditions and medications	Diabetes, heart disease, functional impairment, cognitive impairment. See **Box 2** for a list of medications
Cultural/religious factors	Inhibitions related to prohibitions against sexual activity, discrepant attitudes toward sexuality, especially with a new late-life partner
Social/environmental factors	Lack of privacy caused by living in a nursing home, with adult children, family, or other caregivers

Standardized and internationally validated scales of LUTS and sexual dysfunction were used. Sexual activity was reported by 83% of the sample and decreased with age, whereas the prevalence of moderate to severe LUTS increased, ranging from 22% in men aged 50 to 59 years to 45% in men aged 70 to 80 years. Erectile problems were present in 30%, 51%, and 76% of men aged 50 to 59, 60 to 69, and 70 to 80 years respectively, and were reported by 43%, 66%, and 83% of men with mild, moderate, and severe LUTS, respectively. Within each age category, the frequency of erection difficulties was strongly related to LUTS severity. Furthermore, the relationship between erectile dysfunction and LUTS severity persisted independently of other comorbidities, such as diabetes, hypertension, cardiac disease, and hyperlipidemia, in multivariate analyses. As with erection problems, the prevalence of ejaculatory dysfunction increased significantly with age and severity of LUTS. Ejaculation problems were reported by 30%, 55%, and 74% of men aged 50 to 59 years, 60 to 69 years, and 70 to 80 years, respectively, and by 42%, 61%, and 76% of men with mild, moderate, and severe LUTS. The increased rate of ejaculatory problems in older men and those with more severe LUTS was observed independently of each of the major comorbidities. In the population of sexually active men (n = 8369), intercourse satisfaction declined significantly with age and LUTS severity. Similar results were obtained for sexual desire and overall sexual satisfaction, with significant declines associated with increasing severity of LUTS within each age class.

The EpiLUTS (Epidemiology of Lower Urinary Tract Symptoms) survey queried 11,841 men aged 40 years and older in the United States, the United Kingdom, and Sweden to assess the relationship between lower urinary tract symptoms and decreased sexual activity, erectile dysfunction, and ejaculatory dysfunction.[17] Validated questionnaires for sexual dysfunction and LUTS were used, but these differed from the ones administered in the MSAM-7 study, which partially explains variations in results. The population was also much younger, with a mean age of 56.1 ± 10.8 years, and the data were not analyzed by age category. Overall, only 11% of subjects reported decreased enjoyment or cessation of sexual activity caused by the presence of LUTS. However, almost 30% of men with moderate to severe symptoms, or a greater frequency of combined voiding, storage, and postmicturition symptoms, reported decreased enjoyment, and 25% reported that they had decreased or stopped sexual activity because of their urinary symptoms. Significant associations with decreased sexual enjoyment included weak stream, split stream, perceived urinary frequency, urgency with fear of leaking, leaking during sex, incomplete emptying, bladder area pain, dysuria, bladder and prostate cancer, prostatitis, and reports of pain during sex. As expected, severe erectile dysfunction increased with age, occurring in 10% to 13% of men aged 66 years and older, and also increased with the severity of LUTS. The proportion of men who reported that they could not ejaculate similarly increased with age, ranging from 3.7% among those aged 61 to 65 years to 14% among those aged 76 years and older. Ejaculatory problems were significantly associated with urine leakage during sex and urgency with fear of leaking, as well as depression and prostate cancer. Other studies of aging men in Iran and Taiwan confirm these findings.[18,19] The coexistence of severe LUTS and any degree of erectile dysfunction increases among populations of men seeking treatment of LUTS, compared with community-based studies, and is significantly associated with increasing age and a negative impact on quality of life.[10]

Men with Prostate Cancer Undergoing Radical Prostatectomy

Men undergoing radical prostatectomy for prostate cancer are at a particularly high risk of concomitant erectile dysfunction and stress urinary incontinence caused by surgical damage of the neurovascular bundle located within or adjacent to the prostate.[14,15,20] The neurovascular bundle contains autonomic nerves and vessels that supply both the corpora cavernosa and the external urinary sphincter. Radiation therapy and androgen suppression treatment of prostate cancer can also affect urinary and sexual function.[20] Small retrospective case series have investigated the effect of anti-incontinence surgical procedures (artificial urinary sphincter or male sling) on problems caused by urinary incontinence during sexual activity after radical prostatectomy, with mixed results.[21] Approximately half of patients report improvement.[21] Simultaneous implantation of an inflatable penile prosthesis and a male sling or artificial urinary sphincter to treat concomitant erectile dysfunction and stress urinary incontinence in prostate cancer survivors is another treatment option that offers some efficacy and improves outcomes.[22] Rates of device infection, pain, erosion, or malfunction are significant with these procedures, so the uptake of combination therapy has been slow.[23]

Men with Overactive Bladder and Urgency Incontinence

There is emerging evidence that men with overactive bladder and urgency incontinence are less likely to report being sexually active than men without overactive bladder.[24] A significant association between overactive bladder and erectile dysfunction has also been observed, possibly mediated by depressive symptoms.[24] No studies were found to suggest that treatment of overactive bladder with antimuscarinic agents improves concomitant sexual dysfunction in men.

ASSOCIATION BETWEEN LOWER URINARY TRACT SYMPTOMS AND SEXUAL DYSFUNCTION IN WOMEN
Data from Epidemiologic Studies

Similar to men, sexual and urinary problems are frequently comorbid and possibly synergistic in women.[8] Population-based studies of women with LUTS indicate that women with urinary symptoms are significantly more likely to report decreased sexual satisfaction, although few age group analyses are available.[25] In sexually inactive women, distress may not be present, despite urinary symptoms that would in general portend sexual problems. In 1 Canadian survey of 2361 community-dwelling women aged 55 to 95 years (mean age, 71 ± 7 years), 39% reported urinary incontinence: 29% of continent women versus 25% of incontinent women reported being sexually active.[11] Incontinent women reported worse body image, more medical conditions, and worse physical and mental health than continent women, and these factors have also been associated with sexual function. In women with incontinence, the frequency of urine leakage was not associated with sexual activity; however, higher quantities of urine loss and the presence of nocturnal incontinence were independently associated with lack of sexual activity, even when adjusting for health status. Women with stress incontinence alone were more likely to be sexually active than women with urgency or mixed incontinence subtypes.

A growing body of epidemiologic literature suggests that sexual dysfunction is most common in women with urgency or mixed incontinence subtypes.[24–26] Women with overactive bladder in the presence of incontinence have the highest rates of dissatisfaction, worst quality of life, and highest rates of sexual impairment. As the distribution of incontinence subtypes changes with age, with more women experiencing mixed and urgency incontinence compared with stress urinary incontinence alone, it remains unclear whether poor health and functional impairment mediate the relationship between sexual problems and urinary disorders, or whether there is a direct causal influence.

Coital Incontinence in Women

In younger women, coital incontinence is surprisingly prevalent.[27,28] As many as 40% of women cite sexual intercourse as an inciting or exacerbating event for urinary symptoms. In some series, up to 67% of women seeking treatment of urinary symptoms report coital incontinence.[8,28] Coital incontinence may be subdivided into penetration incontinence (loss of urine with vaginal penetration) and orgasm incontinence (loss of urine at orgasm). Penetration incontinence is more often associated with stress urinary incontinence, whereas orgasm incontinence may occur with either stress incontinence or overactive bladder.[8] There is a lack of data on the prevalence and types of coital incontinence in sexually active women aged 65 years and older.

Sexual Dysfunction and Incontinence After Treatment of Rectal Cancer in Women

A previously unrecognized problem in women is pelvic floor dysfunction, including sexual problems and incontinence, after treatment with surgery or radiotherapy for rectal cancer.[29] Rectal surgery is usually complicated by tissue edema in a restricted space with a high risk of damage to pelvic nerves essential for bladder, bowel, and sexual function. Radiation can also cause vaginal atrophy, fibrosis, adhesions, and shortening of the vagina, leading to problems with lubrication and dyspareunia.[30] In a study of 171 female patients with rectal cancer (mean age, 64 years), 52% had urinary incontinence 5 years after surgery.[31] Difficulties with bladder emptying also occurred. Taken together, patients surviving rectal cancer seem to be a subgroup requiring screening for sexual dysfunction and urinary incontinence, with a view toward future intervention trials.

Improvement of Sexual Function with Treatment of Urinary Symptoms

In cases in which cessation of sexual activity is caused by urinary symptoms, appropriate medical attention may permit an older woman to resume a satisfying sexual life with a partner should she so desire.[8,32] Treatment of urinary incontinence can involve nonsurgical or surgical options. In a multicenter study of women (mean age, 50 years) undergoing nonsurgical treatment of stress urinary incontinence with a combination of pessaries and pelvic floor muscle exercises, successful treatment of urinary incontinence was associated with a significant improvement in sexual function, measured by validated sexual satisfaction questonnaires.[33] Women who were successfully treated for urinary incontinence reported significantly less incontinence with sexual activity and less restriction of sexual activity caused by fear of incontinence compared with women who were not successfully treated. In a different study of sexually active women (mean age, 50 years) who underwent midurethral sling procedures for the correction of stress urinary incontinence, increased coital frequency, decreased fear of incontinence with coitus, and decreased embarrassment caused by incontinence were reported 6 months after surgery.[34] One small uncontrolled study found that tolterodine immediate release improved sexual function in younger women with overactive bladder.[35] These results have yet to be replicated in the older female population.

The female genital and lower urinary tracts share a common embryologic origin, arising from the urogenital sinus, and both are sensitive to the effects of the female sex steroid hormones throughout life. Estrogen is known to have an important role in the function of the lower urinary tract, and estrogen and progesterone receptors have been identified in the vagina, urethra, bladder, and pelvic floor musculature. Symptomatic vulvovaginal atrophy can significantly impair the sexual function of older women and is responsive to vaginal estrogens.[36] Vaginal lubricants and moisturizers are also effective. The choice of therapy should depend on the severity of symptoms, the effectiveness and safety of therapy for the individual patient, and patient preference. Oral estrogens have been found to exacerbate both stress and urgency incontinence in women aged 50 to 79 years.[37] For this reason, treatment of urinary incontinence with vaginal estrogens remains controversial.[38]

PRACTICE IMPLICATIONS

Many older men and women continue to enjoy sexual activity well into their later years. Although sexual dysfunction and LUTS frequently coexist, factors such as partner issues, comorbidities, medication, functional impairment, and mental health may play a contributory role. Taking a complete sexual history, including the timing of sexual dysfunction in relation to the occurrence of urinary symptoms, is a critical part of the evaluation of older men and women with LUTS. Discussing sexual symptoms and their effect on quality of life may prompt a decision to attempt interventions specifically designed to improve function. Treating LUTS has the potential to improve sexual satisfaction. As baby boomers age, clinicians may be asked to focus more on sexual dysfunction in the context of lower urinary tract symptoms. More evidence is required to better inform treatment and prognosis for various categories of sexual dysfunction and different subtypes of lower urinary tract disorders in older men and women.

REFERENCES

1. Lindau ST, Schumm LP, Laumann EO, et al. A study of sexuality and health among older adults in the United States. N Engl J Med 2007;357:762–74.
2. Diagnostic and statistical manual of mental disorders, 5th edition. DSM-5. Arlington (VA): American Psychiatric Association; 2013.
3. Gur S, Kadowitz PJ, Hellstrom WJ. Effects of 5-alpha reductase inhibitors on erectile function, sexual desire and ejaculation. Expert Opin Drug Saf 2013; 12(1):81–90.
4. La Torre A, Giupponi G, Duffy D, et al. Sexual dysfunction related to psychotropic drugs: a critical review–part I: antidepressants. Pharmacopsychiatry 2013;46(5): 191–9.
5. La Torre A, Conca A, Duffy D, et al. Sexual dysfunction related to psychotropic drugs: a critical review part II: antipsychotics. Pharmacopsychiatry 2013;46(6): 201–8.
6. Fogari R, Zoppi A. Effects of antihypertensive therapy on sexual activity in hypertensive men. Curr Hypertens Rep 2002;4(3):202–10.
7. Laumann DO, Das A, Waite LJ. Sexual dysfunction among older adults: prevalence and risk factors from a nationally representative U.S. probability sample of men and women 57-85 years of age. J Sex Med 2008;5(10):2300–11.
8. Chen J, Sweet G, Shindel A. Urinary disorders and female sexual function. Curr Urol Rep 2013;14:298–308.
9. Rosen RC, Link CL, O'Leary MP, et al. Lower urinary tract symptoms and sexual health: the role of gender, lifestyle and medical comorbidities. BJU Int 2009;103: 42–7.
10. Seftel AD, de la Rosette J, Birt J, et al. Coexisting lower urinary tract symptoms and erectile dysfunction: a systematic review of epidemiological data. Int J Clin Pract 2013;67:32–45.
11. Tannenbaum C, Corcos J, Assalian P. The relationship between sexual activity and urinary incontinence in older women. J Am Geriatr Soc 2006;54:1220–4.

12. DuBeau CE, Kuchel GA, Johnson T 2nd, et al, Fourth International Consultation on Incontinence. Incontinence in the frail elderly: report from the 4th International Consultation on Incontinence. Neurourol Urodyn 2010;29(1):165–78.
13. Smith DP, Weber MF, Soga K, et al. Relationship between lifestyle and health factors and severe lower urinary tract symptoms (LUTS) in 106,435 middle-aged and older Australian men: population-based study. PLoS One 2014;9(10):e109278.
14. Wille S, Heidenreich A, Hofmann R, et al. Preoperative erectile function is one predictor for post prostatectomy incontinence. Neurourol Urodyn 2007;26:140–3.
15. Wittmann D, He C, Coelho M, et al. Patient preoperative expectations of urinary, bower, hormonal and sexual functioning do not match actual outcomes 1 year after radical prostatectomy. J Urol 2011;186:494–9.
16. Rosen R, Altwein J, Boyle P, et al. Lower urinary tract symptoms and male sexual dysfunction: the Multinational Survey of the Aging Male (MSAM-7). Eur Urol 2003; 44(6):637–49.
17. Wein AJ, Coyne KS, Tubaro A, et al. The impact of lower urinary tract symptoms on male sexual health: EpiLUTS. BJU Int 2009;103:33–41.
18. Mehraban D, Naderi GH, Yahyazadeh SR, et al. Sexual dysfunction in aging men with lower urinary tract symptoms. Urol J 2008;5:260–4.
19. Tsao CW, Cha TL, Lee SS, et al. Association between lower urinary tract symptoms and sexual dysfunction in Taiwanese men. Andrologia 2008;40:387–91.
20. Sanda MG, Dunn RL, Michalski J, et al. Quality of life and satisfaction with outcome among prostate-cancer survivors. N Engl J Med 2008;358(12):1250–61.
21. Jain R, Mitchell S, Laze J, et al. The effect of surgical intervention for stress urinary incontinence on post-prostatectomy UI during sexual activity. BJU Int 2012;109(8):1208–12.
22. Segal RL, Cabrini MR, Harris ED, et al. Combined inflatable penile prosthesis-artificial urinary sphincter implantation: no increased risk of adverse events compared to single or staged device implantation. J Urol 2013;190(6):2183–8.
23. Lee D, Romero C, Alba F, et al. Simultaneous penile prosthesis and male sling/artificial urinary sphincter. Asian J Androl 2013;15(1):10–5.
24. Coyne K, Sexton CC, Thompson C, et al. The impact of OAB on sexual health in men and women: results from EpiLUTS. J Sex Med 2011;8:1603–15.
25. Coyne KS, Sexton CC, Irwin DE, et al. The impact of overactive bladder, incontinence and other lower urinary tract symptoms on quality of life, work productivity, sexuality and emotional well-being in men and women: results from the EPIC study. BJU Int 2008;101(11):1388–95.
26. Cohen BL, Barboglio P, Gousse A. The impact of lower urinary tract symptoms and urinary incontinence on female sexual dysfunction using a validated instrument. J Sex Med 2008;5:1418–23.
27. Wehbe SA, Whitmore K, Kellogg-Spadt S. Urogenital complaints and female sexual dysfunction. Part 2. J Sex Med 2010;7:2304–17.
28. Serati M, Salvatore S, Uccella S, et al. Female urinary incontinence during intercourse: a review on an understudied problem for women's sexuality. J Sex Med 2009;6:40–8.
29. Panjari M, Bell RJ, Burney S, et al. Sexual function, incontinence, and wellbeing in women after rectal cancer–a review of the evidence. J Sex Med 2012;9(11):2749–58.
30. Lange MM, Marijnen CA, Maas CP, et al. Risk factors for sexual dysfunction after rectal cancer treatment. Eur J Cancer 2009;45:1578–88.
31. Lange MM, Maas CP, Marijnen CA, et al, Cooperative Clinical Investigators of the Dutch Total Mesorectal Excision Trial. Urinary dysfunction after rectal cancer treatment is mainly caused by surgery. Br J Surg 2008;95:1020–8.

32. Ratner ES, Erekson EA, Minkin MJ, et al. Sexual satisfaction in the elderly female population: a special focus on women with gynecologic pathology. Maturitas 2011;70(3):210–5.

33. Handa V, Whitcomb E, Weidner A, et al. Sexual function before and after non-surgical treatment for stress urinary incontinence. J Pelvic Med Surg 2011; 17(1):30–5.

34. Lonnée-Hoffmann RA, Salvesen Ø, Mørkved S, et al. What predicts improvement of sexual function after pelvic floor surgery? A follow-up study. Acta Obstet Gynecol Scand 2013;92(11):1304–12.

35. Hajebrahimi S, Azaripour A, Sadeghi-Bazargani H. Tolterodine immediate release improves sexual function in women with overactive bladder. J Sex Med 2008; 5(12):2880–5.

36. Management of symptomatic vulvovaginal atrophy: 2013 position statement of the North American Menopause Society. Menopause 2013;20(9):888–902.

37. Hendrix SL, Cochrane BB, Nygaard IE, et al. Effects of estrogen with and without progestin on urinary incontinence. JAMA 2005;293(8):935–48.

38. Robinson D, Toozs-Hobson P, Cardozo L. The effect of hormones on the lower urinary tract. Menopause Int 2013;19(4):155–62.

Surgical Risk and Comorbidity in Older Urologic Patients

Nicole T. Townsend, MD, Thomas N. Robinson, MD, MS*

KEYWORDS

- Geriatric surgery • Frailty • Preoperative risk assessment

KEY POINTS

- Urologic surgeons commonly operate on geriatric patients.
- Geriatric patients are at high risk for globally decreased physiologic reserves, a phenomenon described as frailty.
- Geriatric patients are more concerned with functional outcomes than other populations undergoing surgery.
- Frailty can be reliably used to predict risk of postoperative complications and adverse postoperative outcomes, including loss of the ability to live independently.
- Traditional comorbidity-based surgical risk calculators focus on forecasting 30-day morbidity and mortality rather than physical and mental functional outcomes.

INTRODUCTION

The demographic makeup of the surgical population is changing with the overall aging of the population. Older adults are an increasing proportion of surgical care, with greater than 35% of all inpatient operations being performed in adults 65 years or older in the United States.[1] This number is higher in subspecialties, such as urology, where 65% of all operations are performed in adults aged 65 years and older.[2] This proportion is anticipated to increase in the years and decades to come. It is essential to understand the unique physiology, risks, and characteristics of older adults to provide optimal urologic care for these patients.

The geriatric population is at greater risk for postoperative complications than younger adults. This risk is related to the physiologic decline seen in this population known as frailty. Frailty is a state of decreased physiologic reserve that increases the patient's susceptibility to disability.[3] Thus, by definition, frailty increases the risk

Department of Surgery, University of Colorado, 12631 E 17th Avenue, C-305, Aurora, CO 80045, USA
* Corresponding author. 1055 Clermont Street (112), Denver, CO 80220.
E-mail address: thomas.robinson@ucdenver.edu

Clin Geriatr Med 31 (2015) 591–601
http://dx.doi.org/10.1016/j.cger.2015.06.009
0749-0690/15/$ – see front matter Published by Elsevier Inc.
geriatric.theclinics.com

of a poor postoperative outcome.[4,5] Although there are few studies for outcomes specifically in geriatric urologic patients, those that do exist confirm that patterns of worse outcomes in surgical patients are mirrored specifically in the subset of urologic patients. Geriatric urologic patients are at higher risk of delirium, injury, intensive care unit (ICU) admissions, ICU stay, and death than their younger counterparts.[6,7]

Previous models of preoperative risk assessment have focused on single-organ systems to determine risk of adverse postoperative cardiac, renal, pulmonary, or hepatic events.[8–11] Although these algorithms continue to play a role in the preoperative risk assessment of urologic patients, frailty has replaced these strategies as an effective, efficient, global assessment for surgical risk and represents a significant paradigm shift in the preoperative evaluation of surgical patients.

PREOPERATIVE RISK ASSESSMENT IN THE OLDER UROLOGIC PATIENT

Historically, surgeons were primarily responsible for categorizing risk for patients[12]; this reflects a previous era but that emphasized the clinical judgment of an individual surgeon as authoritative that is no longer relevant to current surgical ethics and culture. Initial screening for risk involved taking patient histories, physical examination, and limited laboratory or imaging tests. These approaches were neither sensitive nor specific for actual predictions of risk.[13] Beginning in the 1970s, statistical methodology was applied to provide more quantitative data. These systems focused on single-organ systems, more notably the cardiac risk index, which has evolved into formal recommendations from the American Heart Association.[9–11] Geriatric medicine has continued to define what patient-centric outcomes are important to the older surgical patient to refine a quantitative approach to risk.

The preoperative risk assessment is essential to counseling the older urologic patient. Patients and families need accurate and reliable information about outcomes to make decisions about undergoing surgery and weigh the possible risks and benefits. Older adults can prioritize different outcomes than younger adults and tend to focus on quality-of-life issues rather than longevity. Health-related quality of life is a multidimensional outcome that includes functional independence, cognition, and physiologic health. In fact, living independently and maintaining other measures of functional independence are the most important health outcomes for this population.[4] This information is not reflected in more traditional outcomes from the surgical literature such as 30-day morbidity/mortality and complication rates.

Complications that geriatric patients are at greater risk for include other nontraditional complications, such as delirium. Delirium is more likely in the hospitalized postoperative patient.[14,15] Delirium is common in certain subspecialties, such as orthopedic surgery, which have rates that reach 40% to 60%.[16] Observational studies of urologic patients have demonstrated that, although rates of delirium are not as high as in other specialties, it can occur in 10% of patients.[6] Intraoperative hypotension, previous history of delirium, poor clock-drawing on the Mini-Cog, and inability to perform activities of daily living (ADLs) were all independently related to delirium in this population, although extent of surgery (endoscopic vs open) was not.

Frailty assessments have emerged as a primary way to quantify risk for geriatric patients, as it can predict both the traditional quantitative outcomes of morbidity and mortality as well as the qualitative outcomes of functional independence.

FRAILTY: A SINGLE PREOPERATIVE RISK ASSESSMENT

The American College of Surgeons (ACS) and American Geriatric Society have recommended a frailty assessment as standard of care for the preoperative risk assessment of older surgical patients.[17] Geriatric patients are at increased risk of complications, loss of independence, and death. Instead of a single-organ system assessment, frailty assessments quantify multidimensional, global risk. Frailty represents the risk of inability to tolerate physical stressors (such as surgery) and is a continuous trajectory of decline of multiple systems.

Frailty has been defined in multiple ways, which drive the assessment and diagnostic strategies for patients (**Table 1**). The ACS recommends 2 strategies.[17]

The first way to assess frailty is the multidimensional frailty assessment. Multidimensional frailty has been proved to be an effective (as well as simple and brief) tool to predict poor postoperative outcomes for surgical patients.[18–21] Multiple studies have validated this method to risk stratify patients and identify high-risk preoperative older patients.[22–24] This assessment combines quantification of 7 frailty characteristics: age, mobility (measured by Timed Up-and-Go [TUG] score[25]), dependent function (need for assistance with one or more ADLs), impaired cognition (performance on Mini-Cog test[26]), high chronic disease burden (use of Charlson index score[27] or anemia of chronic disease), poor nutrition (hypoalbuminemia), and presence of a geriatric syndrome (one or more falls in the previous 6 months at the time of assessment).[28] Positivity on each of these assessments is assigned a point value, with greater numbers of points assessing higher levels of frailty. When comparing frail ($\geq$4 points of 7 possible) with nonfrail patients, frail patients were much more likely to experience complications (56% vs 17%; P<.001), discharge to an institutional care facility (47% vs 3%; P<.001), and readmission within 30 days of their operation (28% vs 7%; $P = .014$).[19] The multidimensional frailty assessment can predict 6-month mortality postoperatively with high sensitivity (81%) and specificity (86%).[18]

The Charlson score has been specifically used in urologic patient populations for preoperative risk assessment. The Charlson comorbidity index (**Table 2**) examines comorbidities to calculate overall survival and is predictive of patient frailty.[29] Different iterations of the Charlson score (ie, normal or age adjusted) have been independently associated to be predictive of outcomes.[30,31] One study of patients with transitional cell carcinoma of the bladder and survival after radical cystectomy demonstrated that higher age-adjusted Charlson index was significantly associated with lower overall survival. Patients with Charlson scores of 5 or more had median survival of only 1.7 years compared with patients with low scores of 6.3 years (P<.001).[30]

The second way to assess frailty is by using the phenotypic definition of frailty. This assessment includes 5 characteristics: unintentional weight loss (at least 10 lb [4.5 kg] in the past year), self-reported exhaustion (2-question test), weakness (measured with grip strength), slow walking speed (multiple modes of assessment), and low physical

---

Table 1
Frailty characteristics

Phenotypic Definition of Frailty ($\geq$3 Indicative of Frailty)[4]	Multidimensional Frailty Definition ($\geq$4 Indicative of Frailty)[18,19]
Unintentional weight loss (at least 10 lb in the past year)	Age
Self-reported exhaustion	Slow mobility
Weakness	Dependent function
Slow walking speed	Impaired cognition
Low physical activity	High chronic disease burden
	One or more falls in the past 6 mo
	Poor nutrition

Data from Refs.[4,18,19]

Table 2 Charlson comorbidity index score	
Score	**Condition**
1	Myocardial infarction Congestive heart failure Peripheral vascular disease Cerebrovascular disease Dementia Chronic pulmonary disease Connective tissue disease Peptic ulcer disease Mild liver disease Diabetes without end-organ damage
2	Hemiplegia Moderate or severe renal disease Diabetes with end-organ damage Tumor without metastases Leukemia Lymphoma
3	Moderate or severe liver disease
6	Metastatic solid tumor AIDS

For age adjustment: for each decade greater than 40 years of age, add a score of 1 to the above-mentioned score. Final score must be put into the Charlson probability calculator.

Adapted from Kim SM, Kim MJ, Jung HA, et al. Comparison of the Freiburg and Charlson comorbidity indices in predicting overall survival in elderly patients with newly diagnosed multiple myeloma. Biomed Res Int 2014;2014:437852.

activity (Minnesota Leisure Time Activities Questionnaire).[4] Three or more abnormal domains define frailty in this assessment. Complications after major operations were predicted by frailty with this assessment, with only 19.5% of nonfrail patients experiencing 1 or more complication and 43.5% of frail patients, with an adjusted odds ratio of 2.5 for frail patients when predicting risk of complication.[32]

Frailty can be comprehensively assessed with these simple and reasonable approaches. There are a variety of specific tools to assess these measures (**Table 3**). Frailty, more than the simple number of age, predicts not only both traditional postoperative complications and 30-day morbidity/mortality but also the qualitative aspects of outcomes that matter most to geriatric patients and their families.

Although both these methods of assessment are more rapid than the comprehensive geriatric assessment (which takes several hours), there are practical single tools that are a part of these more complex measures that are as equally predictive as the larger tools. Specifically, grip strength and walking speed are single assessment tools that can be performed in the office to assess a urologic patient's preoperative frailty and risk of adverse postoperative outcome.

Grip strength is an assessment that serves as a marker of frailty via global loss of muscle mass or myopathy associated with decreased physiologic reserve. Handgrip strength is included in several multidimensional frailty measures.[4,33–36] It is also independently predictive of poor postoperative outcome. In a group of cardiac patients, the lowest quartile of geriatric patients' grip strength had higher rates of postoperative bleeding (54% vs 17%; $P<.01$), infection (85% vs 54%; $P = .01$), and death (25% vs 7%; $P = .02$) than the highest quartile. The survival benefit for those with good grip strength was seen up to 3 years postoperatively.[37]

Table 3
Tools to assess frailty

Tool	Description
Mini-Cog[52]	1. Give patient 3 standardized words 2. Ask patient to draw standardized clock 3. Ask patient to recall words
Gait speed[39]	1. Measure 9 m course 2. Instruct patient to walk at usual speed along course 3. Allow 2 m acceleration zone 4. Measure time patient requires to walk 5 m after acceleration zone 5. Allow 2 m deceleration zone
Timed Up-and-Go[25]	1. Measure 10 ft course 2. Instruct patient to sit in chair at beginning of course and walk at usual pace 3. Time patients as they rise from chair, walk course at a usual pace, turn, and return to chair
Grip strength[4]	1. Patient squeezes handgrip dynamometer as hard as possible 2. Repeat 3 times 3. Maximum value recorded 4. Reference to patient body mass index/gender
Knee extensor strength test[53]	1. Seat patient on dynamometer machine 2. Patient extends knee against resistance 3. Maximum force recorded
Low physical activity	Multiple assessment tools 1. Minnesota Leisure Time Activity[54] 2. PASE (Physical Activity Scale for the Elderly)[55] 3. Paffenbarger Physical Activity Questionnaire[56]
Exhaustion[4]	Ask patient 2 questions: 1. How often in the past week did you feel like everything you did was an effort? 2. How often in the past week did you feel like you could not get going? 3. Positive if answer is "Often" ($\geq$3 d) to either question
Weight loss or shrinking[4]	Unintended weight loss $\geq$10 lbs in previous year

Data from Refs.[4,25,39,52–54,56]

Walking speed is another single assessment method to risk stratify frail patients. Slow walking speed has been consistently shown to predict frailty (**Box 1**) and poor postoperative outcomes.[38,39] There are 2 assessment methods for walking speed, the gait speed test and TUG test (see **Table 3**). A prospective cohort study by the authors' group studied adults aged 65 years and older undergoing operations across surgical specialties and grouped them as slow (TUG $\geq$15 seconds), intermediate (11–14 seconds), and fast ($\leq$10 seconds). Outcomes including complications and 1-year mortality declined across the groups.[38] Postoperative complications in the slow group ranged from 52% to 77%, whereas rates in the fast group were 11% to 13%, and 1-year mortality for the slow group was 31% compared with 3% for the fast group.[38]

Frailty is defined as a state of physiologic vulnerability and is associated with worse outcomes for elderly patients across all surgical specialties. Evidence of this increased morbidity is found in both traditional measures of outcomes and in quality-of-life measures more important to this group of patients. Frailty can be measured in a variety of

---

Box 1
Ways in which walking speed alone is representative of the multidimensional frail older adult

Slow walking speed is related to

1. The presence of frailty[50]

2. Impaired cognition[51,52]

3. Future falling episodes[53]

4. Development of functional dependence[53,54]

5. Decreased survival[55,56]

Adapted from Townsend NT, Robinson TN. Does walking speed predict postoperative morbidity? Adv Surg 2014;48:57; with permission.

---

ways. There are several single assessment methods, such as grip strength or walking speed, that can identify and risk stratify frail patients to better inform the surgeon and the patient regarding the risk of postoperative complication in the preoperative assessment.

SINGLE-ORGAN SYSTEMS: IMPORTANT RISK ASSESSMENT ADJUNCTS

Single-organ system assessments have been present since the 1970s with the initiation of an algorithm for cardiac risk.[9] This initial algorithm has been continuously updated, with the American Heart Association releasing routine evidence-based risk algorithms.[10,11] This section explores the role of single-organ system assessment tools. Earlier discussion described how frailty may be used as a global risk assessment. The tools described in this section can be used as adjuncts for the urologic patient depending on an individual's comorbidities. Because urologic patients tend to be older, many of these patients have several comorbidities, increasing their individual risk of poor postoperative outcome.

CARDIAC ASSESSMENT

Older patients are at higher risk of cardiovascular disease and therefore adverse cardiovascular outcomes. Rates of cardiovascular disease, such as myocardial infarction (MI), hypertension, diabetes mellitus, and stroke, are all significantly higher in older adults.[40] Patients older than 65 years are at increased risk of stroke independently of other comorbidities.[41] The American College of Cardiology and American Heart Association Guidelines on Perioperative Cardiovascular Evaluation can be used to risk stratify individual patients based on their specific comorbidities.[11] These guidelines can predict risk of postoperative stroke or MI and can guide the clinician to consult a cardiologist for a more extensive cardiac workup.

NUTRITIONAL ASSESSMENT

In urologic patients, nutritional status can also be used to risk stratify patients. In a prospective cohort study, poor nutritional risk score was independently associated with poor outcomes.[42] Using weight loss, food intake, surgical intensity, and age, a score is created. Individuals with a score 3 or more are considered high risk and have an odds ratio of 2.4 as more likely to experience a complication. However, this study was limited by small patient size and examined only transurethral procedures.

PULMONARY ASSESSMENT

There are also specific risk assessments for pulmonary outcomes, although these have not been specifically validated in a urologic population. Some tests can use as few as 3 variables (age >70 years [2 points], presence of chronic obstructive pulmonary disease [3 points], and preoperative left ventricular ejection fraction <60% [1 point]) to predict postoperative pulmonary infections. This model has been validated to predict increasing rates of infection with each additional point.[43]

RENAL ASSESSMENT

Poor postoperative outcomes are also predicted by the glomerular filtration rate (GFR). Chronic kidney disease is independently associated with morbidity and mortality in the perioperative realm.[44] In addition, GFR has long been proved to steadily decline with age.[45] For patients with decreasing GFR, there is a dose-response effect of increasing risk of all-cause mortality, cardiovascular mortality, and length of hospital stay. The odds ratio for all-cause mortality for an individual with stage 3 (half of normal GFR) kidney disease compared with one with normal GFR is 2.8, whereas for those with stage 4 disease (one-third of normal GFR), it is 11.3. Median length of stay can increase by 3 days across these groups.[46] Assessment of the renal function of older patients is essential for urologic procedures involving kidney resection.

POPULATION-BASED ASSESSMENT

The ACS National Surgical Quality Improvement Program (NSQIP) database can also be used to predict risk of poor postoperative outcome. A public Web site (http://riskcalculator.facs.org/) allows all surgeons to enter the procedure (name or the Current Procedural Terminology code) and information regarding the specific patient, including age, American Society of Anesthesiolgists (ASA) class, functional status, and metrics described in the aforementioned nutritional, cardiac, and pulmonary risk calculators, to provide estimated risk for a variety of complications.[47] These prediction models use a combination of high-risk comorbidities, demographic information, ASA class, body mass index, and other information available in the NSQIP database. Validated studies have shown that these models are as accurate as experienced surgeons in predicting postoperative complications, such as mortality, overall morbidity, and pulmonary, cardiac, thromboembolic, renal, and infectious complications.[48] Although using large databases can help one to quantify how individual patients may be at specific risk, these methods are unable to include the functional and quality-of-life measures that are essential to geriatric patients.

WHAT THE UROLOGIST CAN DO

Preoperative risk assessment is important for the urologist to risk stratify older adults before their planned operation. Surgeons can use single assessment tools, such as walking speed, to assess frailty and thus the global risk of poor postoperative outcomes that are important to both the surgeon and the patient. Further specific evaluations given the patient's comorbidities may contribute additional organ-specific risks for adverse outcomes.

Once the surgeon has determined that the risks of an operation are tolerable for an older patient, high-quality perioperative care of the older patient can improve outcomes. Although large, randomized studies have not validated any specific interventions or techniques, there is some evidence that involvement of geriatric hospital services trend toward improved care. A study of frail Veterans Affairs surgical patients, including urologic patients, indicated a trend toward improved mortality with consultation of a geriatric service and significantly greater adherence to evidence-based recommendations for best practices in geriatric care.[49]

FUTURE DIRECTIONS

Older patients represent a significant proportion of current urologic practice, and will only be increasingly represented with the aging of the American public. Although some evidence exists that outcomes for frail patients can be improved,[50] robust literature on improving postoperative outcomes in the frail older adult population does not exist, and at time of this publication, none exist in the urology literature. By improving a patient's physical and physiologic status before surgery, there is potential to positively modify an older adult's postoperative outcomes. There is evidence that preoperative inspiratory muscle training can improve pulmonary outcomes following cardiothoracic operative procedures.[51] Identifying practical interventions to provide training preoperatively that improve postoperative outcomes could improve the care of the high-risk and vulnerable population of frail surgical patients.

REFERENCES

1. Hall MJ, DeFrances CJ, Williams SN, et al. National Hospital Discharge Survey: 2007 summary. Natl Health Stat Report 2010;(29):1–20, 24.
2. Etzioni DA, Liu JH, O'Connell JB, et al. Elderly patients in surgical workloads: a population-based analysis. Am Surg 2003;69(11):961–5.
3. Buchner DM, Beresford SA, Larson EB, et al. Effects of physical activity on health status in older adults. II. Intervention studies. Annu Rev Public Health 1992;13: 469–88.
4. Fried LP, Tangen CM, Walston J, et al. Frailty in older adults: evidence for a phenotype. J Gerontol A Biol Sci Med Sci 2001;56(3):M146–56.
5. Rockwood K, Song X, MacKnight C, et al. A global clinical measure of fitness and frailty in elderly people. CMAJ 2005;173(5):489–95.
6. Tognoni P, Simonato A, Robutti N, et al. Preoperative risk factors for postoperative delirium (POD) after urological surgery in the elderly. Arch Gerontol Geriat 2011; 52(3):e166–9.
7. Bjurlin MA, Goble SM, Fantus RJ, et al. Outcomes in geriatric genitourinary trauma. J Am Coll Surg 2011;213(3):415–21.
8. Neuman MD, Bosk CL. What we talk about when we talk about risk: refining surgery's hazards in medical thought. Milbank Q 2012;90(1):135–59.
9. Goldman L, Caldera DL, Nussbaum SR, et al. Multifactorial index of cardiac risk in noncardiac surgical procedures. N Engl J Med 1977;297(16):845–50.
10. Fleisher LA, Beckman JA, Brown KA, et al. ACC/AHA 2007 Guidelines on Perioperative Cardiovascular Evaluation and Care for Noncardiac Surgery: Executive Summary: A Report of the American College of Cardiology/American Heart Association Task Force on Practice Guidelines (Writing Committee to Revise the 2002 Guidelines on Perioperative Cardiovascular Evaluation for Noncardiac Surgery) Developed in Collaboration With the American Society of Echocardiography, American Society of Nuclear Cardiology, Heart Rhythm Society, Society of Cardiovascular Anesthesiologists, Society for Cardiovascular Angiography and Interventions, Society for Vascular Medicine and Biology, and Society for Vascular Surgery. J Am Coll Cardiol 2007;50(17):1707–32.
11. Fleisher LA, Fleischmann KE, Auerbach AD, et al. 2014 ACC/AHA guideline on perioperative cardiovascular evaluation and management of patients undergoing

noncardiac surgery: a report of the American College of Cardiology/American Heart Association Task Force on practice guidelines. J Am Coll Cardiol 2014; 64(22):e77–137.

12. Berg JE. Screening for cardiovascular risk: cost-benefit considerations in a comparison of total cholesterol measurements and two compound blood lipid indices. J Cardiovasc Risk 1995;2(5):441–7.

13. Nash GF, Cunnick GH, Allen S, et al. Pre-operative electrocardiograph examination. Ann R Coll Surg Engl 2001;83(6):381–2.

14. Marcantonio ER, Goldman L, Orav EJ, et al. The association of intraoperative factors with the development of postoperative delirium. Am J Med 1998;105(5):380–4.

15. Amador LF, Goodwin JS. Postoperative delirium in the older patient. J Am Coll Surg 2005;200(5):767–73.

16. Papaioannou A, Fraidakis O, Michaloudis D, et al. The impact of the type of anaesthesia on cognitive status and delirium during the first postoperative days in elderly patients. Eur J Anaesthesiol 2005;22(7):492–9.

17. Chow WB, Rosenthal RA, Merkow RP, et al. Optimal preoperative assessment of the geriatric surgical patient: a best practices guideline from the American College of Surgeons National Surgical Quality Improvement Program and the American Geriatrics Society. J Am Coll Surg 2012;215(4):453–66.

18. Robinson TN, Eiseman B, Wallace JI, et al. Redefining geriatric preoperative assessment using frailty, disability and co-morbidity. Ann Surg 2009;250(3): 449–55.

19. Robinson TN, Wu DS, Stiegmann GV, et al. Frailty predicts increased hospital and six-month healthcare cost following colorectal surgery in older adults. Am J Surg 2011;202(5):511–4.

20. Dasgupta M, Rolfson DB, Stolee P, et al. Frailty is associated with postoperative complications in older adults with medical problems. Arch Gerontol Geriatr 2009; 48(1):78–83.

21. Kristjansson SR, Nesbakken A, Jordhøy MS, et al. Comprehensive geriatric assessment can predict complications in elderly patients after elective surgery for colorectal cancer: a prospective observational cohort study. Crit Rev Oncol Hematol 2010;76(3):208–17.

22. Lee JS, He K, Harbaugh CM, et al. Frailty, core muscle size, and mortality in patients undergoing open abdominal aortic aneurysm repair. J Vasc Surg 2011; 53(4):912–7.

23. Podsiadlo D, Richardson S. The timed "Up & Go": a test of basic functional mobility for frail elderly persons. J Am Geriatr Soc 1991;39(2):142–8.

24. Borson S, Scanlan JM, Chen P, et al. The Mini-Cog as a screen for dementia: validation in a population-based sample. J Am Geriatr Soc 2003;51(10):1451–4.

25. Charlson ME, Pompei P, Ales KL, et al. A new method of classifying prognostic comorbidity in longitudinal studies: development and validation. J Chronic Dis 1987;40(5):373–83.

26. Inouye SK, Studenski S, Tinetti ME, et al. Geriatric syndromes: clinical, research, and policy implications of a core geriatric concept. J Am Geriatr Soc 2007;55(5): 780–91.

27. Kim SM, Kim MJ, Jung HA, et al. Comparison of the Freiburg and Charlson comorbidity indices in predicting overall survival in elderly patients with newly diagnosed multiple myeloma. Biomed Res Int 2014;2014:437852.

28. Koppie TM, Serio AM, Vickers AJ, et al. Age-adjusted Charlson comorbidity score is associated with treatment decisions and clinical outcomes for patients undergoing radical cystectomy for bladder cancer. Cancer 2008;112(11):2384–92.

29. Froehner M, Koch R, Litz R, et al. Comparison of the American Society of Anesthesiologists Physical Status classification with the Charlson score as predictors of survival after radical prostatectomy. Urology 2003;62(4):698–701.

30. Makary MA, Segev DL, Pronovost PJ, et al. Frailty as a predictor of surgical outcomes in older patients. J Am Coll Surg 2010;210(6):901–8.

31. Rantanen T, Volpato S, Ferrucci L, et al. Handgrip strength and cause-specific and total mortality in older disabled women: exploring the mechanism. J Am Geriatr Soc 2003;51(5):636–41.

32. Sasaki H, Kasagi F, Yamada M, et al. Grip strength predicts cause-specific mortality in middle-aged and elderly persons. Am J Med 2007;120(4):337–42.

33. Izawa KP, Watanabe S, Osada N, et al. Handgrip strength as a predictor of prognosis in Japanese patients with congestive heart failure. Eur J Cardiovasc Prev Rehabil 2009;16(1):21–7.

34. Chang YT, Wu HL, Guo HR, et al. Handgrip strength is an independent predictor of renal outcomes in patients with chronic kidney diseases. Nephrol Dial Transplant 2011;26(11):3588–95.

35. Chung CJ, Wu C, Jones M, et al. Reduced handgrip strength as a marker of frailty predicts clinical outcomes in patients with heart failure undergoing ventricular assist device placement. J Card Fail 2014;20(5):310–5.

36. Robinson TN, Wu DS, Sauaia A, et al. Slower walking speed forecasts increased postoperative morbidity and 1-year mortality across surgical specialties. Ann Surg 2013;258(4):582–8 [discussion: 588–90].

37. Afilalo J, Eisenberg MJ, Morin JF, et al. Gait speed as an incremental predictor of mortality and major morbidity in elderly patients undergoing cardiac surgery. J Am Coll Cardiol 2010;56(20):1668–76.

38. Schoenborn CA, Heyman KM. Health characteristics of adults aged 55 years and over: United States, 2004-2007. Natl Health Stat Report 2009;(16):1–31.

39. Bateman BT, Schumacher HC, Wang S, et al. Perioperative acute ischemic stroke in noncardiac and nonvascular surgery: incidence, risk factors, and outcomes. Anesthesiology 2009;110(2):231–8.

40. Valerio M, Cerantola Y, Fritschi U, et al. Comorbidity and nutritional indices as predictors of morbidity after transurethral procedures: a prospective cohort study. Can Urol Assoc J 2014;8(9–10):E600–4.

41. Allou N, Bronchard R, Guglielminotti J, et al. Risk factors for postoperative pneumonia after cardiac surgery and development of a preoperative risk score*. Crit Care Med 2014;42(5):1150–6.

42. Mathew S, Tustison KS, Sugatani T, et al. The mechanism of phosphorus as a cardiovascular risk factor in CKD. J Am Soc Nephrol 2008;19(6):1092–105.

43. Glassock RJ, Winearls C. Ageing and the glomerular filtration rate: truths and consequences. Trans Am Clin Climatol Assoc 2009;120:419–28.

44. Mases A, Sabaté S, Guilera N, et al. Preoperative estimated glomerular filtration rate and the risk of major adverse cardiovascular and cerebrovascular events in non-cardiac surgery. Br J Anaesth 2014;113(4):644–51.

45. Glasgow RE, Hawn MT, Hosokawa PW, et al. Comparison of prospective risk estimates for postoperative complications: human vs computer model. J Am Coll Surg 2014;218(2):237–45.e1–4.

46. McRae PJ, Peel NM, Walker PJ, et al. Geriatric syndromes in individuals admitted to vascular and urology surgical units. J Am Geriatr Soc 2014;62(6):1105–9.

47. Hardy SE, Perera S, Roumani YF, et al. Improvement in usual gait speed predicts better survival in older adults. J Am Geriatr Soc 2007;55(11):1727–34.

48. Hulzebos EH, van Meeteren NL, van den Buijs BJ, et al. Feasibility of preoperative inspiratory muscle training in patients undergoing coronary artery bypass surgery with a high risk of postoperative pulmonary complications: a randomized controlled pilot study. Clin Rehabil 2006;20(11):949–59.
49. Townsend NT, Robinson TN. Does walking speed predict postoperative morbidity? Adv Surg 2014;48:53–64.
50. Savva GM, Donoghue OA, Horgan F, et al. Using Timed Up-and-Go to identify frail members of the older population. J Gerontol A Biol Sci Med Sci 2013; 68(4):441–6.
51. Donoghue OA, Horgan NF, Savva GM, et al. Association between Timed Up-and-Go and memory, executive function, and processing speed. J Am Geriatr Soc 2012;60(9):1681–6.
52. Katsumata Y, Todoriki H, Yasura S, et al. Timed Up and Go test predicts cognitive decline in healthy adults aged 80 and older in Okinawa: Keys to Optimal Cognitive Aging (KOCOA) Project. J Am Geriatr Soc 2011;59(11):2188–9.
53. Viccaro LJ, Perera S, Studenski SA. Is Timed Up and Go better than gait speed in predicting health, function, and falls in older adults? J Am Geriatr Soc 2011;59(5): 887–92.
54. Huang SL, Hsieh CL, Wu RM, et al. Minimal detectable change of the Timed "Up & Go" test and the dynamic gait index in people with Parkinson disease. Phys Ther 2011;91(1):114–21.
55. Studenski S, Perera S, Patel K, et al. Gait speed and survival in older adults. JAMA 2011;305(1):50–8.
56. Laukkanen P, Heikkinen E, Kauppinen M. Muscle strength and mobility as predictors of survival in 75–84-year-old people. Age Ageing 1995;24(6):468–73.

Management of Small Renal Masses in the Older Adult

Moben Mirza, MD

KEYWORDS

- Small renal mass • Kidney cancer • Renal cell carcinoma • Active surveillance
- Partial nephrectomy

KEY POINTS

- Small renal masses (SRMs) in older adults are common and usually found incidentally. Although many SRMs are benign, the vast majority are malignant.
- In older patients, the SRM poses a challenge because the treatment paradigm has to strike the balance between competing comorbidities and a lethal cancer.
- Small renal cancers are heterogeneous. The current armament includes nomograms, imaging data, and biopsy data to make clinical decisions. Further genetic research may help differentiate lethal and indolent cancers.
- Active surveillance (AS), partial nephrectomy (PN), radical nephrectomy (RN), cryoablation (CA), and radiofrequency ablation (RFA) are all options in management of SRMs.
- PN confers oncologic outcomes similar to RN and potentially improves survival because of lower risk of chronic renal disease and cardiovascular disease

INTRODUCTION

SRMs in older adults are common and usually found incidentally. They are found on computed tomography (CT), MRI, and renal ultrasonography (RUS). Although many SRMs are benign, the vast majority are malignant. Early detection and treatment is a victory in any cancer scenario. However, in older patients, the SRM poses a challenge because the treatment paradigm has to strike a balance between competing comorbidities and a lethal cancer.

There is relevant debate about the clinical use of percutaneous renal mass biopsy to differentiate benign and malignant tumors, as well as low-grade and high-grade cancers. PN, mainly via robot-assisted technique, has gained favor over RN as the intervention of choice. PN provides similar oncologic outcomes while potentially

Division of Urologic Oncology, Department of Urology, University of Kansas, 3901 Rainbow Boulevard, MS 3016, Kansas City, KS 66160, USA
E-mail address: mmirza@kumc.edu

Clin Geriatr Med 31 (2015) 603–613
http://dx.doi.org/10.1016/j.cger.2015.06.005
0749-0690/15/$ – see front matter © 2015 Elsevier Inc. All rights reserved.
geriatric.theclinics.com

improving survival because of lower risk of renal insufficiency and cardiovascular disease. CA and RFA are also viable treatment options and have a role to play in patients who desire treatment but either are not suitable surgical candidates or prefer not to have a surgical intervention.

AS is gaining favor and will play a stronger role in management of SRMs. This approach is suitable for the older patient as it provides a way to manage risk of a potentially lethal cancer with other competing causes of death. Recognition of tumor heterogeneity has become a marquee stamp of the latest advancements in cancer research. Small renal cancers need such advancement so one is best able to differentiate the patients who benefit most from intervention from those in whom intervention does not affect quality or quantity of life.

This review focuses on the population of adults older than 65 years. For the purposes of this article, a broad definition of SRM is used, which is an incidentally detected, asymptomatic, solid renal mass 4 cm or less. As mentioned, many SRMs can be benign, but most are renal cell cancers with clinical stage T1a (cancer localized to kidney and ≤4 cm). Therefore, when first examined radiographically, the SRM is considered a cancer until proven otherwise. This article considers the epidemiology of renal cancers in general and focuses on the older population, diagnosis and evaluation of a small renal cell cancer, tumor biology and growth kinetics, and treatment.

EPIDEMIOLOGY

Renal cell carcinoma (RCC) represents the eighth most common malignancy and third most common urologic malignancy. The estimated new cases in 2014 were 63,920, accounting for 3.8% of all new cancer cases. The estimated deaths were 13,860, accounting for 2.4% of all cancer deaths. The 5-year survival is 72.4%. But when broken down by stage, it is 92% for localized disease, 65% for regional disease, and 12.1% for distant disease. Median age at diagnosis is 64 years; however, almost 48% of cases are diagnosed in patients 65 years or older. Median age at death is 71 years, with almost 40% of deaths occurring in patients 75 years or older.[1] See **Table 1** for summary.

DIAGNOSIS

The diagnosis of SRMs is generally made on CT, MRI, or RUS. The reason for these examinations may range from abdominal pain to trauma. SRMs are incidental findings, and these tumors are generally asymptomatic and do not cause pain, hematuria, or other constitutional symptoms. Masses showing enhancement on cross-sectional imaging such as CT and MRI or solid echogenicity on ultrasound imaging are considered malignant until proved otherwise. See **Table 2** for percentage of benign pathology based on size.

Table 1		
Renal cell cancer diagnosis and death by age groups		
Age Group (y)	New Cases (%)	Cancer Deaths (%)
65–74	25.2	25.3
75–84	17.4	26.2
>84	5.7	15.0

Data from Surveillance, Epidemiology, and End Results (SEER) Program (www.seer.cancer.gov) SEER*Stat Database: Incidence - SEER 9 Regs Research Data, Nov 2013 Sub (1973–2011) Total U.S., 1969–2012 Counties, National Cancer Institute, DCCPS, Surveillance Research Program, Surveillance Systems Branch, released April 2014, based on the November 2013 submission.

Table 2	
Chances of benign pathology in SRMs based on size	
Size (cm)	Percentage Benign
0–2	21.4
2–3	21.1
3–4	16.7

Data from Duchene DA, Lotan Y, Caddedu JA, et al. Histopathology of surgically managed renal tumors: analysis of a contemporary series. Urology 2003;62:827.

Almost 48% to 66% of all RCC are SRMs.[2] Kunkle and colleagues[3] performed a large review of 99 series representing 6471 SRMs. Mean size at diagnosis is 3.26 cm for compiled series of patients undergoing various treatments modalities. Pathologic findings confirmed RCC in 79.7% of lesions; 12.2% were benign and 8.1% were indeterminate. Local recurrence was reported in 3.7%, and metastatic disease was reported in 4.7%.

Renal Mass Biopsy

Historical beliefs about renal cell cancer are changing and so is the evolving role of renal mass biopsy. Now that most RCCs are diagnosed incidentally, one has to reexamine these previously held ideas that

- Renal masses had a greater than 90% chance of harboring an RCC, so why perform a biopsy?
- Renal biopsy has risk of tumor seeding and high rate of false-negative results.
- Even if biopsy shows benign pathology, the patient may have a hybrid cancer.
- Biopsy does not change what is done, and complete cancer removal is paramount.

Renal mass biopsy has several advantages in this changing landscape:

- Match treatment to tumor biology and reduce therapeutic morbidity.
- Perform risk assessment of cancer without major operation.
- Reduce the number of surgeries on noncancerous masses.
- Reduce RN for low-risk T1 RCC and favor PN or AS when possible.

The following are known about contemporary core renal mass biopsy:

- Greater than 90% are diagnostic.[4]
- Repeat biopsy has 80% success rate.[5]
- The false-positive rate is 1%–2%.[5]
- Tumor seeding risk is low.[4]
- The complication rate is less than 2% (mostly minor).[4]

One of the criticisms of SRM biopsy is its utility in changing clinical management. In the current role, the biggest advantage seems to be in risk stratification based on histologic subtype and grade, which are accurately diagnosed on biopsy (**Box 1**). Rahbar and colleagues[6] showed that up to 50% of high-risk patients (>70 years, ASA (American Society of Anesthesiology) ≥3) based on a biopsy-driven predictive model would have avoided surgical intervention.

Evaluation of Comorbidity

Comorbidities in older patients not only make treatment of the SRMs more challenging but also increase the risk of death from a cause other than malignancy. In a review of

---

Box 1
Indications and contraindications for SRMs biopsy

Indications

Indeterminate SRM

Risk stratify patients undergoing active surveillance or ablative treatments

Confirm success of ablative treatments histologically

Any SRM for risk stratification

Contraindications

Uncorrected coagulopathy

Patient not candidate for any treatment option

7177 Medicare beneficiaries, Patel and colleagues[7] showed that congestive heart failure, chronic kidney disease, peripheral vascular disease, chronic obstructive pulmonary disease, diabetes, and cerebrovascular disease were associated with decreased overall survival (OS).

The current assessment of comorbidity includes a thorough medical history, Eastern Cooperative Oncology Group performance status,[8] Charlson comorbidity index (CCI), and a newly developed simplified cardiovascular index.[7] The CCI was first described in 1987 by Charlson and colleagues.[9,10] The CCI gives a weight of 1 to 6 to different comorbidities ranging from myocardial infarction to metastatic cancer. It has been validated for many disease states. In RCC, it is especially relevant to surgical treatment. Patients older than 75 years and CCI greater than 2 were 1.9 times more likely to have postoperative complications compared with the lower-risk group.

The cardiovascular index may have a more predictive role. The cardiovascular index reclassified 41% of patients with a CCI value of 1 or more to a value of 0, with minimal concession of 5-year survival.[7]

Evaluation of comorbidity is therefore an essential part of risk assessment and should play an important role in guiding discussion and treatment plans.

Nomograms and Risk Assessment Tools

Great effort has been focused on the development of predictive tools, scores, and nomograms to predict malignant potential before surgery. An excellently correlating nomogram could serve as a substitute for core biopsy or surgical excision. Early efforts were not predictive and served as coarse measures using age, gender, smoking, presence of symptoms, and tumor size. Kutikov and colleagues[11] combined individual descriptors of the nephrometry score and individual characteristics such as age and gender to predict malignant RCC histology and high-grade features. This nomogram has been externally validated.[12] The Kutikov nomogram has a predictive capability of malignant potential and tumor grade (high or low) similar to core renal mass biopsy.

What is the likelihood that someone will die from kidney cancer versus other causes, adjusted for other health factors? When the Kutikov nomogram[13] is used for a 70-year-old white man with a 3-cm mass and CCI of 2, the nomogram returns a 2.6% chance of 5-year cancer-specific survival (CSS) and a 17.5% chance of dying of other causes.

Nomograms and risk assessment tools are highly valuable when counseling patients regarding their relative risks. It can help older patients understand that, although their diagnosis of a cancer is significant, other health conditions may be more of a threat to their overall health, quality of life, as well as quantity of life. Using nomograms in the clinical setting also helps patients visualize the predictive risks and educates them of their disease process.

TREATMENT

The treatment options of SRMs include AS, PN, RN, CA, and RFA. All treatment options have advantages, disadvantages, risks, and benefits as pertaining to treatment burden, treatment complications, efficacy, survival benefit, and quality of life. Consideration should be given to treatment goals, tumor biology as predicted by nomogram or renal mass biopsy, patient comorbidities, as well as patient preference. Each treatment option is reviewed.

Active Surveillance

SRMs are heterogeneous, 20% being benign masses, 60% being indolent cancer, and 20% representing potentially aggressive cancers.[14] The premise of AS is that given disease characteristics or patient preference, intervention is not warranted or chosen. During the period of surveillance, interval testing is done to note change and then review options again either to continue AS or to move to treatment based on specific triggers. The idea is that the SRM has a low metastatic potential, is not aggressive, and unlikely to affect any quality-of-life or survival outcome. The potential benefit of treatment may also be outweighed by the competing risks related to medical comorbidities, especially in older patients.

AS in SRM is supported by several studies. Borghesi and colleagues[15] comprehensively reviewed AS. In their report, mean age range was 69 to 81 years and the linear growth rate (LGR) was slow, ranging from 0.1 to 0.4 cm/y. The progression to metastases was low, ranging from 0% to 5.7%. Cancer-related deaths were uncommon.

The first prospective trial evaluating the role and safety of AS was published by Jewett and colleagues.[16] In 178 patients and 209 SRMs with mean age of 73 years, the average growth rate was 0.13 cm/y. About 37% of SRMs showed zero growth. Metastatic progression was reported in 2 patients (1.1%) and accounted for the CSS in the study.

The uncertainty of a cancer spreading can make both patients and physicians reluctant to follow AS. Smaldone and colleagues[17] performed a pooled analysis of AS series. Of 880 patients, 18 (2%) developed metastatic disease after a mean follow-up of 40 months. Characteristics were compared between the group that developed metastasis with the group that did not. Patients who developed metastatic disease had larger tumors (4.1 ± 2.1 cm vs 2.3 ± 1.3 cm; $P<.001$) and a faster LGR (0.8 ± 0.7 cm/y vs 0.3 ± 0.4 cm/y; $P<.001$) than those without systemic progression.

Pierorazio and colleagues[18] have determined the characteristics and clinical outcomes of patients who chose AS for management of their SRM. The registry trial prospectively enrolled patients with SRM who chose AS or immediate treatment. Included in the final analysis were patients who had a delayed intervention after a period of AS. Analyses were performed in an intention to treat manner. About 40% of patients chose AS as the initial management. The OS for the AS and treatment groups was 96% and 98% at 2 years and 75% and 92% at 5 years. CSS was 100% and 99% for the AS and treatment groups, respectively. The investigators conclude that AS with delayed intervention is a noninferior management strategy with regard to oncologic outcomes for selected patients in short to intermediate follow-up. AS patients were older, had higher comorbidities, and smaller tumors, and only 6.7% underwent biopsy in this group.

The existing body of knowledge supports that AS is a safe and viable option in SRMs when disease characteristics and patient comorbidities are taken into account (**Box 2**). The risk of rapid growth, metastasis, and death from SRMs in patients

---

Box 2
Advantages of active surveillance of SRMs

Prevent or delay treatment-related morbidity

Low risk of rapid renal mass growth

Low risk of metastasis

Very low risk of cancer-related death

Noninferior oncologic outcomes for short to intermediate follow-up

---

undergoing AS is low. There is no accepted protocol for AS. All patients should have an initial cross-sectional imaging study (CT or MRI) with contrast media when renal function allows. Otherwise, RUS can be used to differentiate solid from cystic masses. Risk stratification can be done using renal mass biopsy or nomograms. Cross-sectional imaging should be used in short-term follow-up at 6-month intervals. Once stability is demonstrated over a 1- to 2-year period, RUS can be used for continued follow-up and cross-sectional imaging when growth is suspected. Increase in renal mass size or an accelerated LGR can serve as a trigger for renal mass biopsy (if not done initially) and reassessment of treatment options.

Radical Nephrectomy

RN involves removal of the affected kidney without violation of Gerota fascia. As initially described in 1969, it includes the ipsilateral adrenal gland as well as regional lymph nodes.[19] For SRMs or T1a RCC, removal of adrenal gland and lymphadenectomy are not necessary.

RN serves as the historical standard because of its high achievement of cancer control as measured by outcomes of local tumor control, progression-free survival, recurrence-free survival, and CSS rates.[20] Laparoscopic RN was first introduced in the early 1990s. Laparoscopic RN, when feasible, reduces pain, length of hospital stay, and recovery time. The safety, cancer control, and complication rates are equivalent.[21]

Partial Nephrectomy

PN involves complete removal of the tumor while sparing the unaffected part of the kidney, therefore offering functional renal preservation or nephron sparing surgery (NSS). Go and colleagues[22] showed an inverse relationship estimated glomerular filtration rate, incidence of hospitalizations, cardiac events, and overall death, thus highlighting the benefit of NSS. The open technique was first described by Licht and Novick.[23] Since then, laparoscopic PN (LPN) and robot-assisted LPN (RALPN) have been described.

Comparison of these techniques by Benway and colleagues[24] failed to demonstrate difference in operative time, violation of collection system, margin status, conversion to RN, complication rates, and early oncologic outcomes. The study did show decreased estimated blood loss, warm ischemia time, and hospital stay in RALPN. At present, PN by any modality is considered acceptable and represents the standard of care for SRMs. There continues to be increased adoption of PN in the United States.

Partial Nephrectomy Versus Radical Nephrectomy

The debate between PN and RN centers on outcomes of renal function preservation and survival. Is one clearly better than the other? The theoretic advantage of PN is conceptually easy to grasp, preserve unaffected nephrons, maintain better glomerular filtration rate (GFR), and therefore prevent long-term complications of renal dysfunction such as cardiac events (**Box 3**). But does this concept stand the test of scientific rigor and scrutiny? Or is it just better to remove the entire kidney? The theoretic advantage of RN is conceptually easy to grasp as well. If there is a question of cancer, remove the whole kidney, why take a chance? There is a balance because removal of the entire kidney risks overtreatment especially when it comes to benign tumors, indolent cancer, and older patients with comorbidities.

The European Organization for Research and Treatment of Cancer (EORTC) phase 3 trial of NSS and RN was designed to evaluate OS and time to progression of RCC in patients undergoing PN versus RN.[25] The study was closed prematurely because of poor accrual. However, 541 patients with renal tumors less than 5 cm were enrolled and randomized to PN versus RN. Median follow-up was 9.3 years. The investigators concluded that both methods provide excellent oncologic results. In the intention to treat population, NSS seems to be significantly less effective than RN in terms of OS. However, in the targeted population of patients with RCC, the trend in favor of RN is no longer significant.

A follow-up analysis on the same cohort was done to evaluate renal function outcomes. Scosyrev and colleagues[26] concluded that compared with RN, NSS substantially reduced the incidence of at least moderate renal dysfunction (estimated GFR [eGFR] <60). The incidence of advanced kidney disease (eGFR<30) was similar in the 2 treatment arms, and the incidence of kidney failure (eGFR<15) was nearly identical. The beneficial impact of NSS on eGFR did not result in improved survival in this study population.

Capitanio and colleagues[27] published the results of a large multi-institutional collaborative effort to test the correlation between NSS and RN for the long-term risk of postsurgical cardiovascular events (CVEs) after accounting for baseline cardiovascular risk factors. The study cohort was composed of 1331 patients with clinical T1 renal masses and normal preoperative renal function who were treated with NSS and RN. Patients who underwent NSS experienced a statistically significant lower risk of CVEs at 10 years of follow-up (20.2% vs 25.9%) when compared with patients who underwent RN.

There is little doubt based on the available literature that renal function is better preserved with NSS. This improvement results in lower CVEs at 10 years as discussed earlier. Most studies comparing OS between patients who underwent RN and NSS favor NSS.[28] These findings are also demonstrated when comparing OS among patients treated with RN or NSS for benign renal masses.[29] A meta-analysis that included the EORTC 30904 clinical trial results favored OS in the NSS arm.[28] In contrast is EORTC 30904, which is the only randomized trial demonstrating that survival is probably equivalent and may be better for RN. The current thinking therefore is that PN or

---

Box 3
Advantages of partial nephrectomy or nephron sparing surgery

Preservation of renal function

Comparable oncologic efficacy to RN

Lower cardiovascular events

Lower risk of chronic disease

Survival probably better (as shown in meta-analysis, but equivalent in EORTC 30904 RCC population)

NSS remains an important frontline and the standard treatment option for patients with SRM when feasible. The oncologic efficacy is comparable with RN, and the risk of chronic kidney disease is significantly improved.

Thermal Ablative Techniques

CA and RFA were originally developed to manage SRMs in older patients with significant comorbidities or patients electing against surgical removal.[30] Thermal ablative probes are placed on or into the tumor under image guidance using percutaneous techniques. Alternatively, probes can be placed using a laparoscopic approach.

CA has many effects on the affected tissue as temperatures approach -40°C. The important mechanisms and considerations are as follows[31]:

- There is extracellular freezing and targeted tissue desiccation.
- There is intracellular pH alteration and protein denaturation.
- There is destruction of organelles and cell membrane by ice crystal formation.
- Reperfusion of the damaged microcirculation leads to microthrombi formation and occlusion resulting in ischemia and tumor destruction.
- Slow thaw is important.
- Repeated cycles improve odds of complete eradication.
- Ice ball can be visualized on imaging.

RFA relies on alternating radiofrequency energy, which generates heat from the impedance of targeted tissue cells. As temperatures reach 105°C, heating leads to cell death and coagulation necrosis, leaving behind a necrotic lesion.[32]

CA and RFA offer the potential to mitigate many of these risks by avoiding general anesthesia and surgical dissection. However, the oncologic efficacy of focal therapy is generally considered inferior to surgical resection. Kunkle and Uzzo[33] published a meta-analysis of patients undergoing CA and RFA with mean tumor diameter of 2.6 cm. At median follow-up of 18.7 months, 5.2% lesions managed with CA and 12.9% managed with RFA had local progression. The rate of local progression and distant metastasis were 1.8% and 1%, respectively.

Thermal ablation is an available treatment option. It is best suited for the high-surgical-risk patient who prefers active treatment. The following points should be emphasized[30]:

- Tumor biopsy before treatment and possibly after treatment
- Counseling regarding the increased risk of local recurrence
- Difficulty in defining radiologic success
- Limitation in larger tumors (>3.5 cm) and those with irregular shape or infiltrative appearance in terms of increased risk of recurrence

SUMMARY

SRMs in older patients pose a unique challenge. In younger, healthier patients, extirpative treatments are well accepted, as the benefits of immediate intervention outweigh the risks. In contrast, the older patient with comorbidities may be in a situation in which the risks of an immediate intervention can easily outweigh the potential benefits. Despite the understanding that some SRMs are benign and many more are indolent, when patients are told about the potential of cancer, it brings about high anxiety and anguish. Therefore, how patients are counseled is extremely important.

MAJOR SUMMARY POINTS

- Cross-sectional imaging with intravenous enhancing media is the best imaging method for SRMs.
- Enhancing solid masses can be benign but should be considered malignant until proved otherwise.
- Complete evaluation of comorbidities is of paramount importance.
- Risk stratification of tumor potential is important, and renal mass biopsy should be considered to determine histology and grade.
- Renal mass biopsy is safe and accurate.
- Risk stratification with available tools and nomograms is easy to do, provides comparative analysis, and helps guide decision making.
- AS is a reasonable, safe, and well-suited option for older patients with comorbidities who may not benefit from immediate definitive treatment. It is associated with low rates of metastasis and cancer-related mortality.
- PN when feasible is the standard of care for management of healthy patients with SRMs and is associated with excellent cancer control and preserved renal function.
- RN has a limited role in the management of SRMs and should be reserved for healthy patients with anatomically difficult tumors for which PN cannot be performed. Some patients may have relative or imperative indications to avoid RN because it is associated with higher risk of chronic kidney disease.
- Thermal ablation is best suited for high-surgical-risk patients who prefer treatment without the risks associated with major surgical intervention. However, there is an increased risk of local recurrence.

The heterogeneity of renal cancer is well recognized. It is hoped that as the research and understanding of genetic and epigenetic heterogeneity of RCC progresses, one will be better able to sort the potentially lethal cancers from the indolent cancers and benign tumors. Until then, one must use the available tools and knowledge to balance the risk and benefits to come up with a safe and viable treatment plan for each patient.

REFERENCES

1. Surveillance, Epidemiology, and End Results (SEER) Program (www.seer.cancer. gov) SEER*Stat Database: Incidence - SEER 9 Regs Research Data, Nov 2013 Sub (1973-2011) Total U.S., 1969-2012 Counties, National Cancer Institute, DCCPS, Surveillance Research Program, Surveillance Systems Branch, released April 2014, based on the November 2013 submission.
2. Volpe A, Panzarella T, Rendon RA, et al. The natural history of incidentally detected renal masses. Cancer 2004;100:738.
3. Kunkle DA, Egleston BL, Uzzo RG. Excise, ablate, or observe: the small renal mass dilemma – a meta-analysis and review. J Urol 2008;179:1227.
4. Tomaszewski JJ, Uzzo RG, Smaldone MC. Heterogeneity and renal mass biopsy: a review of its role and reliability. Cancer Biol Med 2014;11:162.
5. Leveridge MJ, Finellia A, Kachura JR, et al. Outcomes of small renal mass needle core biopsy, nondiagnostic percutaneous biopsy, and the role of repeat biopsy. Eur Urol 2011;60:578.
6. Rahbar H, Bhayani S, Stifelman M, et al. Evaluation of renal mass biopsy risk stratification algorithm for robotic partial nephrectomy – could a biopsy have guided management? J Urol 2014;192:1337.

7. Patel HD, Kates M, Pierorazio PM, et al. Comorbidities and causes of death in the management of localized T1a kidney cancer. Int J Urol 2014;21:1086.

8. Oken MM, Creech RH, Tormey DC, et al. Toxicity and response criteria of the Eastern Cooperative Oncology Group. Am J Clin Oncol 1982;5:649.

9. Charlson ME, Pompei P, Ales KL, et al. A new method of classifying prognostic comorbidity in longitudinal studies: development and validation. J Chronic Dis 1987;40:373.

10. Tomaszewski JJ, Uzzo RG, Kutikov A, et al. Assessing the burden of complications after surgery for clinically localized kidney cancer by age and comorbidity status. Urology 2014;83:843.

11. Kutikov A, Smaldone MC, Egleston BL, et al. Anatomic features of enhancing renal masses predict malignant and high-grade pathology: a preoperative nomogram using the RENAL nephrometry score. Eur Urol 2011;60:241.

12. Wang HK, Zhu Y, Yao XD, et al. External validation of a nomogram using RENAL nephrometry score to predict high grade renal cell carcinoma. J Urol 2012;187:1555.

13. Kutikov A, Egleston BL, Canter D, et al. Competing risks of death in patients with localized renal cell carcinoma: a comorbidity based model. J Urol 2012;188:2077.

14. Remzi M, Ozsoy M, Klingler HC, et al. Are small renal tumors harmless? Analysis of histopathological features according to tumors 4 cm or less in diameter. J Urol 2006;176:896.

15. Borghesi M, Brunocilla E, Volpe A, et al. Active surveillance for clinically localized renal tumors: an updated review of current indications and clinical outcomes. Int J Urol 2015;22:432–8.

16. Jewett MA, Mattar K, Basiuk J, et al. Active surveillance of small renal masses: progression patterns of early stage kidney cancer. Eur Urol 2011;60:39.

17. Smaldone MC, Kutikov A, Egleston BL, et al. Small renal masses progressing to metastases under active surveillance: a systematic review and pooled analysis. Cancer 2012;118:997.

18. Pierorazio PM, Johnson MH, Ball MW, et al. Five-year analysis of a multi-institutional prospective clinical trial of delayed intervention and surveillance for small renal masses: the DISSRM registry. Eur Urol 2015. http://dx.doi.org/10.1016/j.eururo.2015.02.001.

19. Robson CJ. Radical nephrectomy for renal cell carcinoma. J Urol 1969;89:37–42.

20. Beuthe DD, Spiess PE. Current management considerations for the incidentally detected small renal mass. Cancer Control 2013;20:211.

21. Luo JH, Zhou FJ, Xie D, et al. Analysis of long-term survival in patients with localized renal cell carcinoma: laparoscopic versus open radical nephrectomy. World J Urol 2010;28:289.

22. Go AS, Cherlow GM, Fan D, et al. Chronic kidney disease and the risk of death, cardiovascular events, and hospitalization. N Engl J Med 2004;351:1296.

23. Licht MR, Novick AC. Nephron sparing surgery for renal cell carcinoma. J Urol 1993;149:1.

24. Benway BM, Bhayani SB, Rogers CG, et al. Robot-assisted partial nephrectomy versus laparoscopic partial nephrectomy for renal tumors: a multi-institutional analysis of perioperative outcomes. J Urol 2009;182:866.

25. Von Poppel H, Da Pozzo L, Albrecht W, et al. A prospective, randomized EORTC intergroup phase 3 study comparing the oncologic outcome of elective nephron-sparing surgery and radical nephrectomy for low-stage renal cell carcinoma. Eur Urol 2011;59:543.

26. Scosyrev E, Messing EM, Sylvester R, et al. Renal function after nephron-sparing surgery versus radical nephrectomy: results from EORTC randomized trial 30904. Eur Urol 2014;65:372.

27. Capitanio U, Terrone C, Antonelli A, et al. Nephron-sparing techniques independently decrease the risk of cardiovascular events relative to radical nephrectomy in patients with a T1a-T1b renal mass and normal preoperative renal function. Eur Urol 2015;67:683.

28. Kim SP, Thompson RH, Boorijan SA, et al. Comparative effectiveness for survival and renal function of partial and radical nephrectomy for localized renal tumors: a systematic review and meta-analysis. J Urol 2012;188:51.

29. Kaushik D, Kim SP, Childs MA, et al. Overall survival and development of stage IV chronic kidney disease in patients undergoing partial and radical nephrectomy for benign renal tumors. Eur Urol 2013;64:600.

30. Campbell SC, Novick AC, Belldegrun A, et al. Guideline for management of the clinical T1 renal mass. J Urol 2009;182:1271.

31. Gage AA, Baust J. Mechanisms of tissue injury in cryosurgery. Cryobiology 1998; 37:171.

32. Hwang JJ, Walther MM, Pautler SE, et al. Radio frequency ablation of small renal tumors: intermediate results. J Urol 2004;171:1814.

33. Kunkle DA, Uzzo RG. Cryoablation or radiofrequency ablation of the small renal mass: a meta-analysis. Cancer 2008;113:2671.

Prostate Cancer in Elderly Men

Screening, Active Surveillance, and Definitive Therapy

Breton Roussel, BS[a], Gregory M. Ouellet, MD[b],
Supriya G. Mohile, MD, MS[c], William Dale, MD, PhD[d],*

KEYWORDS

- Prostate cancer • Geriatrics • Shared decision making • CGA • Geriatric oncology
- Aging

KEY POINTS

- Treatment of prostate cancer (PCa) for older men is best considered in the context of one's physiologic and not chronologic age.
- There are resources available to health care providers to best quantify one's physiologic age, including the comprehensive geriatric assessment (CGA).
- In addition to directing candidacy for treatment or modifying treatment, the CGA also identifies areas in which targeted interventions will benefit older men with PCa.
- Most importantly a goal-centric approach to treatment planning is critical in counseling and directing therapy for the older adults in a shared decision-making context.

INTRODUCTION

PCa will be diagnosed in approximately 220,800 men in 2015, and roughly 27,500 will die from the disease.[1] PCa is a common medical condition in the United States, with an estimated 16% of men receiving a diagnosis during their lifetime.[2] Importantly, 57% of those diagnosed with PCa are older than 65 years, so most patients with PCa are considered older men.[3] Although it is the second leading cause of cancer-specific deaths among men, PCa will not be the cause of death for most men who

[a] Robert Wood Johnson Medical School, Rutgers University, 125 Paterson Street, New Brunswick, NJ 08901, USA; [b] Department of Medicine, Yale University School of Medicine, 333 Cedar Street, New Haven, CT 06510, USA; [c] Division of Hematology/Oncology, Department of Medicine, Wilmot Cancer Institute, University of Rochester, 601 Elmwood Avenue, Box 704, Rochester, NY 14642, USA; [d] Section of Geriatrics and Palliative Medicine, Department of Medicine, Specialized Oncology Care & Research in the Elderly (SOCARE) Clinic, University of Chicago, 5841 South Maryland Avenue, MC6098, Chicago, IL 60643, USA
* Corresponding author.
E-mail address: wdale@medicine.bsd.uchicago.edu

Clin Geriatr Med 31 (2015) 615–629
http://dx.doi.org/10.1016/j.cger.2015.07.004
0749-0690/15/$ – see front matter © 2015 Elsevier Inc. All rights reserved.

are diagnosed with it. Still, the lifetime risk for a man to die from PCa is only 3%; however, 70% of those patients who die of PCa are older than 75 years.[2,4] Despite its high prevalence among the older male population, most of the clinical trials conducted on PCa treatment are completed in relatively younger, healthier men.[5] Although there are notable improvements recently, the relative dearth of high-quality data concerning PCa screening and treatment in older men calls for a thoughtful approach to evaluating such men for screening, diagnosis, and treatment options. This article offers guidance to an approach here.

The distinction between chronologic and physiologic age is a crucial one to make when counseling the older adult for screening and management decisions for PCa. There are older adults who stand to benefit from definitive intervention, and there are those whose functional and physiologic condition puts them at undo risk for burdensome side effects and a compromised quality of life (QOL). Increasing evidence suggests that comorbidity and functional loss, rather than chronologic age, best predict outcomes in PCa treatment.[6] Outcomes are best predicted when stratifying patients according to their health status as fit, vulnerable, or frail based on comorbidities, reversibility of health impairments, functional dependency status, and life expectancy.[7] Tools such as the CGA assist in categorizing patients according to their health status based on specific domains including comorbidity, nutritional status, cognition, social support, falls, and functional dependency. This review describes the age-specific considerations in screening practices, treatment options, and management decisions for the older man at risk for or facing a new diagnosis of PCa.

SCREENING

This section addresses the current level of evidence for or against screening for PCa with serum prostate-specific antigen (PSA) testing in older men and discusses issues important for shared decision making between the physician and patient regarding screening.

At present, the American Cancer Society, American Urological Association (AUA), and American College of Physicians recommend against screening in patients with a remaining life expectancy of less than 10 years,[8–10] because the expected mortality benefit from screening is estimated to occur only after approximately 10 years from the initial screening.[11,12] Of these organizations, only the AUA notes that healthy men in their 70s may have a life expectancy of 10 years or more and therefore may still benefit from screening.[10] Based on the recent randomized trials described in the following paragraphs, the United States Preventive Services Task Force currently recommends against routine screening for men of any age group.[4]

Among the major trials studying the efficacy of PSA testing for PCa screening, men older than 70 years have been largely excluded. The 2 very large, major randomized trials with the least risk of bias according to the Cochrane Collaboration are the United States-based Prostate, Lung, Colorectal, and Ovarian Cancer Screening (PLCO) trial (n = 77,000) and the European Randomised Study of Screening for Prostate Cancer (ERSPC) trial (n = 185,000), both of which included men up to the age of 75 years.[13] The PLCO trial, while noting a significant increase in the number of men diagnosed with PCa, did not demonstrate a significant reduction in PCa-specific or all-cause mortality.[14] Of note, over 50% of the men in the control arm of the trial received a PSA test, because that was left to the discretion of providers. The ERSPC trial, conducted in a variety of European countries, demonstrated a 21% relative reduction in PCa mortality at 13 years of follow-up; however, it was noted that the effect was confined to patients younger than 70 years.[11] Importantly, there were very few patients of African dissent in the sample. Meta-analyses including these 2 large trials along with several other smaller ones failed to demonstrate a reduction in either PCa-specific mortality or all-cause mortality.[13,15] As hypothesized, screening did increase the identification of early PCa.[15] However, 2 major trials of radical prostatectomy (RP), while showing overall mortality benefits for early PCa, failed to demonstrate a mortality benefit in men older than 65 years.[16,17]

Clearly, current evidence does not support a population-wide screening program in older men that would reduce mortality. Nevertheless, it is plausible that a subset of older men may derive benefit from screening, specifically patients with aggressive local tumors who would otherwise have a remaining life expectancy of greater than 10 years. Two validated predictive models for life expectancy have been developed in community-dwelling elderly patients, which use age, gender, body mass index, functional status, and comorbidities, but these tools are infrequently used in clinical practice for cancer screening[18–20]; this may be because of the number of elements necessary to calculate these indices. As an alternative, clinicians can consider use of simpler tools from the geriatrics literature including measurement of gait speed,[21] grip strength,[22] or self-assessed health[23] to assist in estimating life expectancy. For men of any age with a life expectancy exceeding 10 years, especially those with known risk factors for high-grade PCa (eg, first-degree relative with PCa, African American race), a shared decision should be made with their physician.

Another consideration is that mortality is unlikely to be the only, or even the most important, outcome that matters to patients. Morbidity due to advanced-stage PCa is typically a significant detriment to QOL. Based on a recent Cochrane Review meta-analysis, screening did reduce the risk of the diagnosis of advanced-stage PCa by 20%[13]; this is another important consideration when contemplating a screening decision for PCa.

In addition to explaining potential benefits to patients, clinicians should also advise their older patients about the potential harms related to screening. False-positive results were found in 12% to 13% of patients after 3 to 4 rounds of PSA testing,[24] which subjects those who opt for a biopsy to the unnecessary risk of fever, bleeding, infection, transient urinary difficulties, and psychological stress. Overdiagnosis, that is, identification of cancers that will not cause symptoms during a patient's lifetime, can range from 5% to 75%, with the percentage increasing with increasing age.[10] Overdiagnosis can result in harms associated with treatment including erectile dysfunction, urinary incontinence, bowel dysfunction, and a small risk of premature death.[4]

Rather limited evidence exists demonstrating ongoing routine screening of elderly patients for PCa, despite current guidelines. For example, a study of Veterans Affairs system patients found PSA screening rates of approximately 56% in men older than 70 years.[25] In a survey of American men screened with PSA, despite relatively high screening rates in older men with limited life expectancies, only 32% reported having a discussion of the risks associated with PSA testing.[26] There continue to be very high rates of screening, even among older men with limited life expectancies, perhaps as a consequence of clinicians emphasizing the benefits of screening over the risks.[27] Given the discrepancy between the current guideline recommendations and ongoing clinical practice, more detailed conversations about likely benefits and harms of screening between physician and patient are needed for achieving true shared decision making as recommended.[28]

LOCALIZED PROSTATE CANCER: MANAGEMENT OPTIONS

It must be kept in mind that although PCa is the second most deadly solid tumor among men, most patients diagnosed with the disease will die from some other cause.[29] Once a diagnosis of PCa has been made from a biopsy, a management strategy must be chosen. This strategy is based on balancing the benefits versus the risks from any intervention against the risks from disease progression. From a cancer perspective, the 2 most important distinctions to be made are: (1) the disease extent, that is whether the cancer is localized or not, and (2) how aggressive is the cancer, which is determined by the Gleason disease grade. From an aging perspective, it is important to determine the likely quality of a patient's survival from engaging in one of the available strategies. First, the management options for localized disease are considered, namely, active surveillance, surgery, and radiation therapy.

ACTIVE SURVEILLANCE

The decision to forgo definitive treatment and initiate a watchful waiting program is an important option for patients of any age with localized PCa, but especially for older, frailer men with limited life expectancies. Most men will not die from their PCa, and the decision to forgo definitive therapy is always made with the intention of maintaining the highest possible QOL, which may otherwise be compromised by overtreatment. However, with active surveillance, which is a program of monitoring disease status and intervening only if disease progresses rapidly, there is some risk of missing an opportunity for definitive therapy or preventing progression to advanced disease when both disease and treatment can be burdensome. In the context of observation, advanced age is shown to be an independent risk factor for disease progression.[30] Both the Prostate Cancer Intervention versus Observation Trial (PIVOT) and Scandinavian Prostate Cancer Group Study Number 4 (SPCG-4) failed to demonstrate significant survival benefit among older men assigned to RP versus surveillance. Furthermore, in the SPCG-4, survival benefit was only observed in men younger than 65 years with intermediate-risk disease after a prolonged follow-up of more than 15 years.[16] These findings provide reassurance on the safety of an active surveillance program.

Another consideration of active surveillance is the impact on a patient's emotions including regret. A systematic review of patients who chose localized treatment of their PCa found an inconsistent relationship between older age and posttreatment regret. There was an increase in feelings of regret in those who reported significant side effects such as sexual dysfunction.[31] It is important to keep in mind that older adults make up a heterogeneous population whose background health status varies significantly across patients, and the presence of age-associated issues such as comorbidities, functional status, frailty, and geriatric syndromes significantly increases the risk for having side effects from intervention. However, for those fit or vulnerable individuals with reversible syndromes or the ability to mitigate toxicities through interventions such as prehabilitation, there is a likely benefit from PCa treatment. Each decision should be made with careful consideration of treatment goals within the context of risks and benefits on a case-by-case basis. To that end, the discussion should include anticipated end points of active surveillance, such as regular monitoring, a plan for initiating definitive treatment with disease progression, or starting a palliative approach with a focus on symptoms management.

PROSTATECTOMY

Choosing definitive therapy for older adults with PCa is a difficult decision given that it is still relatively unclear who will derive benefit from treatment. RP is reserved for patients with localized disease whose life expectancy is estimated to exceed 10 years.[32] The survival benefit associated with RP has been observed only after an extended follow-up of several years.[11] In directing treatment decisions in older adults, emphasis should be placed first on estimating life expectancy in order to best predict who may or may not most likely derive survival benefits from surgery. Walter and Covinsky[33] recommend life-table-based, sex-specific life expectancy based on age and heath status, which is further divided into quartiles for decision making. Other models use functional assessments such as gait speed and grip strength to estimate life expectancy.[21–23]

Although generally well tolerated, RP does not come without the risk of complications and side effects, emphasizing the importance of understanding which older patients are at greatest risks for treatment side effects. Age and comorbidity are considered risk factors for 30-day postoperative complications, which occur in roughly 20% of all patients undergoing RP (odds ratio, 2.04; 95% confidence interval [CI], 1.22–3.39).[34] For other surgical interventions for solid tumors, including elective surgical treatment of colon and rectal tumors, components of the CGA such as instrumental activities of daily living dependency and poor performance status are reported to be predictive of 30-day postoperative complications (relative risk [RR], 1.43; 95% CI, 1.03–1.98 and RR, 1.64; 95% CI, 1.07–2.58, respectively).[35] Historically, chronologic age is used as consideration for candidacy for surgery. These data suggest that functional rather than chronologic age is most relevant for predicting outcomes. The historical reluctance to operate on adults based on high chronologic age contributes to the observation that some groups of fit older adults with low- and (especially) high-grade localized disease are undertreated with RP.[36] This observation even holds for those with similar life expectancies, in which older men with longer life expectancies are much less likely to be offered surgery.[37]

Older adults and those with comorbidities are less likely to receive RP.[38] Large retrospective studies suggest that increasing age is associated with increased overall and cancer-specific mortality among patients undergoing RP or surveillance.[39] Older age is also associated with a higher risk of postoperative biochemical recurrence following RP (hazard ratio [HR], 1.08; 95% CI, 1.03–1.14; P = .004).[40] There is debate regarding the use of RP in older patients. Surveillance Epidemiology and End Results Medicare data examining outcomes in men aged 65 to 80 years who underwent RP versus surveillance reported a 10-year cancer-specific survival benefit of 5.8% in those undergoing RP versus 1.8% in those undergoing observation (P<.001).[39] These results suggest a potential survival advantage for fit older men with long life expectancies from surgery, especially those with high-grade disease.

The 2 largest randomized studies that evaluated RP versus watchful waiting are the SPCG-4 and PIVOT.[16,17] Both studies included men aged up to 75 years with at least a 10-year estimated life expectancy and localized PCa. SPCG-4 reported a reduction in incidence of distant metastasis and requirement for androgen deprivation therapy (ADT) among patients aged 65 to 75 years receiving RP versus watchful waiting at 18-year follow-up (28.3% vs 32.7%, P = .04 and 40.9% vs 62.8%, P<.001, respectively).[16] However, SPCG-4 did not demonstrate an overall and cancer-specific survival benefit in patients aged 65 to 75 years who underwent RP versus watchful waiting at 18 years (69.8% vs 71.7%, P = .52 and 17.3% vs

23.9%, $P = .19$).[16] Similarly, PIVOT did not observe a benefit in overall and cancer-specific mortality among patients randomized to RP versus observation, regardless of age (47.0% vs 49.9%, $P = .22$ and 5.8% vs 8.4%, $P = .09$, respectively).[17] Based on these findings, the default for older men should be no surgery, especially for those with low-grade disease.

There is a dearth of quality data and long-term follow-up examining the efficacy of robot-assisted radical prostatectomy (RARP) in any patient population, including older adults. Early reports on RARP versus open RP (ORP) suggest advantages in several surgical domains including intraoperative transfusion rate, postoperative complications, shorter time to discharge, and time needed to have a catheter postsurgery.[41,42] In addition, in a prospective trial of 120 patients with localized disease randomized to either RARP or laparoscopic radical prostatectomy, a greater percentage of both continence and postsurgical potency were reported in patients undergoing RARP at 1-year follow-up (95% vs 83.3%, $P<.042$ and 80% vs 52.2%, $P<.02$, respectively).[43] Unlike reports in ORP in which older men are more likely to experience long-term post-operative incontinence, early data suggest similar rates of incontinence in older and younger men after RARP.[44] Kumar and colleagues[45] observed similar continence rates among patients aged 70 years or older (median age 72 years) and those aged 70 years or younger (median age 62 years) at 1 year after RARP (87.3% and 91.3%, $P = .07$). Similarly, incidence of biochemical recurrence at 3 and 5 years postoperatively was also observed to be similar, but differences in cancer-specific survival approached statistical significance at 5-year follow-up between patients aged 70 years or older and those aged 70 years or younger (biochemical recurrence: 81.1% and 91.1%, $P = .83$ and cancer-specific survival: 95.3% and 98.2%, $P = .06$, respectively).[45] It should be noted that this study included retrospective analysis from a single institution of 3241 consecutive cases completed by a single surgeon. How this generalizes to other groups and other settings is not clear.

Like most data evaluating efficacy and outcomes of RARP, the studied patient population consists mostly of patients younger than 70 years. Whether or not these results are generalizable to older adults is unknown, but early data are encouraging that RARP may be associated with fewer complications and poor surgical outcomes than open or laparoscopic techniques. High-quality randomized studies are needed to characterize long-term oncologic outcomes, particularly in older adults who would stand to benefit from the potential advantages of this approach.

RADIOTHERAPY

External beam radiation therapy (EBRT) is another option to actively treat localized PCa. Although there are no high-quality head-to-head studies of EBRT versus RP, the general consensus is that they are equivalent with regard to overall survival for localized disease. Therefore, the choice between the 2 now rests on the side effect profile. EBRT is associated with less urinary incontinence and sexual dysfunction than RP; however, rates of bowel and bladder inflammation are higher with EBRT.[46] Adding ADT to radiotherapy augments treatment efficacy with some detriment to QOL, particularly among patients with high-risk local disease.[47] A recent randomized study demonstrated improvement in overall survival on adding long-term (2 years) versus short-term (6 months) adjuvant ADT to radiotherapy over a 63-month follow-up period for patients with intermediate- or high-risk localized disease (HR, 2.48; 95% CI, 1.31–4.68; $P = .009$]).[48] Once again, these data are primarily for fit, younger men; it is less clear what the benefits are for less-fit older men with more indolent disease, given the known risks of ADT, as described below.

Randomized studies are needed to better evaluate differences in efficacy and risks between RP, radiation therapy, and active surveillance. In addition, as new radiation therapy techniques such as intensity-modulated radiotherapy and proton therapy become more ubiquitous, rigorous testing is needed to determine its role in treating localized PCa in older men. For patients with painful osseous metastasis, local targeted radiation therapy serves an important palliative role. As always, the focus in choosing treatment rests on matching the risk/benefit profile to patient preferences to maximize the quality of survival.

ANDROGEN DEPRIVATION THERAPY

PCa is an androgen-dependent tumor. An important strategy for treating PCa, especially high-grade and later-stage disease is to lower the levels of androgens such as testosterone to castrate levels; this can be done though surgery, via orchiectomy, or with endocrine therapies, which lower the levels of downstream androgens such as testosterone through a pituitary-mediated mechanism.[49] ADT is indicated in localized PCa as adjuvant, neoadjuvant, or concomitant along with radiation therapy, or as first-line systemic therapy for advanced disease. ADT is neither shown to be effective nor currently recommended for early, low-stage PCa.[50]

QOL considerations are especially important in older patients considering the use of ADT. Therapy is associated with several well-documented QOL-affecting toxicities including hot flashes, emotional lability, headaches, and nausea and vomiting.[51] In addition, ADT is associated with increased risks for toxicities that are particularly dangerous in elderly patients. For example, men on ADT are at an increased risk for loss of bone mineral density and subsequent fracture. There is a 6.8% ($P<.001$), dose-dependent increase in the osteoporotic fracture incidence in men with PCa on ADT compared with those who did not receive ADT over a 5-year period.[52] Pretreatment assessment of bone mineral density using dual-energy X-ray absorptiometry (DEXA) scans allows practitioners to assess fracture risk and assists in treatment decision making. Calcium and vitamin D supplementation may ameliorate some of this risk, but randomized studies are needed to verify any added benefit. Bone-targeting agents such as bisphosphonates or denosumab are shown to prevent loss of bone mineral density in patients on ADT.[53,54] However, these agents come with the risk of severe hypocalcemia, neutropenia, nephropathy, and osteonecrosis of the jaw and should primarily be used in high-fracture-risk, nonmetastatic disease.[7] Baseline DEXA scans and dental assessments before the initiation of ADT are recommended to avoid these important toxicities.

Bisphosphonates and denosumab also possess an important role in the prevention of pathologic fractures in patients with osseous metastasis. Both denosumab and zolendronic acid have been shown to increase the time to a skeletal-related event such as fracture and lead to improved pain scores, while not impacting overall survival in patients with metastatic PCa.[55,56] However, zolendronic acid does not decrease the time to osseous metastasis in patients with high-risk localized PCa.[57] These bone-modifying agents are important tools in treating the patient with PCa with osseous metastasis, regardless of treatment with ADT. Pain control and prevention of skeletal-related events preserve both QOL and functional independence. Close monitoring of dental hygiene, laboratory values, and side effects are important components of treatment.

There is a growing body of evidence suggesting a link between ADT, heart disease, and diabetes.[58] In a large retrospective study of men older than 66 years (mean 74.2 years), an increase was found in incident diabetes (HR, 1.44; CI,

1.34–1.55; $P<.001$), incident heart disease (HR, 1.16; CI, 1.10–1.21; $P<.001$), myocardial infarction (MI) (HR, 1.11; CI, 1.10–1.21; $P = .03$), and sudden cardiac death (HR, 1.16; CI, 1.05–1.27; $P = .004$).[59] This risk was observed as early as a few months after initiating ADT. Interestingly, in a large retrospective study, patients with high-risk PCa and underlying congestive heart failure or history of MI experienced greater all-cause mortality on ADT + brachytherapy versus brachytherapy alone over a 5-year period (22.7% vs 11.6%, respectively).[60] Furthermore, the association of cardiovascular disease and ADT may be more pronounced in older adults and those with comorbidities.[61] Care must be taken when using ADT in patients with preexisting heart disease or diabetes, and these comorbidities must be actively managed after ADT is started.

Sarcopenia, age-related loss of muscle mass and function, is of growing interest among men being treated with ADT. Within several months of initiating ADT, patients are observed to lose significant mass in lower extremity load-bearing muscles.[62] This decrease in muscle mass contributes, in part, to decreases in physical function, decreased QOL, and reports of fatigue among patients on ADT. In addition, men older than 70 years are at a higher risk of falls when on ADT, which is an important precursor to fractures.[63] For older adults, ADT can accelerate the development of frailty,[64] particularly obese frailty.[65] These observations warrant careful consideration when placing a frail older adult on ADT.

For those adults who are good candidates for ADT, but are vulnerable and exhibit poor functional status, there is increasing evidence that resistance training can ameliorate muscle loss and the symptoms associated with muscle loss during ADT.[66,67] Patients on ADT who were randomized to resistance training versus stretching exercises experienced an improvement in muscle strength ($P<.032$), self-reported physical functioning ($P<.01$), and a trend toward improvement in fatigue ($P = .06$).[68] These data suggest that physical therapy intervention not only improves QOL among older adults on ADT but also aids in the preservation of physical function and independence. Developing a model of team-based care is important for patients on ADT. The participation of occupational and physical therapy is critical not only for identifying those patients at risk for functional decline but also for initiating programs to ameliorate symptoms associated with muscle loss. The emphasis in this care is in proactive and not reactive intervention.

Changes in cognition are common among older adults, and often co-occur with PCa. At present, there is debate regarding changes in cognition in the setting of ADT. Much of the work thus far has been completed within the confines of small sample size and observational design of studies.[69] Using a battery of cognitive tests, a worse performance in memory, attention, and information processing was observed among a small cohort (n = 33) of men on ADT versus patients with PCa who were not on ADT.[70] In a similar-sized cohort, no deficits in verbal or visuospatial functioning were found among a group of patients on ADT over a 6-month follow-up.[71] There are no robust clinical studies to date examining the relationship between ADT and changes in cognition, particularly among older adults with preexisting cognitive impairment. Changes in fatigue and mood, which are documented to worsen in some patients on ADT, may manifest differently in older adults with underlying memory problems.[72] It is important to assess all older patients for preexisting cognitive impairment before starting ADT, in part to compare later concerns with their baseline functioning.

ADT remains a powerful tool in the arsenal of PCa therapy in the older adult. For appropriate patients, it slows the growth of cancer, reduces pain, and delays the progression of disease. However, treatment comes with considerable risk from toxicities. Options for reducing side effects include using an intermittent schedule of therapy, with ADT vacations to recover strength and stamina, which has been shown to improve QOL, but with a possible decrease in survival benefit in the context of metastatic disease.[73] Discussion of risk factors is a critical component of treatment planning in the older adult. Of equal importance is the establishment of supportive care and physical therapy intervention to mitigate risk of treatment, optimize QOL, and ensure treatment benefit.

CHEMOTHERAPY

Systemic chemotherapy is indicated in those with metastatic disease who fail hormonal therapy or is used as first-line treatment for patients with castrate-naive, high-volume metastatic disease.[50] The Tax 327 study observed a 2.9-month increase in median survival in patients with symptomatic metastatic disease who receive a triweekly regimen of docetaxel-based chemotherapy versus mitoxantrone (HR, 0.79; 95% CI, 0.67–0.93; $P = .004$). Subgroup analysis reported similar results in patients aged 75 years and older (HR, 0.80).[74] However, those aged 75 or older were also shown to have higher incidence of infection and need for dose reduction because of toxicity.[74,75]

There are little data examining the benefit and risks associated with docetaxel treatment in octogenarians with metastatic PCa. A small retrospective study of 20 men aged 80 years or older, (median age of 83 years [80–93 years]) with metastatic Castrate-Resistant Prostate Cancer (mCRPC), observed a median overall survival of 13.4 months. Of those treated, 40% completed the full treatment course (60% dose modification) and 45% endured a grade 3 to 4 toxicity.[75] It should be noted that patients included in this study had Eastern Cooperative Oncology Group (ECOG) scores of 0 or 1, highlighting the need for a better understanding of treatment feasibility in vulnerable or frail older adults.

The choice to initiate chemotherapy in an older adult is often a difficult one, because many older adults have comorbidities and geriatric syndromes making them more susceptible to toxicity. For example, older patients on docetaxel are more likely to experience treatment-related febrile neutropenia than younger counterparts (HR, 5.77; $P = .004$).[76,77] Adults aged 75 years or older with poor physical performance (ECOG $\geq$2) experience less overall survival benefit from docetaxel for CRPC than healthier patients of their age group (HR, 3.02; 1.85–4.90; $P<.001$).[78,79] Performance status also predicted a higher incidence of grade 3 and 4 toxicities.[78]

There are several ongoing randomized trials evaluating the efficacy of adding docetaxel to ADT as first-line treatment of metastatic castrate-sensitive PCa or high-risk locally advanced disease. A recent randomized trial demonstrated an improved relapse-free survival among patients (median age 63 years, 47–77 years) with localized high-risk disease treated with docetaxel + ADT versus those treated with ADT alone (adjusted HR, 0.71; 95% CI, 0.54–0.94; $P = .017$). Preliminary data in the Systemic Therapy in Advancing or Metastatic Prostate cancer: Evaluation of Drug Efficacy (STAMPEDE) trial observed a median overall survival benefit of docetaxel + ADT of 10 months (HR, 0.76; 95% CI, 0.63–0.91; $P = .003$) versus standard of care.[80] Of note, the median age of patients in this study is 65 years, and among those randomized to the docetaxel + ADT arm, 50% experienced a grade 3 to 5 toxicity versus 31% patients receiving standard of care (no P value available).[80] Certainly, more work is needed in this area to clarify the benefit of adding docetaxel to ADT for high-risk locally advanced PCa and mCRPC. In addition, it is important to consider the generalizability of such results to older adults, especially considering the high incidence of grade 3 to 5 toxicity reported among a relatively younger, fitter study population.

Treatment side effects and chemotherapy-related toxicity can negatively affect QOL in these patients, and for some, premature discontinuation of treatment regimen is required precluding any benefit. Older patients with dependency in areas of function often also experience further loss of independence while on chemotherapy.[81] Furthermore, neurotoxic effects of docetaxel predisposes older patients to fall-related injury.[82] Frank discussion regarding the patient's own goals of care including level of acceptance to requiring increased level of support and possible institutionalization while on therapy are critical aspects of treatment planning.

The CGA has shown to be an important tool for identifying any areas of vulnerability in patients considering treatment and recommended by the International Society of Geriatric Oncology for all older adults with PCa.[7] The CGA evaluates for several aspects of health and wellness including physical functioning, social support, nutritional status, fall history, depression, cognitive impairment, and level of independence. In addition to identifying geriatric syndromes and revealing potential risk with treatment, the CGA also serves to elucidate areas of opportunity for intervention and support while on treatment.

SUMMARY

Treatment of PCa for older men is best considered in the context of one's physiologic and not chronologic age. There are resources available to health care providers to best quantify one's physiologic age including the CGA. In addition to directing candidacy for treatment or modifying treatment, the CGA also identifies areas in which targeted interventions will benefit the older man with PCa. Most importantly, a goal-centric approach to treatment planning is critical in counseling and directing therapy for the older adult in a shared decision-making context.

REFERENCES

1. Estimated number of new cancer cases and deaths by sex, US. Atlanta, GA: American Cancer Society; 2015. Available at: http://www.cancer.org/research/cancerfactsstatistics/cancerfactsfigures2015/index.
2. Howlader N, Noone AM, Krapcho M, et al. SEER Cancer Statistics Review, 1975-2008. Report based on November 2010 SEER data submission, posted to the SEER web site. Bethesda, MD: National Cancer Institute; 2011. Available at. http://seer.cancer.gov/csr/1975_2008/.
3. Hampson LA, Cowan JE, Zhao S, et al. Impact of age on quality-of-life outcomes after treatment for localized prostate cancer. Eur Urol 2015;68(3):480–6.
4. Moyer VA, U.S. Preventive Services Task Force. Screening for prostate cancer: U.S. Preventive Services Task Force recommendation statement. Ann Intern Med 2012;157(2):120–34.
5. Herrera AP, Snipes SA, King DW, et al. Disparate inclusion of older adults in clinical trials: priorities and opportunities for policy and practice change. Am J Public Health 2010;100(Suppl 1):S105–12.
6. Rider JR, Sandin F, Andrén O, et al. Long-term outcomes among noncuratively treated men according to prostate cancer risk category in a nationwide, population-based study. Eur Urol 2013;63(1):88–96.
7. Droz JP, Aapro M, Balducci L, et al. Management of prostate cancer in older patients: updated recommendations of a working group of the International Society of Geriatric Oncology. Lancet Oncol 2014;15(9):e404–14.

8. Qaseem A, Barry MJ, Denberg TD, et al. Screening for prostate cancer: a guidance statement from the Clinical Guidelines Committee of the American College of Physicians. Ann Intern Med 2013;158(10):761–9.
9. Wolf AM, Wender RC, Etzioni RB, et al. American Cancer Society guideline for the early detection of prostate cancer: update 2010. CA Cancer J Clin 2010;60(2):70–98.
10. Carter HB, Albertsen PC, Barry MJ, et al. Early detection of prostate cancer: AUA Guideline. J Urol 2013;190(2):419–26.
11. Schroder FH, Hugosson J, Roobol MJ, et al. Screening and prostate cancer mortality: results of the European Randomised Study of Screening for Prostate Cancer (ERSPC) at 13 years of follow-up. Lancet 2014;384(9959):2027–35.
12. Hugosson J, Carlsson S, Aus G, et al. Mortality results from the Goteborg randomised population-based prostate-cancer screening trial. Lancet Oncol 2010; 11(8):725–32.
13. Ilic D, Neuberger MM, Djulbegovic M, et al. Screening for prostate cancer. Cochrane Database Syst Rev 2013;(1):CD004720.
14. Andriole GL, Crawford ED, Grubb RL 3rd, et al. Prostate cancer screening in the randomized Prostate, Lung, Colorectal, and Ovarian Cancer Screening Trial: mortality results after 13 years of follow-up. J Natl Cancer Inst 2012;104(2):125–32.
15. Djulbegovic M, Beyth RJ, Neuberger MM, et al. Screening for prostate cancer: systematic review and meta-analysis of randomised controlled trials. BMJ 2010;341. c4543.
16. Bill-Axelson A, Holmberg L, Garmo H, et al. Radical prostatectomy or watchful waiting in early prostate cancer. N Engl J Med 2014;370(10):932–42.
17. Wilt TJ, Brawer MK, Jones KM, et al. Radical prostatectomy versus observation for localized prostate cancer. N Engl J Med 2012;367(3):203–13.
18. Lee SJ, Lindquist K, Segal MR, et al. Development and validation of a prognostic index for 4-year mortality in older adults. JAMA 2006;295(7):801–8.
19. Schonberg MA, Davis RB, McCarthy EP, et al. Index to predict 5-year mortality of community-dwelling adults aged 65 and older using data from the National Health Interview Survey. J Gen Intern Med 2009;24(10):1115–22.
20. Schonberg MA, Davis RB, McCarthy EP, et al. External validation of an index to predict up to 9-year mortality of community-dwelling adults aged 65 and older. J Am Geriatr Soc 2011;59(8):1444–51.
21. Studenski S, Perera S, Patel K, et al. Gait speed and survival in older adults. JAMA 2011;305(1):50–8.
22. Leong DP, Teo KK, Rangarajan S, et al. Prognostic value of grip strength: findings from the Prospective Urban Rural Epidemiology (PURE) study. Lancet 2015;386: 266–73.
23. Kotwal AA, Mohile SG, Dale W. Remaining life expectancy measurement and PSA screening of older men. J Geriatr Oncol 2012;3(3):196–204.
24. Chou R, Croswell JM, Dana T, et al. Screening for prostate cancer: a review of the evidence for the U.S. Preventive Services Task Force. Ann Intern Med 2011; 155(11):762–71.
25. Walter LC, Bertenthal D, Lindquist K, et al. PSA screening among elderly men with limited life expectancies. JAMA 2006;296(19):2336–42.
26. Hoffman RM, Couper MP, Zikmund-Fisher BJ, et al. Prostate cancer screening decisions: results from the National Survey of Medical Decisions (DECISIONS study). Arch Intern Med 2009;169(17):1611–8.
27. Drazer MW, Prasad SM, Huo D, et al. National trends in prostate cancer screening among older American men with limited 9-year life expectancies: evidence of an increased need for shared decision making. Cancer 2014;120(10):1491–8.

28. Dale W. Prostate cancer: PSA testing in older men–are we following the guidelines? Nat Rev Urol 2012;9(7):357–8.

29. Fung C, Dale W, Mohile SG. Prostate cancer in the elderly patient. J Clin Oncol 2014;32(24):2523–30.

30. Margel D, Nandy I, Wilson TH, et al. Predictors of pathological progression among men with localized prostate cancer undergoing active surveillance: a sub-analysis of the REDEEM study. J Urol 2013;190(6):2039–45.

31. Christie DR, Sharpley CF, Bitsika V. Why do patients regret their prostate cancer treatment? A systematic review of regret after treatment for localized prostate cancer. Psychooncology 2015. [Epub ahead of print].

32. Novara G, Ficarra V, D'Elia C, et al. Prospective evaluation with standardised criteria for postoperative complications after robotic-assisted laparoscopic radical prostatectomy. Eur Urol 2010;57(3):363–70.

33. Walter LC, Covinsky KE. Cancer screening in elderly patients. JAMA 2001; 285(21):2750.

34. Alibhai SM, Leach M, Tomlinson G, et al. 30-day mortality and major complications after radical prostatectomy: influence of age and comorbidity. J Natl Cancer Inst 2005;97(20):1525–32.

35. PACE Participants, Audisio RA, Pope D, et al. Shall we operate? Preoperative assessment in elderly cancer patients (PACE) can help. A SIOG surgical task force prospective study. Crit Rev Oncol Hematol 2008;65(2):156–63.

36. Schwartz KL, Alibhai SM, Tomlinson G, et al. Continued undertreatment of older men with localized prostate cancer. Urology 2003;62(5):860–5.

37. Alibhai SM, Krahn MD, Cohen MM, et al. Is there age bias in the treatment of localized prostate carcinoma? Cancer 2004;100(1):72–81.

38. Schymura MJ, Kahn AR, German RR, et al. Factors associated with initial treatment and survival for clinically localized prostate cancer: results from the CDC-NPCR Patterns of Care Study (PoC1). BMC Cancer 2010;10:152.

39. Abdollah F, Sun M, Schmitges J, et al. Cancer-specific and other-cause mortality after radical prostatectomy versus observation in patients with prostate cancer: competing-risks analysis of a large North American population-based cohort. Eur Urol 2011;60(5):920–30.

40. Kane CJ, Im R, Amling CL, et al. Outcomes after radical prostatectomy among men who are candidates for active surveillance: results from the SEARCH database. Urology 2010;76(3):695–700.

41. De Carlo F, Celestino F, Verri C, et al. Retropubic, laparoscopic, and robot-assisted radical prostatectomy: surgical, oncological, and functional outcomes: a systematic review. Urol Int 2014;93(4):373–83.

42. Pilecki MA, McGuire BB, Jain U, et al. National multi-institutional comparison of 30-day postoperative complication and readmission rates between open retropubic radical prostatectomy and robot-assisted laparoscopic prostatectomy using NSQIP. J Endourol 2014;28(4):430–6.

43. Porpiglia F, Morra I, Lucci Chiarissi M, et al. Randomised controlled trial comparing laparoscopic and robot-assisted radical prostatectomy. Eur Urol 2013;63(4):606–14.

44. Basto MY, Vidyasagar C, te Marvelde L, et al. Early urinary continence recovery after robot-assisted radical prostatectomy in older Australian men. BJU Int 2014; 114(Suppl 1):29–33.

45. Kumar A, Samavedi S, Bates AS, et al. Age stratified comparative analysis of perioperative, functional and oncologic outcomes in patients after robot assisted

radical prostatectomy - a propensity score matched study. Eur J Surg Oncol 2015;41(7):837–43.

46. Frank SJ, Pisters LL, Davis J, et al. An assessment of quality of life following radical prostatectomy, high dose external beam radiation therapy and brachytherapy iodine implantation as monotherapies for localized prostate cancer. J Urol 2007;177(6):2151–6 [discussion: 2156].

47. Grant JD, Litwin MS, Kwan L, et al. Does hormone therapy exacerbate the adverse effects of radiotherapy in men with prostate cancer? A quality of life study. J Urol 2011;185(5):1674–80.

48. Zapatero A, Guerrero A, Maldonado X, et al. High-dose radiotherapy with short-term or long-term androgen deprivation in localised prostate cancer (DART01/05 GICOR): a randomised, controlled, phase 3 trial. Lancet Oncol 2015;16(3):320–7.

49. Mohler JL. Concept and viability of androgen annihilation for advanced prostate cancer. Cancer 2014;120(17):2628–37.

50. Mohler J, Bahnson RR, Boston B, et al. NCCN clinical practice guidelines in oncology: prostate cancer. J Natl Compr Canc Netw 2010;8(2):162–200.

51. Cancado BL, Miranda LC, Madeira M, et al. Importance of bone assessment and prevention of osteoporotic fracture in patients with prostate cancer in the gonadotropic hormone analogues use. Rev Col Bras Cir 2015;42(1):62–6.

52. Shahinian VB, Kuo YF, Freeman JL, et al. Risk of fracture after androgen deprivation for prostate cancer. N Engl J Med 2005;352(2):154–64.

53. Smith MR, Saad F, Egerdie B, et al. Effects of denosumab on bone mineral density in men receiving androgen deprivation therapy for prostate cancer. J Urol 2009;182(6):2670–5.

54. Klotz LH, McNeill IY, Kebabdjian M, et al. A phase 3, double-blind, randomised, parallel-group, placebo-controlled study of oral weekly alendronate for the prevention of androgen deprivation bone loss in nonmetastatic prostate cancer: the Cancer and Osteoporosis Research with Alendronate and Leuprolide (CORAL) study. Eur Urol 2013;63(5):927–35.

55. Saad F, Gleason DM, Murray R, et al. A randomized, placebo-controlled trial of zoledronic acid in patients with hormone-refractory metastatic prostate carcinoma. J Natl Cancer Inst 2002;94(19):1458–68.

56. Henry D, Vadhan-Raj S, Hirsh V, et al. Delaying skeletal-related events in a randomized phase 3 study of denosumab versus zoledronic acid in patients with advanced cancer: an analysis of data from patients with solid tumors. Support Care Cancer 2014;22(3):679–87.

57. Wirth M, Tammela T, Cicalese V, et al. Prevention of bone metastases in patients with high-risk nonmetastatic prostate cancer treated with zoledronic acid: efficacy and safety results of the Zometa European Study (ZEUS). Eur Urol 2015; 67(3):482–91.

58. Bosco C, Bosnyak Z, Malmberg A, et al. Quantifying observational evidence for risk of fatal and nonfatal cardiovascular disease following androgen deprivation therapy for prostate cancer: a meta-analysis. Eur Urol 2014;14:1222–6.

59. Keating NL, O'Malley AJ, Smith MR. Diabetes and cardiovascular disease during androgen deprivation therapy for prostate cancer. J Clin Oncol 2006;24(27):4448–56.

60. Nguyen PL, Chen MH, Beckman JA, et al. Influence of androgen deprivation therapy on all-cause mortality in men with high-risk prostate cancer and a history of congestive heart failure or myocardial infarction. Int J Radiat Oncol Biol Phys 2012;82(4):1411–6.

61. Morgans AK, Fan KH, Koyama T, et al. Influence of age on incident diabetes and cardiovascular disease in prostate cancer survivors receiving androgen deprivation therapy. J Urol 2015;193(4):1226–31.
62. Chang D, Joseph DJ, Ebert MA, et al. Effect of androgen deprivation therapy on muscle attenuation in men with prostate cancer. J Med Imaging Radiat Oncol 2014;58(2):223–8.
63. Bylow K, Dale W, Mustian K, et al. Falls and physical performance deficits in older patients with prostate cancer undergoing androgen deprivation therapy. Urology 2008;72(2):422–7.
64. Bylow K, Mohile SG, Stadler WM, et al. Does androgen-deprivation therapy accelerate the development of frailty in older men with prostate cancer?: a conceptual review. Cancer 2007;110(12):2604–13.
65. Bylow K, Hemmerich J, Mohile SG, et al. Obese frailty, physical performance deficits, and falls in older men with biochemical recurrence of prostate cancer on androgen deprivation therapy: a case-control study. Urology 2011;77(4):934–40.
66. Galvao DA, Taaffe DR, Spry N, et al. Combined resistance and aerobic exercise program reverses muscle loss in men undergoing androgen suppression therapy for prostate cancer without bone metastases: a randomized controlled trial. J Clin Oncol 2010;28(2):340–7.
67. Gardner JR, Livingston PM, Fraser SF. Effects of exercise on treatment-related adverse effects for patients with prostate cancer receiving androgen-deprivation therapy: a systematic review. J Clin Oncol 2014;32(4):335–46.
68. Winters-Stone KM, Dobek JC, Bennett JA, et al. Resistance training reduces disability in prostate cancer survivors on androgen deprivation therapy: evidence from a randomized controlled trial. Arch Phys Med Rehabil 2015;96(1):7–14.
69. Jamadar RJ, Winters MJ, Maki PM. Cognitive changes associated with ADT: a review of the literature. Asian J Androl 2012;14(2):232–8.
70. Yang J, Zhong F, Qiu J, et al. Cognitive function in Chinese prostate cancer patients on androgen-deprivation therapy: a cross-sectional study. Asia Pac J Clin Oncol 2015. [Epub ahead of print].
71. Mohile SG, Lacy M, Rodin M, et al. Cognitive effects of androgen deprivation therapy in an older cohort of men with prostate cancer. Crit Rev Oncol Hematol 2010; 75(2):152–9.
72. Bourke L, Boorjian SA, Briganti A, et al. Survivorship and improving quality of life in men with prostate cancer. Eur Urol 2015. [Epub ahead of print].
73. Alva A, Hussain M. Intermittent androgen deprivation therapy in advanced prostate cancer. Curr Treat Options Oncol 2014;15(1):127–36.
74. Berthold DR, Pond GR, Soban F, et al. Docetaxel plus prednisone or mitoxantrone plus prednisone for advanced prostate cancer: updated survival in the TAX 327 study. J Clin Oncol 2008;26(2):242–5.
75. Wong H-L, Lok SW, Wong S, et al. Docetaxel in very elderly men with metastatic castration-resistant prostate cancer. Prostate Int 2015;3(2):42–6.
76. Shigeta K, Kosaka T, Yazawa S, et al. Predictive factors for severe and febrile neutropenia during docetaxel chemotherapy for castration-resistant prostate cancer. Int J Clin Oncol 2015;20(3):605–12.
77. Leibowitz-Amit R, Templeton AJ, Alibhai SM, et al. Efficacy and toxicity of abiraterone and docetaxel in octogenarians with metastatic castration-resistant prostate cancer. J Geriatr Oncol 2015;6(1):23–8.
78. Italiano A, Ortholan C, Oudard S, et al. Docetaxel-based chemotherapy in elderly patients (age 75 and older) with castration-resistant prostate cancer. Eur Urol 2009;55(6):1368–75.

79. Fizazi K, Faivre L, Lesaunier F, et al. Androgen deprivation therapy plus docetaxel and estramustine versus androgen deprivation therapy alone for high-risk localised prostate cancer (GETUG 12): a phase 3 randomised controlled trial. Lancet Oncol 2015;16(7):787–94.

80. James ND, Mason SM, Clarke NW, et al. Docetaxel and/or zoledronic acid for hormone-naïve prostate cancer: first overall survival results from STAMPEDE (NCT00268476). J Clin Oncol 2015;33(15 Suppl):2001, 2015 ASCO Annual Meeting. [abstract: 5001].

81. Hoppe S, Rainfray M, Fonck M, et al. Functional decline in older patients with cancer receiving first-line chemotherapy. J Clin Oncol 2013;31(31):3877–82.

82. Ward PR, Wong MD, Moore R, et al. Fall-related injuries in elderly cancer patients treated with neurotoxic chemotherapy: a retrospective cohort study. J Geriatr Oncol 2014;5(1):57–64.

Late-Onset Hypogonadism and Testosterone Replacement in Older Men

 CrossMark

Rajib K. Bhattacharya, MD[a],*, Shelley B. Bhattacharya, DO, MPH[b]

KEYWORDS

- Hypogonadism • Osteoporosis • Geriatric • Testosterone • Management
- Treatment

KEY POINTS

- Late-onset hypogonadism is defined as a syndrome in men of advancing age. This syndrome is underdiagnosed, often untreated and is characterized by a deficiency of serum testosterone.
- Testosterone level decline begins at the age of 30, with a 1% annual gradual, age-related process. Men older than 65 have an age-associated increase in levels of sex-hormone-binding globulin (SHBG), which results in a disproportionately faster decline in free testosterone levels.
- Having clinical signs of low testosterone levels does not necessarily correlate to hypogonadal laboratory levels. Multiple comorbidities such as polypharmacy, depression, social isolation, recent loss, thyroid, and cardiovascular disease can affect the clinical presentation.
- The most widely accepted biochemical evaluation of male hypogonadism is from the Endocrine Society guidelines published in 2010. These guidelines do not recommend routine testing of older men for low testosterone levels without clinical signs or symptoms.
- The initiation of treatment of late-onset hypogonadism should be considered at or below a testosterone level of 200 ng/dL. The target for older men's total testosterone levels should be between 300 and 400 ng/dL. This target is lower than the traditional targets recommended for younger men of 500 to 600 ng/dL.
- The major goal of treatment in this population is to treat some of the symptoms related to hypogonadism, but recent concerns related to side effects of testosterone replacement need to be considered.

[a] Department of Internal Medicine, Division of Endocrinology and Metabolism, University of Kansas School of Medicine, 4023 Wescoe, Mailstop 2024, 3901 Rainbow Boulevard, Kansas City, KS 66160, USA; [b] Department of Family Medicine, Division of Geriatric Medicine, University of Kansas School of Medicine, 3901 Rainbow Boulevard, Kansas City, KS 66160, USA
* Corresponding author.
E-mail address: rbhattacharya@kumc.edu

Clin Geriatr Med 31 (2015) 631–644
http://dx.doi.org/10.1016/j.cger.2015.07.001
0749-0690/15/$ – see front matter © 2015 Elsevier Inc. All rights reserved.
geriatric.theclinics.com

INTRODUCTION

Late-life-onset hypogonadism (LLOH) is defined as a syndrome in men of advancing age. This syndrome is underdiagnosed and often untreated, and it is characterized by a deficiency in serum testosterone levels.[1] The clinical signs of relative androgen loss in older men are a decrease in muscle mass and strength, a decrease in bone mass, osteoporosis, and an increase in central body fat. These signs are not specific to androgen loss but can be markers to suggest testosterone deficiency. Additional symptoms include decreased libido, insomnia, difficulty concentrating, loss of memory, and depression. Consequently, these can result in a reduced quality of life and can adversely affect the function of multiple organ systems.[2] This situation is especially concerning because this cohort is rising dramatically. It is estimated that only 5% of affected men are currently treated.[3] LLOH is an easily treated condition, and, when treated, dire consequences can be prevented or reduced. Prospective population-based studies show that in the past decade, low testosterone levels have been associated with an increased risk for developing type 2 diabetes mellitus and manifestations of the metabolic syndrome.[4]

DEMOGRAPHY

By 2020, approximately 20% of the United States population will be older than 65 years and the size of the population older than 85 years is expected to double to 7 million.[5] The population older than 65 years will rise from 40 million in 2010, to 55 million in 2020, and 72 million by 2030.[6]

Decline in testosterone levels begins at the age of 30 years, with a 1% annual gradual, age-related process. Men older than 65 years have an age-associated increase in levels of SHBG, which results in a disproportionately faster decline in free testosterone levels. In the largest cross-sectional study to date, the European Male Aging Study (EMAS), 3220 men aged 40 to 79 years had an annual decline in their serum total testosterone levels of 0.4% and free testosterone levels of 1.3%.[7] According to the Baltimore Longitudinal Study, by the age of 80 years, 30% of men had total testosterone values in the hypogonadal range and 50% had low free testosterone values (**Fig. 1**).[8] The rate of age-related decline varies and is affected by multiple factors including medications and chronic disease.

Having clinical signs of low testosterone levels does not necessarily correlate to hypogonadal laboratory levels. Many men are not symptomatic with low testosterone levels, and men with normal levels may exhibit decreased libido or other signs of hypogonadism.[9] Multiple comorbidities such as depression, social isolation, recent loss, thyroid abnormalities, and cardiovascular disease can affect the clinical presentation.

EVALUATION

The evaluation for late-onset hypogonadism is initiated when signs and symptoms suggesting testosterone deficiency are apparent.[10,11] These symptoms usually are low libido, decrease in muscle mass, mild anemia, fatigue, decrease in erections, and others.[11] Clinically, this information can be gathered easily from the Androgen Deficiency in Aging Males (ADAM) questionnaire (**Box 1**).[12,13]

The patient needs to be evaluated for several other syndromes with similar side effects such as hypothyroidism, depression, nephrotic syndrome, long-term glucocorticoid use, and other long-term illnesses.[11,14] There are medications that have been

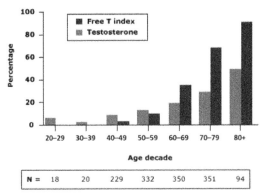

Fig. 1. Incidence of hypogonadism with each 10-year interval. Bar height indicates the percentage of men in each 10-year interval, from the third to the ninth decades, with at least one total testosterone (T) level less than 325 ng/dL (11.3 nmol/L) (*light bars*) or T/SHBG (free T index) less than 0.153 nmol/L (*dark bars*). The fraction of men who are hypogonadal increases progressively after the age of 50 years by either criterion. More men are hypogonadal by free T index than by total T after the age of 50 years. The number of men studied in each decade is noted below the graph. (*Adapted from* Harman SM, Metter EJ, Tobin JD, et al. Longitudinal effects of aging on serum total and free testosterone levels in healthy men. Baltimore Longitudinal Study of Aging. J Clin Endocrinol Metab 2001;86(2):727.)

associated with adverse affects on the hypothalamic-pituitary-gonadal axis, which include opiates, high-dose glucocorticoids, methadone, gonadotropin-releasing hormone, and others. These drugs need be evaluated and discussed with the patient before initiating the hypogonadal evaluation of patients.[11,14]

Box 1
Androgen Deficiency in Aging Males (ADAM) questionnaire

1. Do you have a decrease in libido or sex drive?

2. Do you have a lack of energy?

3. Do you have a decrease in strength or endurance?

4. Have you lost weight?

5. Have you noticed a decreased enjoyment of life?

6. Are you sad or grumpy?

7. Are your erections less strong?

8. Have you noticed a recent deterioration in your ability to play sports?

9. Are you falling asleep after dinner?

10. Has there been a recent deterioration in your work performance?

A positive result in ADAM questionnaire was defined as "Yes" for questions 1 or 7, or any 3 other questions.

From Morley JE, Charlton E, Patrick P, et al. Validation of a screening questionnaire for androgen deficiency in aging males. Metabolism 2000;49(9):1240; with permission.

The most widely accepted biochemical evaluation of male hypogonadism is from the Endocrine Society Guidelines published in 2010. These guidelines do not recommend routinely testing older men for low testosterone levels without clinical signs or symptoms. Initial evaluation begins with the measurement of baseline morning testosterone level and a repeat measurement of testosterone level with follicle-stimulating hormone (FSH) and luteinizing hormone (LH) levels 3 to 6 months later, depending on the clinical scenario. This procedure helps to diagnose primary versus secondary disease.[10] Further details of this process are described in **Fig. 2**. As mentioned earlier, it is crucial to address reversible causes before initiating testosterone replacement.

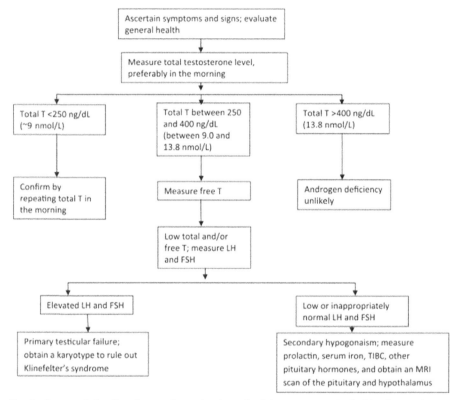

Fig. 2. Approach for the diagnostic evaluation of adult men suspected of having androgen deficiency. SDA, seminal fluid analysis; T, testosterone. In some laboratories, the lower limit of the normal T range in healthy young men is approximately 280 to 300 ng/dL (9.8–10.4 nmol/L); however, this range may vary in different laboratories. Use the lower limit of the range established in your reference laboratory. In some reference laboratories, the lower limit of the normal free T range in healthy young men is approximately 5 to 9 ng/dL (0.17–0.31 nmol/L) using equilibrium dialysis or calculated from total T and SHBG levels; however, this range may vary in different laboratories, depending on the specific equilibrium dialysis or calculated from total T and SHBG assays and the reference population used. Use the lower limit of the range established in your reference laboratory. [c] Perform pituitary MRI to exclude pituitary and/or hypothalamic tumor or infiltrative disease, if severe secondary hypogonadism (serum T <150 ng/dL), panhypopituitarism, persistent hyperprolactinemia, or symptoms or signs of tumor mass effect, such as headache, visual impairment, or visual field defect, are present. (*From* Bhasin S, Basaria S. Diagnosis and treatment of hypogonadism in men. Best Pract Res Clin Endocrinol Metab 2011;25(2):251–70; with permission.)

The diagnosis of hypogonadism is an evaluation of laboratory values and validated symptoms. The other important aspect in the diagnosis is to exclude individuals with transient decreases in serum testosterone levels. This transient decrease occurs in individuals who are in acute distress, malnourished, or take certain concomitant medications. As described in **Fig. 2**, there are generally 2 categories of hypogonadism: primary and secondary hypogonadism. Primary hypogonadism is the elevation of LH and FSH levels in the setting of a low testosterone level.[10] Secondary hypogonadism is characterized by a low LH and FSH level with a correspondingly low testosterone level. In older men, it is sometimes unclear as to what the true category is. In general, individuals have multiple comorbidities that together contribute to an idiopathic hypogonadal hypogonadotropic state.[2,15]

There is substantial diurnal variation in the level of serum testosterone in men. The highest level of testosterone is generally in the morning from 7 to 9 AM.[16] A large report from the EMAS of 3000 healthy men older than 65 years showed that 2.1% of men had testosterone levels less than 317 ng/dL with 3 concomitant sexual complaints.[17] This observation is in contrast to the observation of Baltimore Longitudinal Study mentioned earlier, in which by the age of 80 years, 30% of men had total testosterone values in the hypogonadal range and 50% had low free testosterone values.[8] In addition, more severe hypogonadism, defined as testosterone levels less than 230 ng/dL, was associated with insulin resistance.[8,18]

There is some controversy about the general threshold for treatment of hypogonadism in older men. If they have symptoms suggesting hypogonadism such as decreased libido, energy, and mood, then measurements of testosterone levels are warranted. If the total testosterone level is less than 200 ng/dL, testosterone replacement should be considered after evaluating for pituitary or testicular disease. If the persistent levels of total testosterone are less than 200 ng/dL, then testosterone replacement should be considered. The target for older men's total testosterone levels should be between 300 and 400 ng/dL. This value is lower than the traditional targets recommended for younger men of 500 to 600 ng/dL.[10]

PHARMACOLOGIC STRATEGIES

In men the most important androgen is testosterone. Most of the naturally occurring testosterone is bound to SHBG. The remaining testosterone is bound to albumin, and only 2% of testosterone is free and available to enter into tissue.[19] The major goal of treatment in this population is to treat some of the symptoms related to hypogonadism, but recent concerns related to side effects of testosterone replacement need to be considered.[20–24] Therefore some experts who are contributing to the guidelines recommend a target testosterone level for older men to be between 300 and 400 ng/dL.

There are multiple treatment options in terms of testosterone replacement therapy in the United States (**Table 1**).

Intramuscular Injections

Testosterone cypionate and enanthate are the most common forms of intramuscular short-acting testosterone supplements used in United States. In general, these medications are used every 2 to 3 weeks with dosing ranging from 100 to 300 mg every 2 weeks.[19] The new alternative testosterone replacement is testosterone undecanoate; this medication after reaching steady state can be injected every 10 weeks.[25,26] It is important to recognize that these medications reduce gonadotropin levels and therefore reduce spermatogenesis and may cause testicular atrophy.

Table 1		
Androgen preparations for replacement therapy		
Drug	**Route of Administration**	**Dosage**
Testosterone	Sublingual (buccal)	30 mg every 12h
Testosterone enanthate	Intramuscular	See text
Testosterone cypionate	Intramuscular	See text
Testosterone undecanoate	Intramuscular	750 mg/3 mL
Testosterone	Transdermal patch	2.5–10 mg/d
	Topical gel (1%, 1.62%, and 2%)	5–10 g/d

Adapted from Chrousos GP. The Gonadal Hormones & Inhibitors. In: Katzung BG, Trevor AJ, editors. Basic & Clinical Pharmacology. 13th edition. New York: McGraw-Hill; 2015.

Transdermal Delivery

Testosterone can also be administered transdermally; skin patches or gels are available for application to scrotal or other skin areas. Most applications provide continuous delivery of testosterone for 24 hours. Daily use of these medications is required and usually is initiated at 5 to 10 g of testosterone per day.[19] In general, scrotal patches are no longer favored in the United States. The major side effect of transdermal delivery is skin irritation, especially in testosterone patches, but there is also evidence of skin irritation, at lower rates, with the gel formulations.[27–31]

Buccal

A mucoadhesive buccal testosterone sustained-release tablet delivering 30 mg of testosterone is currently available. This tablet is known to restore testosterone concentrations within 4 hours of application. The dosing is twice daily.[32] This tablet is not a commonly used option in the United States most likely due to the complex administration to the gums.[33]

Subdermal Implants

Subdermal testosterone implants offer a long duration of delivery. The standard dosage is 200-mg pellets (800 mg) implanted subdermally. The pellets are usually replaced within 5 to 7 months. There is risk of infection at the implant site in up to 5% to 10% of cases.[34]

With all these preparations, the development of polycythemia, edema, urinary obstruction, and hypertension may require some reduction in dose.

EFFECTS OF TESTOSTERONE REPLACEMENT

There has not been any clear evidence of universally giving older men with low serum testosterone levels and hypogonadal symptoms testosterone replacement. The Endocrine Society's 2010 hypogonadal guidelines recommended that testosterone therapy has a role in selected patients.

Bone Density

Testosterone does have an effect in increasing osteoblast activity through the aromatization to estrogen and reducing osteoclast activity. There have been mixed results in individuals placed on testosterone therapy with regard to bone mineral density (BMD).[35–37] In an initial study comparing testosterone treatment for 3 years with administration of a placebo, there was not a substantial increase in BMD in the spine and hip, but a secondary analysis showed that individuals with lower testosterone levels did have increases in bone density.[38] A meta-analysis suggests that the benefit occurs in the lumbar spine bone density and that there is no clear benefit in the femoral neck BMD. There does seem to be evidence from trials that intramuscular testosterone injections have a more significant impact on bone density than transdermal testosterone administration. None of the studies were powered to show fracture benefit.[39]

Body Composition and Muscle Strength

It is generally accepted that the decline in testosterone levels that occur in aging contribute to the redistribution of fat mass and reduction in muscle mass.[11] There are direct effects of testosterone leading to increase in muscle protein synthesis and growth. In a systematic review conducted by the Endocrine Society, testosterone therapy significantly increased lean body mass (generally 2.7 kg) and led to a reduction in fat mass by 2 kg compared with placebo.[10,40,41] There was no substantial change in the overall weight.

A limited number of studies have shown direct effects of muscle strength caused by testosterone replacement. These studies have shown benefits of testosterone in terms of knee extension and flexion, handgrip strength and leg press strength.[40,42] It is premature to state whether there can be a benefit in frail older men.

Mood and Quality of Life

The overall presentations of older men with hypogonadism include complaints of a loss of libido and fatigue.[8] Clinically, these symptoms can overlap with the presentation of depression. This overlap makes it difficult for us to have good qualitative studies to differentiate treatment benefit. There are two placebo-controlled trials that were rather small that showed improvement in depression scores when comparing testosterone with placebo treatment.[43,44] There is some evidence that there is augmented benefit of testosterone in patients who were also on a selective serotonin reuptake inhibitor.[45] There needs to be larger placebo-controlled trials for a longer duration to confirm true benefit. There has been some benefit linked with improved libido after testosterone replacement. This improvement did not correlate to better sexual function or satisfaction.

Cognitive Function

There has been evidence of a decrease in predicted testosterone levels and age-related decline in cognitive performance such as visual and verbal memory as well as spatial and mathematical reasoning. Small and short-duration trials have been used for evaluating testosterone replacement in older men. There is some evidence of benefit in spatial cognition and verbal fluency in men without dementia. Intramuscular testosterone improved verbal and spatial memory and constructional abilities in nonhypogonadal men with mild cognitive impairment. In randomized placebo-controlled trials with crossover design, intramuscular testosterone therapy resulted in decreased verbal memory.[44] In another placebo-controlled trial, patients with Alzheimer's disease and low testosterone levels reported no significant changes in cognition.[3]

Effects on Metabolic Syndrome and Type 2 Diabetes

Obesity decreases the level of total testosterone in the body by directly decreasing the level of SHBG. There is some controversy regarding whether there can be true effect of testosterone replacement on reducing insulin resistance and therefore improving metabolic status.[4,46,47] One placebo-controlled trial showed a 15.2% reduction in the homeostatic model of assessment-insulin resistance in 6 months.[48] However, another trial has not shown such clinical effect.[49] Therefore it is premature to state that testosterone replacement can overall benefit metabolic syndrome or diabetes.

RISK OF TESTOSTERONE REPLACEMENT
Cardiovascular Risk

There have been well-done epidemiologic studies associating low testosterone levels with an increase in all-cause mortality and cardiovascular disease.[17,24] As with all epidemiologic literature, it is not clear if the testosterone is the cause or the result of a perceived good health status.

A meta-analysis of 51 trials encompassing 1053 patients was carried out. This trial showed that the relative risk reduction was 0.91 with no significant effect on cardiovascular mortality. This study was done in variable ages and at different baseline cardiovascular risks.[22]

There has been some recent research in a randomized controlled study entitled Testosterone in Older Men with Sarcopenia (TOM). In this frail older population where the mean age was 74, the trial was stopped prematurely because of self-reported cardiovascular adverse events. There were a total of 209 men in this trial, and of those, 23 subjects on testosterone had cardiovascular-related events compared with 5 in the placebo group.[21]

A retrospective cohort of 8709 men aged 60 to 64 years with low serum testosterone concentrations who were undergoing coronary angiography were randomly initiated on testosterone therapy and then followed up longitudinally. This study observed composite end points of all-cause mortality, myocardial infarction (MI), and stroke. The study subjects were compared with other individuals not taking testosterone therapy. The hazard ratio calculated by the study was 1.29 (95% confidence interval, 1.04–1.58). The absolute difference between the 2 groups was 1.3% after 1 year. These patients had an overwhelming high percentage of a history of coronary artery disease (80%).[50]

A separate retrospective cohort study examined records of 55,593 men who were prescribed testosterone therapy in a total population of 167,279 patients taking phosphodiesterase 5 inhibitors. The investigators found an increased rate of MIs 3 months after starting testosterone when compared with the rate of MIs in the prior year (rate ratio [RR], 1.36). This increase led to an increased number of 1.25 cases per 1000 patient-years. This effect was more pronounced in individuals older than 65 years (RR, 2.19; absolute increase of 6.25 additional cases per 1000 patient-years). It is important to note that the comparison group was on phosphodiesterase E5 inhibitors (**Table 2**).[23] Also, baseline testosterone levels and reason for the testosterone prescription were not obtained during the study. This fact is important to note because 25% of individuals who are started on testosterone therapy in the United States do not have a baseline testosterone level drawn before initiating therapy.[51]

These retrospective trials prompt important questions about testosterone use in older men. Most importantly, they raise concerns in individuals who are being placed on this therapy inappropriately without a proper diagnosis of true hypogonadism.[33] In light of this data, the US Food and Drug Administration (FDA) established an advisory committee and published a briefing document. The FDA concluded that there was a relative absence of large controlled long-term studies in regard to cardiovascular

Table 2
Rates of MI per 1000 PY in men younger than 65 years and those aged 65 years and older, in preprescription and postprescription intervals for an initial prescription of PDE5I with adjusted RR and 95% CI

	All Ages	Age <65 y	Age ≥65 y
Patients (N)	167,279[a]	141,512[a]	25,767[a]
Preprescription			
Cases	695	556	139
Rate per 1000 PY (95% CI)	3.48 (3.02, 4.01)	3.22 (2.75, 3.77)	5.27 (3.81, 7.27)
Postprescription			
Cases	152	119	33
Rate per 1000 PY (95% CI)	3.75 (3.19, 4.40)	3.42 (2.76, 4.24)	6.06 (4.26, 8.63)
RR (post/pre) (95% CI)	1.08 (0.93, 1.24)	1.06 (0.91, 1.24)	1.15 (0.83, 1.59)

Adjusted for age and preexisting medical conditions and medication use associated with MI or its risk factors.
Abbreviations: CI, confidence interval; PDE5I, phosphodiesterase 5 inhibitor; PY, persons per year; RR, rate ratio.
[a] Effective sample sizes of PDE5I cohorts after weighting:
All ages: 141,671.
Age less than 65 years: 121,696.
Age 65 years or greater: 19,505.
From Finkle WD, Greenland S, Ridgeway GK, et al. Increased risk of non-fatal myocardial infarction following testosterone therapy prescription in men. PLoS One 2014;9(1):e85805.

safety. However, a systematic review did not link testosterone replacement with cardiovascular events.[20,22] The FDA summarized that there was a concern regarding the inconsistency of monitoring of free and/or posttreatment testosterone levels after the initiation of testosterone replacement.[51] Also, the FDA mentioned that ongoing clinical trials designed to characterize the benefits of testosterone in older men will provide relevant safety information.

Fertility

Testosterone is not appropriate in individuals who seek to have continued fertility regardless of age. Exogenous testosterone suppresses the gonadotropic hormones and thus reduces spermatogenesis.[37,52]

Prostate Cancer

Prostate cancer is an androgen-sensitive disease, therefore androgen replacement therapy is contraindicated in men with a history of this malignancy.[10] There is currently no conclusive evidence that testosterone therapy increases the risk of prostate cancer. In many studies with testosterone replacement therapy, the prevalence of prostate cancer was not higher than in the general population.[20] If individuals present for the initiation of testosterone therapy, then a baseline prostate-specific antigen (PSA) level and a digital rectal examination (DRE) should be performed.[53] Individuals with a baseline PSA of greater than 4.0 ng/mL or abnormal findings on the DRE require additional assessment by a urologist and potentially a prostate biopsy.[3,10,54]

Polycythemia

Testosterone stimulates erythropoiesis. Therefore erythrocytosis can occur during treatment with testosterone, especially if administered through injections. Erythrocytosis increases the risk of stroke and other thromboembolic events in older adults. Individuals who present with a hematocrit of greater than 51% should be evaluated for untreated obstructive sleep apnea or untreated severe congestive heart failure.[3,10]

Other Potential Effects of Testosterone Replacement

Testosterone replacement has been associated with gynecomastia; it is related to the aromatization of testosterone into estradiol in adipose tissues. Dose adjustment may be needed. Testosterone replacement therapy has shown to exacerbate sleep apnea. It appears that testosterone does not directly diminish function of the upper airway, but rather most likely contributes to sleep-disordered breathing by a central mechanism. A formal sleep study may be beneficial in individuals with an elevated hematocrit.[10]

MONITORING STRATEGIES

In 2010, the Endocrine Society developed a set of clinical guidelines to follow-up a patient on testosterone replacement. Before initiating replacement, a DRE should be performed and serum PSA should be measured. In men who have a prostate nodule or a PSA over 4.0 ng/mL without identifiable risk factors, or 3.0 ng/mL with increased risk, a urologic evaluation should be performed before testosterone treatment is started. Risk factors include African American descent, men with a first-degree relative with prostate cancer or men with a personal history of prostate or breast cancer, hematocrit over 50%, untreated severe obstructive sleep apnea and severe lower urinary tract symptoms with International Prostate Symptom Score over 19, or uncontrolled heart failure.

Once testosterone therapy is initiated, the Endocrine Society recommends achieving midnormal testosterone levels during treatment with formulations chosen based on the patient's preference, financial limitations, and pharmacokinetic considerations.

Three to six months after initiating testosterone replacement, the DRE and measurement of PSA levels should be repeated. If a new nodule has developed or if the PSA level has increased by over 1.4 ng/mL from baseline (confirmed with a second measurement), a urologic evaluation is warranted.[10] No evidence exists for or against the need to maintain the circadian rhythm of serum testosterone. The span of 3 to 6 months is adequate to assess for benefit in clinical manifestations such as libido, muscle mass, and body fat improvement.[16]

Laboratory tests that should be performed before and during treatment include measurement of PSA levels, lipid panel, liver function tests, hemoglobin levels, and hematocrit. Clinically, men should also be monitored for edema, gynecomastia, sleep apnea, lower urinary tract symptoms, and low BMD. The Endocrine Society suggests that PSA levels, testosterone levels, DRE, hematocrit, BMD, and lipid levels be checked at baseline, 3 and 6 months after treatment starts, and then annually thereafter. The annual assessments are to determine if symptoms have responded to treatment and if any adverse effects are becoming apparent.[3]

The testosterone levels measured at 3 months should be a midmorning level. A target goal of 400 to 500 ng/dL (14.0–17.5 nmol/L) is recommended. However, if there is no symptomatic response, higher goals may be necessary. For men treated with a transdermal testosterone patch, the level should be obtained 3 to 12 hours after the patch is applied. If patients are receiving buccal tablets, the level should be measured immediately before application of a fresh system. Patients on the transdermal gel may have levels checked anytime after at least 1 week of therapy.[53] In all cases, free bioavailable testosterone levels should also be monitored because testosterone therapy reduces SHBG levels.

As mentioned earlier, hematocrit should be checked at baseline and at 3 and 6 months. If the hematocrit is over 54%, therapy should be stopped until hematocrit decreases to a safe level. Meanwhile, the patient should be evaluated for sleep apnea and hypoxia. When appropriate, therapy should be reinitiated at a reduced dose.

BMD measurements should be conducted at baseline and every 1 to 2 years of testosterone therapy.

SUMMARY/DISCUSSION

The evaluation of late-onset hypogonadism is a clinical diagnosis based on clinical signs of low testosterone and laboratory levels. Multiple comorbidities such as polypharmacy, depression, social isolation, recent loss, thyroid, and cardiovascular disease can affect the clinical presentation. The most widely accepted biochemical evaluation of male hypogonadism is from the Endocrine Society Guidelines published in 2010.[10] Expert opinion suggests that initiation of treatment of late-onset hypogonadism should be considered at a testosterone level of 200 ng/dL. The target for older men's total testosterone levels should be between 300 and 400 ng/dL. There has been a great deal of controversy in regard to the cardiovascular side effects related to exogenous testosterone treatment especially in older adults. Owing to this recent literature, it is important to consider individualized therapy incorporating patients' goals. Proper evaluation and monitoring related to replacement should always be advised. Before the initiation of treatment, patients and their families need to be familiar with the potential risks related to testosterone treatment and the limitations of the current understanding of this disease process.

REFERENCES

1. Nieschlag E, Swerdloff R, Behre HM, et al. Investigation, treatment and monitoring of late-onset hypogonadism in males. ISA, ISSAM, and EAU recommendations. Eur Urol 2005;48(1):1–4.
2. Morales A, Schulman CC, Tostain J, et al. Testosterone Deficiency Syndrome (TDS) needs to be named appropriately–the importance of accurate terminology. Eur Urol 2006;50(3):407–9.
3. Bassil N, Morley JE. Late-life onset hypogonadism: a review. Clin Geriatr Med 2010;26(2):197–222.
4. Ding EL, Song Y, Malik VS, et al. Sex differences of endogenous sex hormones and risk of type 2 diabetes: a systematic review and meta-analysis. JAMA 2006;295(11):1288–99.
5. Census.gov. Aging in the United States. Available at: http://www.census.gov/.../files/97agewc.pdf%5D. Accessed December 2, 2014.
6. A profile of Older Americans: 2011. Washington, DC: Administration for Community Living, US Department of Health and Human Services; 2011. Available at: http://www.aoa.acl.gov/Aging_Statistics/Profile/2011/4.aspx%5D. Accessed December 2, 2014.
7. Wu FC, Tajar A, Pye SR, et al. Hypothalamic-pituitary-testicular axis disruptions in older men are differentially linked to age and modifiable risk factors: the European Male Aging Study. J Clin Endocrinol Metab 2008;93(7):2737–45.
8. Harman SM, Metter EJ, Tobin JD, et al. Longitudinal effects of aging on serum total and free testosterone levels in healthy men. Baltimore Longitudinal Study of Aging. J Clin Endocrinol Metab 2001;86(2):724–31.

9. Travison TG, Morley JE, Araujo AB, et al. The relationship between libido and testosterone levels in aging men. J Clin Endocrinol Metab 2006;91(7): 2509–13.

10. Bhasin S, Cunningham GR, Hayes FJ, et al. Testosterone therapy in men with androgen deficiency syndromes: an Endocrine Society clinical practice guideline. J Clin Endocrinol Metab 2010;95(6):2536–59.

11. Morley JE. Anorexia, sarcopenia, and aging. Nutrition 2001;17(7–8):660–3.

12. Morley JE, Charlton E, Patrick P, et al. Validation of a screening questionnaire for Androgen deficiency in aging males. Metabolism 2000;49(9):1239–42.

13. Morley JE, Perry HM 3rd, Kevorkian RT, et al. Comparison of screening questionnaires for the diagnosis of hypogonadism. Maturitas 2006;53(4):424–9.

14. Abellan van Kan G, Rolland YM, Morley JE, et al. Frailty: toward a clinical definition. J Am Med Dir Assoc 2008;9(2):71–2.

15. Matsumoto AM, Paulsen CA, Hopper BR, et al. Human chorionic gonadotropin and testicular function: stimulation of testosterone, testosterone precursors, and sperm production despite high estradiol levels. J Clin Endocrinol Metab 1983;56(4):720–8.

16. Singh P. Andropause: current concepts. Indian J Endocrinol Metab 2013; 17(Suppl 3):S621–9.

17. Corona G, Lee DM, Forti G, et al. Age-related changes in general and sexual health in middle-aged and older men: results from the European Male Ageing Study (EMAS). J Sex Med 2010;7(4 Pt 1):1362–80.

18. Tajar A, Huhtaniemi IT, O'Neill TW, et al. Characteristics of androgen deficiency in late-onset hypogonadism: results from the European Male Aging Study (EMAS). J Clin Endocrinol Metab 2012;97(5):1508–16.

19. Chrousos GP. The Gonadal Hormones & Inhibitors. In: Katzung BG, Trevor AJ, editors. Basic & Clinical Pharmacology. 13th edition. New York: McGraw-Hill; 2015. Available at: http://accessmedicine.mhmedical.com/content.aspx?bookid=1193&Sectionid=69110111. Accessed August 9, 2015.

20. Shores MM, Smith NL, Forsberg CW, et al. Testosterone treatment and mortality in men with low testosterone levels. J Clin Endocrinol Metab 2012;97(6):2050–8.

21. Basaria S, Coviello AD, Travison TG, et al. Adverse events associated with testosterone administration. N Engl J Med 2010;363(2):109–22.

22. Fernández-Balsells MM, Murad MH, Lane M, et al. Clinical review 1: adverse effects of testosterone therapy in adult men: a systematic review and meta-analysis. J Clin Endocrinol Metab 2010;95(6):2560–75.

23. Finkle WD, Greenland S, Ridgeway GK, et al. Increased risk of non-fatal myocardial infarction following testosterone therapy prescription in men. PLoS One 2014; 9(1):e85805.

24. Pye SR, Huhtaniemi IT, Finn JD, et al. Late-onset hypogonadism and mortality in aging men. J Clin Endocrinol Metab 2014;99(4):1357–66.

25. Conaglen HM, Paul RG, Yarndley T, et al. Retrospective investigation of testosterone undecanoate depot for the long-term treatment of male hypogonadism in clinical practice. J Sex Med 2014;11(2):574–82.

26. Wang C, Harnett M, Dobs AS, et al. Pharmacokinetics and safety of long-acting testosterone undecanoate injections in hypogonadal men: an 84-week phase III clinical trial. J Androl 2010;31(5):457–65.

27. Dobs AS, Meikle AW, Arver S, et al. Pharmacokinetics, efficacy, and safety of a permeation-enhanced testosterone transdermal system in comparison with biweekly injections of testosterone enanthate for the treatment of hypogonadal men. J Clin Endocrinol Metab 1999;84(10):3469–78.

28. Wang C, Berman N, Longstreth JA, et al. Pharmacokinetics of transdermal testosterone gel in hypogonadal men: application of gel at one site versus four sites: a General Clinical Research Center Study. J Clin Endocrinol Metab 2000;85(3): 964–9.

29. Wang C, Swerdloff RS, Iranmanesh A, et al. Transdermal testosterone gel improves sexual function, mood, muscle strength, and body composition parameters in hypogonadal men. J Clin Endocrinol Metab 2000;85(8):2839–53.

30. Yu Z, Gupta SK, Hwang SS, et al. Transdermal testosterone administration in hypogonadal men: comparison of pharmacokinetics at different sites of application and at the first and fifth days of application. J Clin Pharmacol 1997;37(12): 1129–38.

31. Yu Z, Gupta SK, Hwang SS, et al. Testosterone pharmacokinetics after application of an investigational transdermal system in hypogonadal men. J Clin Pharmacol 1997;37(12):1139–45.

32. Salehian B, Wang C, Alexander G, et al. Pharmacokinetics, bioefficacy, and safety of sublingual testosterone cyclodextrin in hypogonadal men: comparison to testosterone enanthate–a clinical research center study. J Clin Endocrinol Metab 1995;80(12):3567–75.

33. Handelsman DJ. Global trends in testosterone prescribing, 2000–2011: expanding the spectrum of prescription drug misuse. Med J Aust 2013;199(8): 548–51.

34. Kelleher S, Conway AJ, Handelsman DJ. Influence of implantation site and track geometry on the extrusion rate and pharmacology of testosterone implants. Clin Endocrinol (Oxf) 2001;55(4):531–6.

35. Anderson FH. Osteoporosis in men. Int J Clin Pract 1998;52(3):176–80.

36. Center JR, Nguyen TV, Sambrook PN, et al. Hormonal and biochemical parameters in the determination of osteoporosis in elderly men. J Clin Endocrinol Metab 1999;84(10):3626–35.

37. Matsumoto AM. Reproductive endocrinology: estrogens–not just female hormones. Nat Rev Endocrinol 2013;9(12):693–4.

38. Behre HM, Kliesch S, Leifke E, et al. Long-term effect of testosterone therapy on bone mineral density in hypogonadal men. J Clin Endocrinol Metab 1997;82(8): 2386–90.

39. Rolland Y, Abellan van Kan G, Bénétos A, et al. Frailty, osteoporosis and hip fracture: causes, consequences and therapeutic perspectives. J Nutr Health Aging 2008;12(5):335–46.

40. Chu LW, Tam S, Kung AW, et al. Serum total and bioavailable testosterone levels, central obesity, and muscle strength changes with aging in healthy Chinese men. J Am Geriatr Soc 2008;56(7):1286–91.

41. Harman SM, Blackman MR. The effects of growth hormone and sex steroid on lean body mass, fat mass, muscle strength, cardiovascular endurance and adverse events in healthy elderly women and men. Horm Res 2003;60(Suppl 1):121–4.

42. Page ST, Amory JK, Bowman FD, et al. Exogenous testosterone (T) alone or with finasteride increases physical performance, grip strength, and lean body mass in older men with low serum T. J Clin Endocrinol Metab 2005;90(3):1502–10.

43. Seidman SN, Spatz E, Rizzo C, et al. Testosterone replacement therapy for hypogonadal men with major depressive disorder: a randomized, placebo-controlled clinical trial. J Clin Psychiatry 2001;62(6):406–12.

44. Barrett-Connor E, Goodman-Gruen D, Patay B. Endogenous sex hormones and cognitive function in older men. J Clin Endocrinol Metab 1999;84(10):3681–5.

45. Seidman SN, Miyazaki M, Roose SP. Intramuscular testosterone supplementation to selective serotonin reuptake inhibitor in treatment-resistant depressed men: randomized placebo-controlled clinical trial. J Clin Psychopharmacol 2005; 25(6):584–8.

46. Gray A, Feldman HA, McKinlay JB, et al. Age, disease, and changing sex hormone levels in middle-aged men: results of the Massachusetts Male Aging Study. J Clin Endocrinol Metab 1991;73(5):1016–25.

47. Kapoor D, Aldred H, Clark S, et al. Clinical and biochemical assessment of hypogonadism in men with type 2 diabetes: correlations with bioavailable testosterone and visceral adiposity. Diabetes Care 2007;30(4):911–7.

48. Jones TH, Arver S, Behre HM, et al. Testosterone replacement in hypogonadal men with type 2 diabetes and/or metabolic syndrome (the TIMES2 study). Diabetes Care 2011;34(4):828–37.

49. Gianatti EJ, Dupuis P, Hoermann R, et al. Effect of testosterone treatment on glucose metabolism in men with type 2 diabetes: a randomized controlled trial. Diabetes Care 2014;37(8):2098–107.

50. Vigen R, O'Donnell CI, Barón AE, et al. Association of testosterone therapy with mortality, myocardial infarction, and stroke in men with low testosterone levels. JAMA 2013;310(17):1829–36.

51. Braun SR. Promoting "low T": a medical writer's perspective. JAMA Intern Med 2013;173(15):1458–60.

52. Snyder PJ. Hypogonadism in elderly men–what to do until the evidence comes. N Engl J Med 2004;350(5):440–2.

53. Parsons JK, Carter HB, Platz EA, et al. Serum testosterone and the risk of prostate cancer: potential implications for testosterone therapy. Cancer Epidemiol Biomarkers Prev 2005;14(9):2257–60.

54. Holzbeierlein JM, Castle E, Thrasher JB. Complications of androgen deprivation therapy: prevention and treatment. Oncology (Williston Park) 2004;18(3):303–9 [discussion: 310, 315, 319–21].

Contemporary Systemic Therapy for Urologic Malignancies in Geriatric Patients

Bo Zhao, MD[a], Petros D. Grivas, MD, PhD[b],*

KEYWORDS

- Geriatric oncology • Urothelial carcinoma • Bladder cancer • Renal cell carcinoma
- Kidney cancer • Prostate cancer • Systemic therapy • Geriatric assessment tools

KEY POINTS

- Geriatric patients represent a highly heterogeneous population; the life expectancy, functional status, and disease-related prognosis at a given age is highly variable among same-age individuals.
- Treatment decisions for geriatric patients with urologic (genitourinary) malignancies should be based on a comprehensive evaluation of several factors in addition to chronologic age, including clinical disease status and characteristics; life expectancy; medical comorbidities; organ function; performance, nutritional, cognitive, and emotional status; concomitant medications; psychosocial support; and patient preference, beliefs, goals, and expectations.
- Chronologic age alone should not be an absolute barrier or contraindication to systemic therapy.
- Validated assessment tools can be useful for the integrated evaluation of geriatric patients and can aid in the decision-making process; prospective evaluation of such tools in clinical trials is recommended.

INTRODUCTION

Aging is increasingly becoming a global issue, in both developed and developing countries. By 2050, the number of people older than 60 years is expected to be 2 billion worldwide.[1] In the United States, people greater than or equal to 65 years of age represented 12.4% of the population in the year 2000 but are expected to increase to 19% by 2030.[2] Aging is the single most important risk factor for developing

Disclosure: Dr. P.D. Grivas has done consulting with Genentech/Roche, and Valeant/Dendreon. Dr. B. Zhao has nothing to disclose.
[a] Department of Hematology/Oncology, Taussig Cancer Institute, Cleveland Clinic, Desk R30, 9500 Euclid Avenue, Cleveland, OH 44195, USA; [b] Department of Hematology/Oncology, Taussig Cancer Institute, Cleveland Clinic, Desk R35, 9500 Euclid Avenue, Cleveland, OH 44195, USA
* Corresponding author.
E-mail address: grivasp@ccf.org

cancer, and numbers of older patients with cancer continue to increase.[3] Cancer is the leading cause of death among people greater than or equal to 65 years of age.[4] In the United States, urologic malignancies (cancers of the kidney, ureter, bladder, urethra, prostate, testes, and penis) account for 23% of all types of cancer and for more than 50,000 deaths in 2014.[5] Most of them were diagnosed in older individuals. The management of these patients becomes a major public health concern and clinical challenge. This article summarizes data regarding systemic therapy in geriatric populations with urologic malignancies, referencing data primarily from recently published clinical trials. When prospective evidence is not sufficient, retrospective data are included. Testicular cancer typically develops in young men, and penile cancer and other urinary tract cancers are rare, therefore this article focuses on prostate cancer, kidney cancer, and bladder cancer.

PROSTATE CANCER

Prostate cancer is the most common cause of nonskin cancer and the second leading cause of cancer death in US men. In 2014, there were an estimated 233,000 new diagnoses of prostate cancer and 29,480 deaths from the disease.[5] Prostate cancer is most frequently diagnosed among men aged 65 to 74 years, and the median age of diagnosis is 66 years. More than 55% of diagnoses occur in patients older than or equal to 65 years.[6] Prostate cancer is largely an androgen-driven disease, and androgen deprivation therapy (ADT) with medical or surgical castration remains part of the first-line therapy for metastatic prostate cancer. Despite tumor responses in 80% to 90% of treated patients and median response durations of 14 to 20 months, metastatic disease almost always eventually progresses in the form of castration-resistant prostate cancer (CRPC).[7] Data on ADT and agents currently approved for metastatic CRPC, including docetaxel, cabazitaxel, sipuleucel-T, abiraterone acetate, enzalutamide, and radium-223 are summarized later. Bone targeting agents, including zoledronic acid and denosumab, are not discussed, because these agents are generally well tolerated even in older individuals, but have not been shown to offer overall survival (OS) benefit.

Androgen Deprivation Therapy

Two recent large studies, NCIC-CTG PR.7 and SWOG-9346, have provided prospective data on quality of life (QoL) for patients receiving ADT. Both studies compared intermittent ADT (IAD) with continuous ADT (CAD); the former was conducted in patients with increasing prostate-specific antigen (PSA) levels after definitive radiotherapy,[8] and the latter was conducted in patients with newly diagnosed metastatic prostate cancer.[9] Although no age-specific outcomes were reported, both studies had enrolled primarily older patients: median age was 74 years in the NCIC-CTG study, the oldest patient was 89 years; median age of patients in the SWOG-9346 study was 70 years, and the oldest patient was 97 years. Common side effects of ADT, including sarcopenia, metabolic syndrome, and cardiovascular disease, were comparable in patients received IAD versus CAD in both studies. For QoL, hot flashes, libido, and urinary symptoms were better in the IAD arm in the NCIC-CTG study, as well as at 3-month and 9-month analyses in the SWOG-study[8,9] (**Table 1**). In the absence of OS benefit,[8] ADT should not be encouraged in patients with increasing PSA syndrome without detectable metastasis, unless progressive shortening of PSA doubling time predicts the impending emergence of overt metastases.[10] Primary ADT alone in older patients with localized disease should be discouraged because this practice has not been shown to improve survival.[11] When prolonged ADT is being

Table 1
Summary of age, benefit, and adverse effects of ADT in NCIC-CTG PR.7 and SWOG-9346

Trial, Disease	Arm, Median Age (Range) (y)	Survival Benefit	QoL Outcomes	Serious AEs
NCIC-CTGPR.7 PSA-only disease	IAD, 74.2 (29.4–89.7) CAD, 74.4 (45.3–88.9)	IAD noninferior to CAD	Hot flashes, libido, urinary symptoms were better in IAD arm	≥Grade 4: 9.4% IAD; 12.3% CAD
SWOG-9346 Metastatic disease	IAD, 70 (39–97) CAD, 70 (39–92)	IAD not non-inferior to CAD	Erectile function, libido, and vitality were better at 3-mo and 9-mo analysis, but not at 15-mo analysis	≥Grade 3: 30.4% IAD; 32.7% CAD

Abbreviation: AEs, adverse events.

used, careful assessment of bone health should be considered; this is more of a concern in older patients.[12]

Abiraterone Acetate and Enzalutamide

Abiraterone acetate (AA) is a potent oral inhibitor of CYP17A1, a critical enzyme converting steroidal precursors to testosterone. Side effects of AA are primarily related to the accumulation of upstream steroid precursors and mineralocorticoid excess, including hypertension, fluid retention, and hypokalemia.[13] Addition of prednisone can mitigate such side effects. Two phase III trials, COU-AA-301 and COU-AA-302, compared AA plus prednisone (AA/P) with prednisone in patients with metastatic CRPC after and before receiving docetaxel, respectively.[14,15] In COU-AA-301, median age of patients receiving AA/P was 69 years, the oldest patient was 95 years old, and 28% of patients were aged greater than or equal to 75 years.[14] A post-hoc analysis of COU-AA-301 showed that patients greater than or equal to 75 years old experienced significant OS benefit, just like their younger counterparts, with comparable side effects (**Table 2**).[16] In COU-AA-302, median age was 71 years in patients receiving AA/P, the oldest patient was 95 years old, and more than 30% of patients were aged greater than or equal to 75 years.[15] In a prespecified subgroup analysis, patients greater than or equal to 75 years old achieved similar radiographic progression-free survival (rPFS) to younger patients.[15]

Enzalutamide is a potent oral androgen receptor (AR) antagonist[17]; concurrent steroids are not required. Two phase III trials (AFFIRM and PREVAIL) compared enzalutamide with placebo in patients with metastatic CRPC in the postdocetaxel and predocetaxel settings, respectively.[18,19] The most common side effect was fatigue.[18] In the AFFIRM trial, median age was 69 years, the oldest patient was 92 years old, and nearly 25% of patients were aged greater than or equal to 75 years.[18] A post-hoc analysis showed that patients greater than or equal to 75 years old enjoyed significant OS benefit, just like their younger counterparts, with more fatigue, peripheral edema, and diarrhea. However, rates of adverse events (AEs) of grades greater than or equal to 3 were comparable in the 2 age groups (see **Table 2**).[20] In the PREVAIL trial, median age was 72 years, the oldest patient was 93 years old, and nearly 35% of patients were aged greater than or equal to 75 years.[19] In a prespecified subgroup analysis, patients greater than or equal to 75 years old received similar survival benefit to younger patients (see **Table 2**).[19]

Table 2
Summary of age groups, survival, adverse effects from studies on AA/prednisone and enzalutamide

Agents	Trial, Patients	Median Age (Range) (y), Patients ≥Age 75 y	Benefit for Older Patients	AEs Specific for Older Patients
Abiraterone/ prednisone	COU-AA-301 (post-hoc analyses), 1195	69 (42–95), 27.6%	HR for OS compared with prednisone: 0.78 for patients aged <75 y, 0.64 for patients aged ≥75 y	Grade 3/4 AEs: 62% for patients aged ≥75 y, 60% for <75 y. Incidence of hypertension and hypokalemia similar in both age subgroups
Abiraterone/ prednisone	COU-AA-302, 1088	71 (44–95), 33.9%	HR for rPFS compared with prednisone, age groups: 0.48 <65 y; 0.55 ≥65 y; 0.64 ≥75 y	NA
Enzalutamide	AFFIRM (post-hoc analyses), 1199	69 (41–92), 24.9%	HR for OS compared with placebo: 0.63 for patients aged <75 y, 0.61 for ≥75 y	Grade ≥3 AEs: no difference between age groups. More frequent peripheral edema, fatigue, diarrhea for patients aged ≥75 y
Enzalutamide	PREVAIL, 1717	72 (43–93), 36.4%	HR for OS vs placebo. Age groups: 0.77 for <75 y; 0.60 for ≥75 y	NA

Abbreviations: HR, hazard ratio; NA, not available; rPFS, radiographic progression-free survival.

Chemotherapy

The approval of docetaxel in patients with CRPC was based on 2 pivotal trials published in 2004: TAX-327 and SWOG-9916.[21,22] Although there were no stratified data according to age groups, both studies enrolled a significant portion of older patients. In the TAX-327 study, median age of patients receiving docetaxel every 3 weeks was 68 years, the oldest patient was 92 years old, and 20% patients were aged greater than or equal to 75 years. In the SWOG-9916 study, median age of patients receiving docetaxel/estramustine was 70 years, and the oldest patient was 88 years old.[21] No significant increase of AEs in older group was reported. In an updated survival analysis of the TAX-327 study, older patients seemed to benefit from docetaxel the same as younger patients (**Table 3**).[23] ECOG 3805 (CHAARTED) study evaluated the role of docetaxel started within 4 months of ADT initiation for treatment-naive metastatic prostate cancer.[24] Median age of patients receiving docetaxel/ADT was 64 years, and the oldest patient was 88 years old. Subgroup analysis showed that patients aged greater than or equal to 70 years had OS benefit the same as younger patients (see **Table 3**).[24]

Table 3
Summary of age groups, OS, and adverse effects from studies on docetaxel and cabazitaxel

Agents	Trial, Patients	Median Age (Range) (y)	Benefit for Older Patients	AEs Specific for Older Patients
Docetaxel every 3 wk	TAX 327, 1006	68 (42–92) 20% ≥75	HR for OS vs prednisone: 0.77 for ≥69 y; 0.81 for <69 y	NA
Docetaxel/ ADT	ECOG 3805, 790	64 (36–88)	HR for OS compared with ADT: 0.43 for ≥70 y; 0.68 for <70 y	NA
Docetaxel	NePro (retrospective) 568	≥80 (18); 75–79 (85); 70–74 (150); <70 (315)	OS similar up to age 80 y	Grade 3/4 AEs: age <70 y (18.5%); 70–74 y (23.3%), 75–79 y (21.2%), ≥80 y (44%)
Cabazitaxel	TROPIC, 755	68 (62–73), 18% ≥75	HR for OS vs mitoxantrone: 0.62 for ≥65; 0.81 for <65	NA
Cabazitaxel	European CUPs/ EAPs (retrospective), 746	≥75 (145); 70–74 (180); <70 (421)	NA	Age ≥75 y was associated with increased risk of grade ≥3 neutropenia; otherwise tolerability was similar in the 3 age groups

In addition to data from prospective studies, 2 large retrospective reviews specifically analyzed docetaxel in older patients.[25,26] The first study reviewed patients aged greater than or equal to 70 years from the Netherlands Prostate Study, which accounts for 44.5% of the 568 patients (see **Table 3**).[25] There was neither a relationship between dosage and age identified nor significant difference between the number of dose reductions, time to progression, OS, chemotherapy tolerance, and toxicities in the 3 groups up to the age of 80 years. However, men aged greater than or equal to 80 years experienced more frequent grade 3 to 4 toxicity (odds ratio, 5.34; $P = .0052$), and had decreased survival (15.3 months vs 24.5 months; $P = .020$).[25] In contrast, in 175 patients aged greater than or equal to 75 years treated with frontline docetaxel in France, only performance status (PS) greater than or equal to 2 and the presence of visceral disease were negative prognostic factors for OS.[26] These findings suggest that it may be fragility rather than chronologic age that predicts benefit and toxicities from docetaxel.

Cabazitaxel was approved in the postdocetaxel setting based on the TROPIC study.[27] Median age of patients was 68 years in the cabazitaxel arm, the oldest patient was 73 years old, with 18% of patients aged greater than or equal to 75 years. Subgroup analysis showed that patients aged greater than or equal to 65 years had OS benefit the same as younger patients (see **Table 3**).[27] No specific data on AEs were reported regarding older age. A retrospective review analyzed 746 patients treated in the European CUP/EAP program with cabazitaxel, and number of cycles, dose reductions/delays, and tolerability were similar in patients aged less than 70 years, 70 to 74 years, or greater than or equal to 75 years.[28] In multivariate analysis, age greater than or equal to 75 years was associated with increased risk of developing grade 3 or 4 neutropenia and/or neutropenic complications. Prophylactic use of granulocyte colony-stimulating factor (G-CSF) significantly reduced this risk by 30%.

Sipuleucel-T

Sipuleucel-T was approved based on a 4.1-month improvement in median OS versus placebo shown in the IMPACT study. Median age of patients receiving sipuleucel-T was 72 years, and the oldest patient was 91 years old.[29] Adverse events were mild to moderate, including fever, chills, headache, influenzalike illness, myalgia, hypertension, and hyperhidrosis. There were no specific data regarding toxicities in the older subpopulation; subgroup analysis showed that patients older than the median age still benefited from therapy.[29] There was no clear evidence of measurable antitumor effects, such as time to progression, objective response, and PSA response rates; the role of this vaccine is being further evaluated in the era of other effective agents (eg, AA, enzalutamide, radium-223). Retrospective analysis of subsets within the IMPACT trial showed that patients with lower baseline PSA levels achieved greater survival benefit from sipuleucel-T, suggesting that, if used, this agent should probably be used early in the clinical course.[30]

Radium-223

Radium-223 was approved based on the ALSYMPCA study, which showed a 2.8-month improvement in OS versus placebo.[31] Median age of patients receiving radium-223 was 71 years, the oldest patient was 90 years old, and 28% of patients were greater than or equal to 75 years old. Adverse events were mild to moderate, including thrombocytopenia and diarrhea, with no significant grade 3 or 4 events. There were no specific data regarding survival or toxicity in the older subpopulation.[31]

BLADDER CANCER

In 2014, there were an estimated 74,690 new diagnoses of bladder cancer and 15,580 related deaths in the United States.[5] Bladder cancer is most frequently diagnosed among men aged 75 to 84 years, the median age of diagnosis is 73 years, and more than 70% of diagnoses occur in patients aged greater than or equal to 65 years.[6] The percentage of bladder cancer deaths is highest among people aged 75 to 84 years, and more than half of deaths occur in patients more than 75 years old.[6] Urothelial carcinoma (UC) accounts for most bladder cancer, and platinum-based chemotherapy is generally used in muscle-invasive perioperative and advanced disease settings. Because chemotherapy is a physiologic stressor that can unmask the declining physiologic reserve of older patients, this population is largely underrepresented in clinical trials.[32] Applying the available evidence to older patients with UC requires careful assessment of the benefit and risks. This article summarizes data on age groups, efficacy, and adverse effects from major clinical trials and meta-analyses primarily on bladder UC.

Concurrent Chemoradiation

The National Cancer Institute (NCI) of Canada trial first prospectively studied the role of concurrent chemoradiation for bladder preservation in patients with muscle-invasive bladder cancer (MIBC).[33] The regimen for cisplatin was 100 mg/m^2 at

2-week intervals for 3 cycles.[33] The BC2001 study used a regimen that consisted of fluorouracil (500 mg/m^2) and mitomycin C (12 mg/m^2).[34] Both studies showed significant improvement in locoregional disease-free survival (DFS) but not OS. Neither of them reported specific data regarding age groups, the median age at enrollment for the NCI-Canada study was 65 years, and the oldest patient was 75 years old. Specific AEs, including renal insufficiency and anemia, were more common in patients receiving cisplatin. Patients in the BC 2001 study were older, their median age was 72 years, and the oldest patient was 77 years old. The addition of chemotherapy to radiation had a nonsignificant trend toward more grade 3 to 4 AEs during treatment (36% vs 27.5%; P = .07), especially gastrointestinal toxicity (9.6% vs 2.7%; P = .007), but not during follow-up (8.3% vs 15.7%; P = .07) (**Table 4**).

Perioperative Chemotherapy

Data from 2 large phase III randomized trials and meta-analyses[35–37] showed OS benefit with cisplatin-based neoadjuvant chemotherapy in MIBC (level I evidence), which is clearly underused, especially in elderly patients. Benefit from adjuvant chemotherapy is less definitive (possibly because of underpowered studies with methodological issues); a meta-analysis of 9 clinical trials showed DFS prolongation (hazard ratio [HR], 0.66; P = .014) and possible OS benefit (HR, 0.77; P = .049)[38]; however, the evidence is not as robust as for neoadjuvant chemotherapy. The recent EORTC30994 trial (median age, 61 years; range, 35–82 years) showed significant DFS benefit (HR, 0.54; 95% confidence interval [CI], 0.4–0.73; $P<.0001$), but no significant OS benefit (HR, 0.78; 95% CI, 0.56–1.08; P = .13) with immediate (adjuvant) versus deferred chemotherapy (the trial closed early because of slow accrual). Grade 3 to 4 myelosuppression was reported in 26% of patients getting immediate chemotherapy versus 35% with deferred chemotherapy; neutropenia occurred in 38% versus 53% of patients, and thrombocytopenia in 28% versus 38%, respectively. Two patients died of toxicity, 1 in each arm.[39] In the neoadjuvant setting, both the BA06 30,894 trial and SWOG-8710 trials enrolled a significant portion of patients 65 years of age or older (**Table 5**). In the BA06 30,894 trial, CMV (cisplatin, methotrexate, vinblastine) was used, the median age was 64 years, and 17% of patients were greater than 70 years old. Histologic grade and renal function, but not age, were associated

---

Table 4
Summary of age, DFS, and AEs from studies on chemoradiotherapy in MIBC for bladder preservation

Therapy	Trial, No. of Patients	Median Age (Range) (y)	Benefit for Older Patients	AEs
Cis/RT (40–60 Gy)	Canadian NCI, 99	65 (43–75)	Pelvic first recurrence favored Cis/RT (HR, 0.50; P = .036)	More creatinine level increase (P = .01) and anemia (P = .0001) in Cis/RT vs RT
5-FU/mitomycin C/ 55–64 Gy	BC2001, 360	72.3 (65.1–76.6)	NA (2-year pelvic DFS with 5-FU/mitomycin/RT vs RT [67% vs 54%, P = .03])	NA

Abbreviations: Cis, cisplatin; DFS, disease-free survival; FU, fluorouracil; RT, radiation therapy.

Table 5
Summary of age groups, DFS, and AEs from studies on neoadjuvant chemotherapy for bladder UC

Therapy	Trial, Patients	Median Age (Range) (y)	Benefit for Older Patients	AEs Specific for Older Patients
CMV	BA06 30894, 976	64 (NA), 17% >70	No interaction among age groups (<55, 55–65, >65 y), P = .38	NA
MVAC	SWOG-8710, 317	63 (36–79), 44.4% ≥65	OS for MVAC vs control (mo): <65 y: 104 vs 43; ≥65 y: 61 vs 30. P = .74 for age groups	NA

Abbreviations: CMV, cisplatin, methotrexate, vinblastine; MVAC, methotrexate, vinblastine, doxorubicin, cisplatin.

with survival (see **Table 5**).[35] In the SWOG-8710 study, MVAC (methotrexate, vinblastine, doxorubicin, cisplatin) was used, and 44.4% of patients were greater than or equal to 65 years old. Older age did not correlate with OS benefit (see **Table 5**).[36] Gemcitabine/cisplatin (GC) has been increasingly used because of its similar efficacy and favorable toxicity compared with MVAC in metastatic disease.[40] However, these regimens have not been prospectively compared with each other in the neoadjuvant setting. Several retrospective data sets suggest that pathologic complete response rates are comparable between neoadjuvant GC and MVAC.[41–44] Encouraged by the longer progression-free survival (PFS) with dose-dense MVAC versus conventional MVAC in advanced UC,[45] 3 phase II studies explored the role of dose-dense/accelerated MVAC in the neoadjuvant setting with promising results.[46–48] Two of these studies reported enrollment of patients aged greater than or equal to 65 years old; toxicities greater than or equal to grade 3 were observed in 10% to 20% of patients with no treatment-related death.[47,48] In summary, neoadjuvant cisplatin-based combination chemotherapy offers a real but modest OS improvement and is strongly recommended in cisplatin-eligible patients with cT2-T4aN0 MIBC. The underrepresentation for patients greater than or equal to 80 years old in trials and the risks of cisplatin may limit its use in this subset of geriatric patients. In patients who are cisplatin ineligible, noncisplatin neoadjuvant chemotherapy has been studied in phase II trials,[49,50] but no level I evidence from prospective phase III trials is available.

Metastatic Disease: Cisplatin-based First-line Therapy

The MVAC regimen for metastatic UC was first reported in 1985 with nearly half of patients achieving complete response.[51] The European Cooperative Group study then established the superior OS with MVAC compared with single-agent cisplatin.[52,53] However, AEs were significant, 10% of patients had neutropenic fever, the treatment-related death rate was 4%, and mucositis and nausea/vomiting were common.[52] Neutropenic fever and mucositis have been improved by the use of G-CSF,[45,54] allowing patients to tolerate dose-dense MVAC with improved PFS (9.1 vs 8.2 months for conventional MVAC; P = .037).[45] Information on age in these trials is summarized in **Table 6**. Although the oldest patient in these trials was 82 years old, range of median ages was 61 to 66 years, suggesting that a younger population was enrolled.[45] Because of toxicities with MVAC other regimens have been studied. A phase III trial compared GC with MVAC.[55] Response rates, time to progression, and OS were comparable in both arms; and GC was better tolerated than MVAC, with

Table 6
Summary of age groups, OS, AEs from studies on MVAC and GC for metastatic bladder cancer

Agents	Trial, Patients	Median Age (Range), Arm, Age (y)	Benefit for Older Patients	AEs Specific for Older Patients
MVAC vs Cis	European Cooperative Group Study, 269	64 (?-82), Cis, 42% ≥65 66 (30–79), MVAC, 46% ≥65	Median OS (mo), <65 vs ≥65: 9 vs 11, $P = .76$	NA
DD-MVAC vs MVAC	EORTC 30924, 263	61 (36–76) DD-MVAC 62 (32–81) MVAC	NA	NA
GC vs MVAC	Netherlands, 426	63 (NA), GC; MVAC, 21% >70	OS for ≤70 vs >70 (mo): GC 160 vs 43; MVAC: 159 vs 43 HR 1.05, $P = .6927$	NA

significantly fewer side effects.[55] In an updated analysis, patients more than 70 years old seemed to have a similar degree of OS benefit (see **Table 6**).[40] As a result, GC has become the preferred first-line treatment of patients with advanced UC. The addition of paclitaxel to GC resulted in more toxicity without significant OS improvement.[56] Note that, for patients who are cisplatin eligible, age alone has not been shown to have prognostic value. Bajorin and colleagues[57] retrospectively analyzed factors predicting survival in 203 patients with UC who received first-line MVAC (median age, 63 years; the oldest patient was 83 years old); PS ECOG greater than 1 and visceral metastasis, instead of chronologic age, were identified as negative prognostic factors for OS. In another large retrospective review of 381 patients with UC who received platinum-based first-line chemotherapy, patients greater than or equal to 70 years old experienced more frequent neutropenic infections and renal toxicity; PS less than 2 and hemoglobin level greater than or equal to 10 g/dL were associated with longer survival.[58]

Metastatic Disease: Cisplatin-ineligible or Second-line Therapy

There is no standard treatment of patients with advanced UC who are ineligible for or have progressed on cisplatin-based chemotherapy, thus clinical trials should be considered. In patients with reduced functional status or comorbidities, such as renal impairment, significant hearing loss, cardiovascular disease, or neuropathy, who are deemed cisplatin ineligible, substitution with carboplatin is a common practice.[59] Only 1 phase III trial compared a cisplatin-based regimen with A carboplatin-based regimen in advanced UC (MVAC vs carboplatin/paclitaxel), and this showed a nonsignificant trend toward shorter survival with carboplatin/paclitaxel; however, the study was closed early and was underpowered. Patients treated with carboplatin/paclitaxel had less severe toxicities.[60] One randomized phase II trial compared GC with carboplatin/gemcitabine (GCa); response rates were 49% for GC and 40.0% for GCa, and median survival was 12.8 months for GC and 9.8 months for GCa.[61] These results suggest that carboplatin/paclitaxel and GCa are active in UC and can be considered in cisplatin-ineligible patients. The EORTC 30986 study prospectively evaluated GCa with M-CaVI (methotrexate, carboplatin, vinblastine) in patients who were unfit for cisplatin (**Table 7**). The studied population was older, median age was greater than or equal to 70 years, both arms comprised patients less than or equal to 86 years old. No survival or AE data specific for age groups were reported; subgroup analysis showed that Bajorin risk group 2 was associated with increased toxicity.[62] Another phase II study specifically evaluated first-line biweekly GCa in patients who were unfit for cisplatin (median age, 75.5 years). Patients were stratified to 3 geriatric groups based on combining activities of daily living (ADL) and instrumental ADL.[63] Response rate was 24%; patients in group 1 and 2 had significantly longer median PFS versus group 3 (6.9 vs 1.9 months; $P = .005$).[63] In those patients with borderline renal function and potentially curable disease (T4b and/or lymph node–only disease), the use of carboplatin-based versus cisplatin-based combinations largely relies on clinical judgment and careful evaluation for cisplatin candidacy.[64] A shared medical decision should be made based on thorough discussions regarding the risks and benefits of therapy. Creatinine alone is not adequate for renal function assessment; creatinine clearance should be calculated, especially in borderline cases.

For patients with advanced UC who progressed on first-line platinum-based treatment clinical trials should be considered; various single agents and combination regimens have been studied. Response rates of singles agents are ~20%, combination regimens are associated with greater response rates and toxicities, but not necessarily longer survival.[65] As a result, single-agent chemotherapy with a goal of palliation is commonly used. Taxanes, gemcitabine, and pemetrexed are among the most commonly used agents.[66–69] Vinflunine is the only agent approved in Europe but is not approved in the United States based on a phase III trial that compared it with best supportive care only (see **Table 7**). More than 45% of enrolled patients were 65 years of age or older. Again, age was not prognostic for OS, which was significantly higher with vinflunine in the eligible patients (6.9 vs 4.3 months; $P = .036$) but not in the intention-to-treat population ($P = .287$).[70] Major AEs include neutropenia (50%), anemia (19%), fatigue (19%), and constipation (16%). Occasionally, in selected patients who have achieved a very good response to first-line chemotherapy (eg, ≥12-month response duration), rechallenge with platinum-based therapy may be considered. The AUO AB 20/99 phase III study evaluated 6 cycles of gemcitabine/paclitaxel (GP) versus GP maintenance until progression in 102 patients in the second-line setting, and both arms enrolled patients less than or equal to 79 years old. Response rates were close to 40% in both arms; prolonged treatment did not improve outcomes and was associated with significant toxicities, including 2 toxic deaths.[71] These results

Table 7
Summary of age and adverse events from EORTC 30986 and vinflunine/best supportive care (BSC) versus BSC phase III studies for UC

Therapy	Trial, No. of Patients	Median Age (Range), Arm, Age (y)	Benefit for Older Patients	AEs
GCa vs M-CaVI	EORTC 30986, 238	70 (36–87), GCa 72 (34–86), M-CaVI	NA	More toxicities in patients receiving M-CaVI or in Bajorin risk group 2
VFL/BSC vs BSC	Phase III, 370	NA, VFL + BSC, 47% ≥65 NA, BSC, 49% ≥65	NA	Grade 3/4 toxicities associated with VFL: neutropenia, anemia, fatigue, constipation.

Abbreviation: VFL, vinflunine.

suggest that maintenance chemotherapy in UC should not be a standard practice outside of a clinical trial. Results from a phase I expansion study on MPDL3280A, an immune checkpoint inhibitor (anti-PDL1), in patients with advanced UC showed very promising results, including rapid and durable responses. Median age for efficacy-evaluable patients was 65 years (36–86) years; toxicity profile was favorable without renal toxicity, grade 4 or 5 treatment-related AEs, or investigator-assessed immune-related events; and no specific data in older patients were reported.[72]

RENAL CELL CARCINOMA

In 2014, there were an estimated 63,920 new diagnoses of kidney and renal pelvis cancer in the United States, and 13,860 deaths from the disease.[5] Renal cell carcinomas (RCC) are responsible for 80% to 85% of all primary renal neoplasms. Kidney and renal pelvis cancer are most frequently diagnosed among people aged 55 to 64 years, the median age of diagnosis is 64 years, and nearly half of diagnoses occur in patients aged greater than or equal to 65 years.[5] To date, most randomized clinical trials on RCCs enrolled patients with clear cell histology, but therapies for RCCs with non–clear cell histology are not a focus of this article.

RCCs have been considered highly insensitive to conventional chemotherapy. Historically, high-dose interleukin-2 (IL-2) was the standard care, with 5% to 10% durable response rates,[73,74] and several predictive factors of response to IL-2 have been proposed.[75] Acute toxicities are significant, such as hypotension and capillary leak syndrome; treatment-related mortality can be high.[73,74] Although age was not a prognostic factor, offering this therapy to older patients or those with major comorbidities is not advised. Better understanding of the underlying mechanisms of RCC has led to the development and US Food and Drug Administration (FDA) approval of 7 agents, primarily targeting vascular endothelial growth factor (VEGF) receptor and the mammalian target of rapamycin (mTOR) pathways. Sunitinib, pazopanib, sorafenib, bevacizumab (with interferon [IFN] alpha), and temsirolimus are FDA approved and used for first-line treatment; axitinib and everolimus are used for second-line treatment. Tolerability and AEs specifically for older patients are scant in prospectively conducted trials. However, many trials enrolled octogenarians, patients greater than or equal to 65 years old accounted for 20% to 35% of the studied population, and the median age of patients at enrollment in these studies ranged from 58 to 64 years (**Table 8**). Efficacy specifically related to age groups from major clinical trials is generally derived from subgroup analysis; almost all of these trials showed that patients aged greater than or equal to 65 years (in CALGB 90206, age $\geq$44.8 years) experienced similar benefit to younger patients based on HR for PFS (see **Table 8**). The only exception is the ARCC trial, in which temsirolimus was evaluated against IFN-alpha; the effect of temsirolimus on OS was greater in patients aged less than 65 years. However, interpretation of the data from exploratory subgroup analyses should always be cautious.

Because there are no prospective data on the benefit and toxicity profiles of sunitinib in older patients,[76] a large retrospective review evaluated 1059 patients pooled from 6 clinical trials; patients greater than or equal to 70 years old were specifically analyzed. PFS remained significantly different in older patients, but AEs occurred more frequent in this population (see **Table 8**).[77] The standard sunitinib schedule is 4 weeks on and 2 weeks off (schedule 4/2), which is often associated with toxicity necessitating dose reduction. However, maintaining drug exposure with proper/adequate AE management is essential for optimizing clinical efficacy.[78] Alternatively, 2 weeks on and 1 week off (schedule 2/1) has been used at some centers.

Table 8
Summary of benefit and adverse events related to age groups for agents in metastatic RCC

Treatment Arm	Trial/No. of Patients	Median Age (Range) (y)	Benefit for Older Patients	Most Common ≥Grade 3 AEs Overall, Unless Specifically Indicated for Older Patients
Sunitinib (4/2[a])	Phase III, 750	62 (27–87), 37% ≥65	PFS: similar HR in patients ≥65 y old	Hypertension (12%), fatigue (11%), diarrhea (9%), HFS (9%)
Sunitinib (4/2)	Pooled data from 6 trials, 1059, 26% after cytokine	73 (70–87) for ≥70, 57 (24–69) for <70	PFS (month): sunitinib vs IFN-alpha <70 y old: 9.9 vs 5.0, $P = .000$ ≥70 y old: 11.0 vs 7.9, $P = .0197$	AEs more frequent in patients ≥70 vs <70 y old ($P<.05$): fatigue, cough, edema, anemia, decreased appetite, thrombocytopenia
Pazopanib	Phase III, 435	59 (28–85), 35% ≥65	PFS: similar HR in patients ≥65	Diarrhea (4%), hypertension (4%), increased ALT level (12%)
Sorafenib	TARGET, 903	58 (19–86)	PFS: similar HR in patients ≥65	HFS (6%), diarrhea (2%), hypertension (4%), fatigue (5%)
Sorafenib	Pooled data from 6 trials, 4684 (52.4% after cytokines)	<55: 49 (13–54) 55–65: 59 (55–64) 65–75: 69 (65–74) ≥75: 78 (75–100)	NA	No substantial differences among age groups; treatment duration ~30% shorter in patients ≥75 y old
Bevacizumab/IFN	CALGB 90206, 732	61 (56–70)	PFS: HR similar in patients ≥44.8 y old	Hypertension (11%), anorexia (7%), proteinuria (15%)
Bevacizumab/IFN	AVOREN, 649	61 (30–82), 37% ≥65	PFS: HR similar in patients ≥65 y old	Hypertension (3%), bleeding (3%), proteinuria (7%)
Temsirolimus	ARCC, 626	58 (32–81) 30% ≥65	OS: greater benefit in patients <65 y old	Hyperglycemia (11%), hyperlipidemia (3%), asthenia (11%), anemia (30%), dyspnea (9%)

Treatment	Study	Age	Outcome	Toxicity
Pazopanib vs sunitinib (4/2)	COMPARZ, 1110	61 (18–88), pazopanib 62 (23–86), sunitinib	OS and PFS: pazopanib noninferior to sunitinib	NA for age-specific groups, QoL better with pazopanib. Sunitinib vs pazopanib: fatigue (63% vs 55%), HFS (50% vs 29%), thrombocytopenia (78% vs 41%), transaminitis (43% vs 60%)
Pazopanib vs sunitinib (4/2)	PISCES, phase IIIb, 114	62, sunitinib > pazopanib 64, pazopanib > sunitinib	Patients preference: 70% vs 22% Physician preference: 61% vs 22% (Both favoring pazopanib)	NA for age-specific groups QoL better with pazopanib
Axitinib vs sorafenib	AXIS, 723 (35% received prior cytokines)	61 (20–82), axitinib 61 (22–80), sorafenib 34.2% ≥65	PFS: HR similar in patients ≥65 y old favoring axitinib	Axitinib: hypertension (16%), diarrhea (11%), fatigue (10%), HFS (5%), increased lipase level (5%), hypophosphatemia (2%) Sorafenib: HFS (16%), hypertension (11%), diarrhea (7%), fatigue (5%), increased lipase level (15%), hypophosphatemia (16%)
Everolimus	RECORD-1, 410	61 (27–85), 36.8% ≥65	PFS: HR similar in patients ≥65 y old	Stomatitis (3%), fatigue (3%), pneumonitis (3%), anemia (9%), hyperglycemia (12%), lymphopenia (14%), hypophosphatemia (4%)

Abbreviations: ALT, alanine aminotransferase; HFS, hand-foot syndrome.
[a] The numbers *"4/2"* indicate 4 weeks of treatment followed by 2 weeks of rest.

Retrospective experience from the Cleveland Clinic suggests that the 2/1 schedule is associated with significantly decreased toxicity in patients who experienced toxicity greater than or equal to grade 3 on a 4/2 schedule, and can extend treatment duration considerably.[79] Experience from MD Anderson suggests that the 2/1 schedule achieves comparable outcomes with the 4/2 schedule.[80] The safety and efficacy of the sunitinib 2/1 schedule is being prospectively investigated in an ongoing multicenter phase II clinical trial.

The FDA approval of pazopanib was based on a 5-month improvement in median PFS versus placebo.[81] Importantly, the QoL measurements were not significantly different for pazopanib versus placebo.[81] Subsequently, the COMPARZ study compared pazopanib with sunitnib (4/2 schedule) regarding efficacy and QoL[82]; 39% of patients in this study were greater than or equal to 65 years old. Pazopanib was noninferior to sunitinib with respect to PFS, but QoL domains were significantly better in patients on pazopanib (see **Table 8**).[82] The phase IIIb PISCES study compared patient preference between pazopanib and sunitinib. Median age at enrollment was 62 years, and significantly more patients preferred pazopanib (70%) to sunitinib (22%); less fatigue and better overall QoL were the main reasons favoring pazopanib, with less diarrhea being the most cited reason for preferring sunitinib (see **Table 8**).[83] Note that the schedule of sunitinib used in these studies was 4/2; QoL on a sunitinib 2/1 schedule versus pazopanib is not known. In addition, although well tolerated, the drug discontinuation rate for pazopanib in the COMPARZ study was not lower than the rate for sunitinib (24% vs 20%), primarily because of abnormalities in liver function tests.[82] According to these results, pazopanib or sunitinib can be considered in older patients; local experience with AE management may influence the selection of agent.

Bevacizumab in metastatic RCC was developed in combination with IFN-alpha,[84,85] but, because of the significant AEs from IFN-alpha, this combination is not commonly used, and bevacizumab is often used as a single agent. Hypertension, thromboembolism, hemorrhage, and proteinuria are some of the potential side effects, but there are no specific data regarding toxicities of bevacizumab in older patients with RCC.[84,85] However, AEs from bevacizumab in the older population with metastatic colorectal cancer did not differ significantly from those in younger patients when given as a single agent or in combination with chemotherapy.[86] In patients who cannot take (or absorb) oral medications or who have significant AEs (eg, hand-foot syndrome, fatigue, diarrhea) with different oral agents, bevacizumab could be considered. Temsirolimus is another agent that is administered intravenously. Although well tolerated overall, especially in patients with poor PS, subanalysis comparing temsirolimus with IFN-alpha showed that its effect on OS was greater in patients less than 65 years old.[87] For sorafenib, a large retrospective review analyzed 4684 patients from 6 clinical trials, and suggested that sorafenib was well tolerated in older patients; there were no substantial differences in drug-related AEs among the age groups less than 55 years, 55 to 65 years, 65 to 75 years, and greater than 75 years old, although treatment duration was ~30% shorter in patients greater than or equal to 75 years old.[88] Note that sorafenib was initially approved as a first-line agent,[89] but it is now more commonly used beyond third line (when it is used).

In the second-line setting, the phase III AXIS trial showed superior PFS with axitinib versus sorafenib (8.3 vs 5.7 months; $P<.0001$); 34% of patients were aged greater than or equal to 65 years, and no AEs specific for age groups were reported. The most common AEs with axitinib are diarrhea, hypertension, fatigue, anorexia, and dysphonia.[90] The INTORSECT study compared the efficacy of temsirolimus and sorafenib as second-line therapy in patients with metastatic RCC after progression on sunitinib.

PFS was similar between treatment arms; however, OS was significantly longer with sorafenib. The incidence of serious AEs was higher with temsirolimus (41%) than with sorafenib (34%).[91] Therefore, second-line use of VEGF tyrosine kinase inhibitor may be favored by physicians, especially in patients whose response to a frontline VEGF inhibitor was favorable and prolonged. However, more commonly used second-line agents are axitinib or everolimus. The RECORD-1 study established the role of everolimus in patients with metastatic RCC in the second-line setting[92]; 36% of patients were greater than or equal to 65 years old and 17.5% were greater than or equal to 70 years old. PFS, OS, and overall response rate were similar in the older patients and the overall RECORD-1 population.[93] Stomatitis, rash, and fatigue were the most common AEs associated with everolimus; grade 3 hyperglycemia was 12%; and pneumonitis was 8% (3% grade 3).[93] Notably, the immune checkpoint inhibitor nivolumab (anti-PD1) showed antitumor activity in a phase II study in metastatic RCC. Median age was 61 years, overall response rate was 20%, and 11% of patients experienced grade 3 or 4 treatment-related AEs. There were no specific data available regarding older patients.[94]

SUMMARY AND FUTURE

Current data on systemic therapy in geriatric populations with genitourinary malignancies are largely derived from retrospective analyses of prospectively conducted trials or retrospective reviews. Although extrapolation of the data to real-world patients should be cautious, patients greater than or equal to 65 years old with good functional status and minimal comorbidities seem to enjoy similar survival benefit from therapy to their younger counterparts. Chronologic age alone should generally not be used to guide management decisions. Physicians' recommendations should be based on disease status, drug efficacy and toxicity profiles, the patient's physiologic reserve, psychosocial support, PS, medical comorbidities, and life expectancy. Cognitive function, nutritional status, visual/hearing status, history of falls, polypharmacy, and transportation are other parameters to consider in the geriatric population. Interventions to improve age-related concomitant issues may help and influence candidacy for therapy. Use of geriatric assessment tools and prospective studies in older adults integrating comprehensive geriatric assessment can shed light on the optimal management of urologic malignancies in this population.[95]

REFERENCES

1. World population ageing report. 2013. Available at: http://www.un.org/en/development/desa/population/publications/pdf/ageing/WorldPopulationAgeing2013.pdf. Accessed November 18, 2014.
2. Ortman JM, Velkoff VA, Hogan H. An aging nation: the older population in the United States. Current Population Reports, P25-1140. Washington, DC: U.S. Census Bureau; 2014.
3. Yancik R. Population aging and cancer: a cross-national concern. Cancer J 2005; 11(6):437–41.
4. Muss HB. Cancer in the older: a societal perspective from the United States. Clin Oncol (R Coll Radiol) 2009;21(2):92–8.
5. Siegel R, Ma J, Zou Z, et al. Cancer statistics, 2014. CA Cancer J Clin 2014;64(1): 9–29.
6. Howlader N, Noone AM, Krapcho M, et al, editors. SEER cancer statistics review, 1975–2011. Bethesda, MD: National Cancer Institute; 2014. Available at: http://

seer.cancer.gov/csr/1975_2011/. based on November 2013 SEER data submission, posted to the SEER Web site.

7. Scher HI, Sawyers CL. Biology of progressive, castration-resistant prostate cancer: directed therapies targeting the androgen-receptor signaling axis. J Clin Oncol 2005;23:8253–61.

8. Crook JM, O'Callaghan CJ, Duncan G, et al. Intermittent androgen suppression for rising PSA level after radiotherapy. N Engl J Med 2012;367(10):895–903.

9. Hussain M, Tangen CM, Berry DL, et al. Intermittent versus continuous androgen deprivation in prostate cancer. N Engl J Med 2013;368(14):1314–25.

10. Slovin SF, Wilton AS, Heller G, et al. Time to detectable metastatic disease in patients with rising prostate-specific antigen values following surgery or radiation therapy. Clin Cancer Res 2005;11(24 Pt 1):8669–73.

11. Lu-Yao GL, Albertsen PC, Moore DF, et al. Fifteen-year survival outcomes following primary androgen-deprivation therapy for localized prostate cancer. JAMA Intern Med 2014;174(9):1460–7.

12. Smith MR, Egerdie B, Hernández Toriz N, et al. Denosumab in men receiving androgen-deprivation therapy for prostate cancer. N Engl J Med 2009;361(8): 745–55.

13. Bryce A, Ryan CJ. Development and clinical utility of abiraterone acetate as an androgen synthesis inhibitor. Clin Pharmacol Ther 2012;91(1):101–8.

14. de Bono JS, Logothetis CJ, Molina A, et al, COU-AA-301 Investigators. Abiraterone and increased survival in metastatic prostate cancer. N Engl J Med 2011; 364(21):1995–2005.

15. Ryan CJ, Smith MR, de Bono JS, et al, COU-AA-302 Investigators. Abiraterone in metastatic prostate cancer without previous chemotherapy. N Engl J Med 2013; 368(2):138–48.

16. Mulders PF, Molina A, Marberger M, et al. Efficacy and safety of abiraterone acetate in an older patient subgroup (aged 75 and older) with metastatic castration-resistant prostate cancer after docetaxel-based chemotherapy. Eur Urol 2014; 65(5):875–83.

17. Tran C, Ouk S, Clegg NJ, et al. Development of a second-generation antiandrogen for treatment of advanced prostate cancer. Science 2009;324(5928):787–90.

18. Scher HI, Fizazi K, Saad F, et al, AFFIRM Investigators. Increased survival with enzalutamide in prostate cancer after chemotherapy. N Engl J Med 2012; 367(13):1187–97.

19. Beer TM, Armstrong AJ, Rathkopf DE, et al, PREVAIL Investigators. Enzalutamide in metastatic prostate cancer before chemotherapy. N Engl J Med 2014;371(5): 424–33.

20. Sternberg CN, de Bono JS, Chi KN, et al. Improved outcomes in older patients with metastatic castration-resistant prostate cancer treated with the androgen receptor inhibitor enzalutamide: results from the phase III AFFIRM trial. Ann Oncol 2014;25(2):429–34.

21. Tannock IF, de Wit R, Berry WR, et al, TAX 327 Investigators. Docetaxel plus prednisone or mitoxantrone plus prednisone for advanced prostate cancer. N Engl J Med 2004;351(15):1502–12.

22. Petrylak DP, Tangen CM, Hussain MH, et al. Docetaxel and estramustine compared with mitoxantrone and prednisone for advanced refractory prostate cancer. N Engl J Med 2004;351(15):1513–20.

23. Berthold DR, Pond GR, Soban F, et al. Docetaxel plus prednisone or mitoxantrone plus prednisone for advanced prostate cancer: updated survival in the TAX 327 study. J Clin Oncol 2008;26(2):242–5.

24. Sweeney C, Chen YH, Carducci MA, et al. Impact on overall survival (OS) with chemohormonal therapy versus hormonal therapy for hormone-sensitive newly metastatic prostate cancer (mPrCa): an ECOG-led phase III randomized trial. J Clin Oncol 2014;32(Suppl 5) [abstract: LBA2].

25. Gerritse FL, Meulenbeld HJ, Roodhart JM, et al, NePro Study Investigators. Analysis of docetaxel therapy in older (≥70 years) castration resistant prostate cancer patients enrolled in the Netherlands Prostate Study. Eur J Cancer 2013;49(15): 3176–83.

26. Italiano A, Ortholan C, Oudard S, et al. Docetaxel-based chemotherapy in older patients (age 75 and older) with castration-resistant prostate cancer. Eur Urol 2009;55(6):1368–75.

27. de Bono JS, Oudard S, Ozguroglu M, et al, TROPIC Investigators. Prednisone plus cabazitaxel or mitoxantrone for metastatic castration-resistant prostate cancer progressing after docetaxel treatment: a randomised open-label trial. Lancet 2010;376(9747):1147–54.

28. Heidenreich A, Bracarda S, Mason M, et al. European investigators. Safety of cabazitaxel in senior adults with metastatic castration-resistant prostate cancer: results of the European compassionate-use programme. Eur J Cancer 2014; 50(6):1090–9.

29. Kantoff PW, Higano CS, Shore ND, et al, IMPACT Study Investigators. Sipuleucel-T immunotherapy for castration-resistant prostate cancer. N Engl J Med 2010; 363(5):411–22.

30. Schellhammer PF, Chodak G, Whitmore JB, et al. Lower baseline prostate-specific antigen is associated with a greater overall survival benefit from sipuleucel-T in the Immunotherapy for Prostate Adenocarcinoma Treatment (IMPACT) trial. Urology 2013;81(6):1297–302.

31. Parker C, Nilsson S, Heinrich D, et al, ALSYMPCA Investigators. Alpha emitter radium-223 and survival in metastatic prostate cancer. N Engl J Med 2013; 369(3):213–23.

32. Hutchins LF, Unger JM, Crowley JJ, et al. Underrepresentation of patients 65 years of age or older in cancer-treatment trials. N Engl J Med 1999;341: 2061–7.

33. Coppin CM, Gospodarowicz MK, James K, et al. Improved local control of invasive bladder cancer by concurrent cisplatin and preoperative or definitive radiation. The National Cancer Institute of Canada Clinical Trials Group. J Clin Oncol 1996;14:2901–7.

34. James ND, Hussain SA, Hall E, et al, BC2001 Investigators. Radiotherapy with or without chemotherapy in muscle-invasive bladder cancer. N Engl J Med 2012; 366(16):1477–88.

35. International Collaboration of Trialists, Medical Research Council Advanced Bladder Cancer Working Party (now the National Cancer Research Institute Bladder Cancer Clinical Studies Group), European Organisation for Research and Treatment of Cancer Genito-Urinary Tract Cancer Group, et al. International phase III trial assessing neoadjuvant cisplatin, methotrexate, and vinblastine chemotherapy for muscle-invasive bladder cancer: long-term results of the BA06 30894 trial. J Clin Oncol 2011;29:2171–7.

36. Grossman HB, Natale RB, Tangen CM, et al. Neoadjuvant chemotherapy plus cystectomy compared with cystectomy alone for locally advanced bladder cancer. N Engl J Med 2003;349:859–66.

37. Advanced Bladder Cancer Meta-analysis Collaboration. Neoadjuvant chemotherapy in invasive bladder cancer: update of a systematic review and meta-

analysis of individual patient data advanced bladder cancer (ABC) meta-analysis collaboration. Eur Urol 2005;48:202–5.

38. Leow JJ, Martin-Doyle W, Rajagopal PS, et al. Adjuvant chemotherapy for invasive bladder cancer: a 2013 updated systematic review and meta-analysis of randomized trials. Eur Urol 2014;66(1):42–54.

39. Sternberg CN, Skoneczna I, Kerst JM, et al. Immediate versus deferred chemotherapy after radical cystectomy in patients with pT3-pT4 or N+ M0 urothelial carcinoma of the bladder (EORTC 30994): an intergroup, open-label, randomised phase 3 trial. Lancet Oncol 2015;16(1):76–86.

40. von der Maase H, Sengelov L, Roberts JT, et al. Long-term survival results of a randomized trial comparing gemcitabine plus cisplatin, with methotrexate, vinblastine, doxorubicin, plus cisplatin in patients with bladder cancer. J Clin Oncol 2005;23(21):4602–8.

41. Yeshchina O, Badalato GM, Wosnitzer MS, et al. Relative efficacy of perioperative gemcitabine and cisplatin versus methotrexate, vinblastine, adriamycin, and cisplatin in the management of locally advanced urothelial carcinoma of the bladder. Urology 2012;79(2):384–90.

42. Zaid HB, Patel SG, Stimson CJ, et al. Trends in the utilization of neoadjuvant chemotherapy in muscle-invasive bladder cancer: results from the National Cancer Database. Urology 2014;83:75–80.

43. Dash A, Pettus JA 4th, Herr HW, et al. A role for neoadjuvant gemcitabine plus cisplatin in muscle-invasive urothelial carcinoma of the bladder: a retrospective experience. Cancer 2008;113(9):2471–7.

44. Lee FC, Harris W, Cheng HH, et al. Pathologic response rates of gemcitabine/cisplatin versus methotrexate/vinblastine/adriamycin/cisplatin neoadjuvant chemotherapy for muscle invasive urothelial bladder cancer. Adv Urol 2013; 2013:317190.

45. Sternberg CN, de Mulder PH, Schornagel JH, et al, European Organization for Research and Treatment of Cancer Genitourinary Tract Cancer Cooperative Group. Randomized phase III trial of high-dose-intensity methotrexate, vinblastine, doxorubicin, and cisplatin (MVAC) chemotherapy and recombinant human granulocyte colony-stimulating factor versus classic MVAC in advanced urothelial tract tumors: European Organization for Research and Treatment of Cancer Protocol no. 30924. J Clin Oncol 2001;19(10):2638–46.

46. Choueiri TK, Jacobus S, Bellmunt J, et al. Neoadjuvant dose-dense methotrexate, vinblastine, doxorubicin, and cisplatin with pegfilgrastim support in muscle-invasive urothelial cancer: pathologic, radiologic, and biomarker correlates. J Clin Oncol 2014;32(18):1889–94.

47. Plimack ER, Hoffman-Censits JH, Viterbo R, et al. Accelerated methotrexate, vinblastine, doxorubicin, and cisplatin is safe, effective, and efficient neoadjuvant treatment for muscle-invasive bladder cancer: results of a multicenter phase II study with molecular correlates of response and toxicity. J Clin Oncol 2014; 32(18):1895–901.

48. Siefker-Radtke AO, Kamat AM, Corn PG, et al. Neoadjuvant chemotherapy with DD-MVAC and bevacizumab in high-risk urothelial cancer: results from a phase II trial at the M. D. Anderson Cancer Center. J Clin Oncol 2012;30(Suppl 5) [abstract: 261].

49. Smith DC, Mackler NJ, Dunn RL, et al. Phase II trial of paclitaxel, carboplatin and gemcitabine in patients with locally advanced carcinoma of the bladder. J Urol 2008;180(6):2384–8.

50. Grivas PD, Hussain M, Hafez K, et al. A phase II trial of neoadjuvant nab-paclitaxel, carboplatin, and gemcitabine (ACaG) in patients with locally advanced carcinoma of the bladder. Urology 2013;82(1):111–7.
51. Sternberg CN, Yagoda A, Scher HI, et al. Preliminary results of M-VAC (methotrexate, vinblastine, doxorubicin and cisplatin) for transitional cell carcinoma of the urothelium. J Urol 1985;133:403–7.
52. Loehrer PJ, Einhorn LH, Elson PJ, et al. A randomized comparison of cisplatin alone or in combination with methotrexate, vinblastine, and doxorubicin in patients with metastatic urothelial carcinoma: a cooperative group study. J Clin Oncol 1992;10:1066–73.
53. Saxman SB, Propert KJ, Einhorn LH, et al. Long-term follow-up of a phase III intergroup study of cisplatin alone or in combination with methotrexate, vinblastine, and doxorubicin in patients with metastatic urothelial carcinoma: a cooperative group study. J Clin Oncol 1997;15:2564–9.
54. Gabrilove JL, Jakubowski A, Scher H, et al. Effect of granulocyte colony-stimulating factor on neutropenia and associated morbidity due to chemotherapy for transitional-cell carcinoma of the urothelium. N Engl J Med 1998; 318:1414–22.
55. von der Maase H, Hansen SW, Roberts JT, et al. Gemcitabine and cisplatin versus methotrexate, vinblastine, doxorubicin, and cisplatin in advanced or metastatic bladder cancer: results of a large, randomized, multinational, multicenter, phase III study. J Clin Oncol 2000;18(17):3068–77.
56. Bellmunt J, von der Maase H, Mead GM, et al. Randomized phase III study comparing paclitaxel/cisplatin/gemcitabine and gemcitabine/cisplatin in patients with locally advanced or metastatic urothelial cancer without prior systemic therapy: EORTC Intergroup Study 30987. J Clin Oncol 2012;30(10):1107–13.
57. Bajorin DF, Dodd PM, Mazumdar M, et al. Long-term survival in metastatic transitional-cell carcinoma and prognostic factors predicting outcome of therapy. J Clin Oncol 1999;17(10):3173–81.
58. Bamias A, Efstathiou E, Moulopoulos LA, et al. The outcome of older patients with advanced urothelial carcinoma after platinum-based combination chemotherapy. Ann Oncol 2005;16(2):307–13.
59. Galsky MD, Hahn NM, Rosenberg J, et al. Treatment of patients with metastatic urothelial cancer "unfit" for cisplatin-based chemotherapy. J Clin Oncol 2011; 29(17):2432–8.
60. Dreicer R, Manola J, Roth BJ, et al. Phase III trial of methotrexate, vinblastine, doxorubicin, and cisplatin versus carboplatin and paclitaxel in patients with advanced carcinoma of the urothelium. Cancer 2004;100:1639–45.
61. Dogliotti L, Carteni G, Siena S, et al. Gemcitabine plus cisplatin versus gemcitabine plus carboplatin as first-line chemotherapy in advanced transitional cell carcinoma of the urothelium: results of a randomized phase 2 trial. Eur Urol 2007;52: 134–41.
62. De Santis M, Bellmunt J, Mead G, et al. Randomized phase II/III trial assessing gemcitabine/carboplatin and methotrexate/carboplatin/vinblastine in patients with advanced urothelial cancer "unfit" for cisplatin-based chemotherapy: phase II-results of EORTC study 30986. J Clin Oncol 2009;27(33):5634–9.
63. Bamias A, Lainakis G, Kastritis E, et al. Biweekly carboplatin/gemcitabine in patients with advanced urothelial cancer who are unfit for cisplatin-based chemotherapy: report of efficacy, quality of life and geriatric assessment. Oncology 2007;73(5–6):290–7.

64. Yafi FA, North S, Kassouf W. First- and second-line therapy for metastatic urothelial carcinoma of the bladder. Curr Oncol 2011;18(1):e25–34.

65. Dreicer R. Second-line chemotherapy for advanced urothelial cancer: because we should or because we can? J Clin Oncol 2009;27(27):4444–5.

66. McCaffrey JA, Hilton S, Mazumdar M, et al. Phase II trial of docetaxel in patients with advanced or metastatic transitional-cell carcinoma. J Clin Oncol 1997;15(5): 1853–7.

67. Vaughn DJ, Broome CM, Hussain M, et al. Phase II trial of weekly paclitaxel in patients with previously treated advanced urothelial cancer. J Clin Oncol 2002; 20(4):937–40.

68. Lorusso V, Pollera CF, Antimi M, et al. A phase II study of gemcitabine in patients with transitional cell carcinoma of the urinary tract previously treated with platinum. Italian Co-operative Group on Bladder Cancer. Eur J Cancer 1998;34(8): 1208–12.

69. Sweeney CJ, Roth BJ, Kabbinavar FF, et al. Phase II study of pemetrexed for second-line treatment of transitional cell cancer of the urothelium. J Clin Oncol 2006;24(21):3451–7.

70. Bellmunt J, Théodore C, Demkov T, et al. Phase III trial of vinflunine plus best supportive care compared with best supportive care alone after a platinum-containing regimen in patients with advanced transitional cell carcinoma of the urothelial tract. J Clin Oncol 2009;27(27):4454–61.

71. Albers P, Park SI, Niegisch G, et al, AUO Bladder Cancer Group. Randomized phase III trial of 2nd line gemcitabine and paclitaxel chemotherapy in patients with advanced bladder cancer: short-term versus prolonged treatment [German Association of Urological Oncology (AUO) trial AB 20/99]. Ann Oncol 2011;22(2): 288–94.

72. Powles T, Eder JP, Fine GD, et al. MPDL3280A (anti-PD-L1) treatment leads to clinical activity in metastatic bladder cancer. Nature 2014;515(7528):558–62.

73. Fyfe G, Fisher RI, Rosenberg SA, et al. Results of treatment of 255 patients with metastatic renal cell carcinoma who received high-dose recombinant interleukin-2 therapy. J Clin Oncol 1995;13(3):688–96.

74. Negrier S, Escudier B, Lasset C, et al. Recombinant human interleukin-2, recombinant human interferon alfa-2a, or both in metastatic renal-cell carcinoma. Groupe Français d'Immunothérapie. N Engl J Med 1998;338(18):1272–8.

75. Grivas PD, Redman BG. Immunotherapy of kidney cancer. Curr Clin Pharmacol 2011;6(3):151–63.

76. Motzer RJ, Hutson TE, Tomczak P, et al. Sunitinib versus interferon alfa in metastatic renal-cell carcinoma. N Engl J Med 2007;356(2):115–24.

77. Hutson TE, Bukowski RM, Rini BI, et al. Efficacy and safety of sunitinib in elderly patients with metastatic renal cell carcinoma. Br J Cancer 2014; 110(5):1125–32.

78. Motzer RJ, Hutson TE, Olsen MR, et al. Randomized phase II trial of sunitinib on an intermittent versus continuous dosing schedule as first-line therapy for advanced renal cell carcinoma. J Clin Oncol 2012;30(12):1371–7.

79. Najjar YG, Mittal K, Elson P, et al. A 2 weeks on and 1 week off schedule of sunitinib is associated with decreased toxicity in metastatic renal cell carcinoma. Eur J Cancer 2014;50(6):1084–9.

80. Atkinson BJ, Kalra S, Wang X, et al. Clinical outcomes for patients with metastatic renal cell carcinoma treated with alternative sunitinib schedules. J Urol 2014; 191(3):611–8.

81. Sternberg CN, Davis ID, Mardiak J, et al. Pazopanib in locally advanced or metastatic renal cell carcinoma: results of a randomized phase III trial. J Clin Oncol 2010;28(6):1061–8.

82. Motzer RJ, Hutson TE, Cella D, et al. Pazopanib versus sunitinib in metastatic renal-cell carcinoma. N Engl J Med 2013;369(8):722–31.

83. Escudier B, Porta C, Bono P, et al. Randomized, controlled, double-blind, crossover trial assessing treatment preference for pazopanib versus sunitinib in patients with metastatic renal cell carcinoma: PISCES Study. J Clin Oncol 2014; 32(14):1412–8.

84. Rini BI, Halabi S, Rosenberg JE, et al. Bevacizumab plus interferon alfa compared with interferon alfa monotherapy in patients with metastatic renal cell carcinoma: CALGB 90206. J Clin Oncol 2008;26(33):5422–8.

85. Escudier B, Pluzanska A, Koralewski P, et al, AVOREN Trial investigators. Bevacizumab plus interferon alfa-2a for treatment of metastatic renal cell carcinoma: a randomised, double-blind phase III trial. Lancet 2007;370(9605):2103–11.

86. Sclafani F, Cunningham D. Bevacizumab in elderly patients with metastatic colorectal cancer. J Geriatr Oncol 2014;5(1):78–88.

87. Hudes G, Carducci M, Tomczak P, et al, Global ARCC Trial. Temsirolimus, interferon alfa, or both for advanced renal-cell carcinoma. N Engl J Med 2007; 356(22):2271–81.

88. Procopio G, Bellmunt J, Dutcher J, et al. Sorafenib tolerability in elderly patients with advanced renal cell carcinoma: results from a large pooled analysis. Br J Cancer 2013;108(2):311–8.

89. Escudier B, Eisen T, Stadler WM, et al, TARGET Study Group. Sorafenib in advanced clear-cell renal-cell carcinoma. N Engl J Med 2007;356(2):125–34.

90. Rini BI, Escudier B, Tomczak P, et al. Comparative effectiveness of axitinib versus sorafenib in advanced renal cell carcinoma (AXIS): a randomised phase 3 trial. Lancet 2011;378(9807):1931–9.

91. Hutson TE, Escudier B, Esteban E, et al. Randomized phase III trial of temsirolimus versus sorafenib as second-line therapy after sunitinib in patients with metastatic renal cell carcinoma. J Clin Oncol 2014;32(8):760–7.

92. Motzer RJ, Escudier B, Oudard S, et al, RECORD-1 Study Group. Efficacy of everolimus in advanced renal cell carcinoma: a double-blind, randomised, placebo-controlled phase III trial. Lancet 2008;372(9637):449–56.

93. Porta C, Calvo E, Climent MA, et al. Efficacy and safety of everolimus in elderly patients with metastatic renal cell carcinoma: an exploratory analysis of the outcomes of elderly patients in the RECORD-1 Trial. Eur Urol 2012;61(4):826–33.

94. Motzer RJ, Rini BI, McDermott DF, et al. Nivolumab for metastatic renal cell carcinoma: results of a randomized phase II trial. J Clin Oncol 2015;33(13):1430–7.

95. Hurria A, Togawa K, Mohile SG, et al. Predicting chemotherapy toxicity in older adults with cancer: a prospective multicenter study. J Clin Oncol 2011;29(25): 3457–65.

Palliative Care of Urologic Patients at End of Life

Christian T. Sinclair, MD[a],*, Jessica L. Kalender-Rich, MD[a], Tomas L. Griebling, MD, MPH[b], Karin Porter-Williamson, MD[a]

KEYWORDS

- Palliative care • End-of-life care • Urinary symptoms • Urology • Geriatrics
- Chronic illness • Hospice • Death

KEY POINTS

- For patients and families facing serious illness, they and their providers need to have a good understanding of how that patient's illness trajectory is likely to manifest itself; with this information, patients and providers can work together to formulate treatment plans that fit with what is most important to the patient and family as the illness changes over time.
- Palliative care integrated along the trajectory of illness improves patient care, family coping, and professional satisfaction with work.
- Excellent management of urologic symptoms (pain, spasm, bladder outlet obstruction, spinal cord compression, hematuria, delirium) is paramount to the palliative approach in advanced illness.
- There are common urologic issues that may be faced by all patients in the late terminal stage of illness, known as the active dying process; excellent management of these symptoms is important to ensure quality of care at the end of life.
- An understanding of caregiver burden for loved ones of those with advanced urologic illness is important; physical care burdens, emotional issues, spiritual needs, intimacy, and practical issues of the health care system all weigh heavily on patients and their families.

INTRODUCTION

This article focuses on the issues facing patients with advanced and ultimately terminal urologic illness, including a framework of care planning based on defining patient and family goals of care, as well as palliative management strategies for common symptoms and syndromes that these patients and their families experience. It also focuses on the management of common urologic issues that may arise in the course of care for all patients at the end of life, as well as the impact on caregivers.

[a] Division of Palliative Medicine, University of Kansas School of Medicine, 3901 Rainbow Boulevard, MS 1020, Kansas City, KS 66160, USA; [b] Department of Urology, The Landon Center on Aging, School of Medicine, The University of Kansas, 3901 Rainbow Boulevard, Kansas City, KS 66160, USA
* Corresponding author.
E-mail address: csinclair@kumc.edu

Clin Geriatr Med 31 (2015) 667–678
http://dx.doi.org/10.1016/j.cger.2015.07.002   geriatric.theclinics.com

EPIDEMIOLOGY

For patients who will die of urologic illnesses, prostate, bladder, and renal cell cancer are the most common causes, with these cancers accounting for 10.1% of all cancer deaths annually.[1] However, people can live with these conditions for an extended period of time, and can experience related symptoms. In addition, these patients may be dealing with progression of comorbid conditions. Such factors should be considered when considering the risks and benefits of possible treatment options.

In general, people do not die of noncancer urologic issues. However urologic symptoms can play a prominent role in several illnesses as they approach the terminal stage, including multiple sclerosis, amyotrophic lateral sclerosis, Alzheimer disease, tuberculosis, and stroke. Many patients facing the end of life, regardless of the terminal diagnosis, may experience urologic symptoms that need to be recognized and appropriately addressed.

TREATMENT PLANNING IN ADVANCED ILLNESS: PROGNOSTICATION

It is hard to know exactly who is dying. Doctors tend to overestimate how long a patient has, even by as much as 5 times the prognosis.[2] However, an understanding of time frame is often one of the most important pieces of information that patients and families want to know. Although median survival data for patients with a particular type and stage of cancer can be helpful to provide a general understanding, no individual prognosis should be derived from those data. Studies to identify factors that clarify individual prognosis have found that markers of core functional status, including the ability for self-care, ambulation, nutritional intake, and level of consciousness, play pivotal roles in determining treatment candidacy as well as survival.[3] Even more simply, a study in which providers were asked "Would it surprise you if your patient were to die in the next year?" found that a provider's answer of "No" had a positive predictive value of 83.8% for who would die in the following 12 months.[4] Clinical recommendations for estimating prognosis in patients with advanced cancer ultimately conclude that a combination of clinical prediction of survival and prognostic scores such as the Palliative Prognostic Score (PPS) are best.[5]

TREATMENT PLANNING IN ADVANCED ILLNESS: UNDERSTANDING ILLNESS TRAJECTORIES

Lunney and colleagues[6] sought to better understand the patterns of functional decline at the end of life. They studied markers of core functional decline over time and found that there are 4 fairly predictable patterns: the cancer, organ failure, frailty, and sudden illness trajectories (**Fig. 1**).[6] The cancer trajectory is characterized by a more predictable, steady loss in function, likely as tumor burden not responsive to interventions increases. Approximately 30% of patients have this pattern of functional decline. The organ failure trajectory is characterized by recurrent, sudden episodes of decline and partial recovery in function, in an unpredictable fashion. On the frailty trajectory, patients may live for an extended period of time, even years, with a low level of functional independence, with the organ failure trajectory pattern becoming more prominent in the end. Together the organ failure and frailty patterns account for about 60% of deaths in the United States.

TREATMENT PLANNING IN ADVANCED ILLNESS: DEFINING AND DISCUSSING GOALS OF CARE

Where a patient is along the illness trajectory is an important facet in answering the question noted earlier about prognostication, and should factor into discussions of

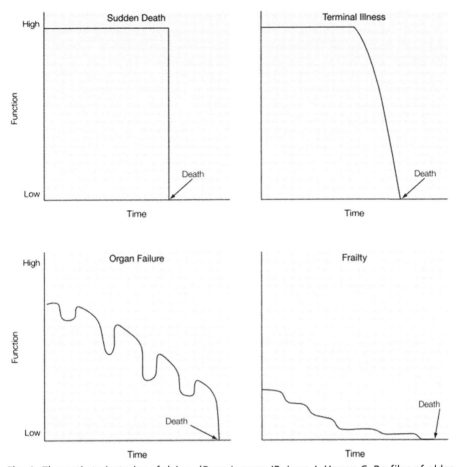

Fig. 1. Theoretic trajectories of dying. (*From* Lunney JR, Lynn J, Hogan C. Profiles of older Medicare decedents. J Am Geriatr Soc 2002;50(6):1109; with permission.)

goals of care and expectations for treatment. Framing treatment options around patient preferences, with a good understanding of trajectory, can help patients and families understand and prepare for the progression of illness over time. In order for patients and families to develop rational goals for their care, they need:

- Information, to understand their conditions and the expected course of illness over time.
- Details regarding the risks and benefits of all of their treatment options, including the options of supportive care and comfort measures as valid choices when appropriate.
- An ability to reflect and match potential treatment options with who they are as people, and how they want the medical system to approach their treatment as individuals over time.[7]

As a framework for discussion about goals of care, it can be useful to describe 3 categories for global treatment focus. These categories are, first, doing every treatment that might possibly be helpful to keep the patient alive; second, doing treatments that are simple and noninvasive for reversible conditions; and third, doing treatments that will maximize the patient's comfort through symptom management only, even if the patient is dying. This framework for goals of care and levels of intervention can help people identify how they would like their providers to respond if the illness changes over time. Because the patient's experience of the illness evolves over time as well, it is important that goals of care be discussed periodically and altered as necessary in order to ensure that the patient's preferences regarding approach to treatment continue to be accurately understood and implemented.[8]

It is important that all medical providers be competent in discussing illness trajectory and goals of care with their patients and families who face advanced illness. Studies show that patients often want to talk with their physician about these things but are waiting for the physician to bring it up.[9] However, doctors often do not start these conversations because of time constraints, fear of abolishing hope, or a feeling of not knowing what to say. It is an important area in which to gain confidence. Studies show that when physicians have good conversations with their patients regarding goals of care, those patients are much more likely to have their end of life play out in a way that is congruent with their unique goals and preferences.[10]

TREATMENT PLANNING IN ADVANCED ILLNESS: TIMING OF PALLIATIVE CARE

Any time a clinician is caring for a patient with advance illness, the core principles of palliative care are important to consider, and the earlier the better. Active treatments can be paired with palliative treatments, and can be offered simultaneously (**Fig. 2**).[11] Several studies show that early integration of palliative care into the treatment plan improves symptoms, improves quality of life, and can even improve survival.[12]

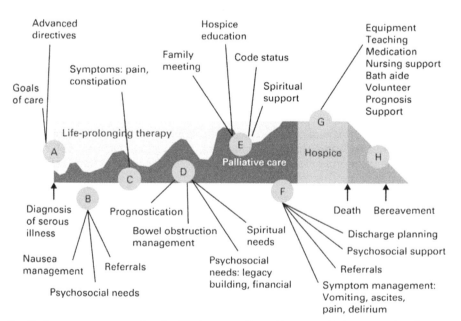

Fig. 2. Common components of palliative care. (*From* Hennessy JE, Lown BA, Landzaat L, et al. Practical issues in palliative and quality-of-life care. J Oncol Pract 2013;9(2):79; with permission.)

SYMPTOM MANAGEMENT
Management Goals

How to approach urinary tract symptoms for someone with very advanced disease who is possibly near the end of life often depends on both the current goals of care and the estimated prognosis. Knowing when to apply any of the approaches listed later in this article requires clinicians to make an honest appraisal of expected outcomes and prognosis so they can adequately weigh the risks and benefits. The clinician may even decide to choose different strategies for the same symptom in a patient who has days to live compared with one who has a few weeks. In addition, if the goals of care are focused on avoiding the hospital, certain procedures are likely to be ruled out.

General Symptoms in Patients with Advanced Urinary Tract Disease

The symptoms of patients with advanced disease that primarily stems from the urinary system are the focus here. In particular, cancers of the prostate, bladder, and kidney are the most common primary diseases that may be seen in a practice, but there may be some rarer disease, such as penile cancer and vulvar cancer, that may present similar issues. When cancer becomes systemic, a wide range of symptoms may be present. Some of the more common key symptoms that clinicians may see are discussed here.

Bone Pain/Spinal Cord Compression

Bone metastases are common in cases of advanced prostate and renal cancer, but less likely to occur with bladder cancer. Pain results from direct tumor invasion of the bone, although some bone metastasis can be pain free. The triad of movement-related pain, spontaneous pain at rest, and background pain is classic for bone pain. It is often localized to the site of the metastatic tumor, but occasionally can radiate along nerve paths. Patients frequently describe the background pain as a dull ache and the movement-related pain as sharp.[13]

The palliation of bone pain is critical because if left untreated it can lead to a precipitous decline in functional status and quality of life for both patients and caregivers. Because of the inflammatory nature of the pain and the quick onset of relief, nonsteroidal antiinflammatory drugs (NSAIDs) and steroids tend to be the mainstay of drug treatment in the short term. Addition of 4 to 12 mg daily of oral dexamethasone may be adequate to improve functional status and quality of life. However, the effect of the dexamethasone may only last a few weeks. NSAIDs can be used at low doses for a longer period, but the typical risks of these medications force them to be used sparingly in most palliative situations. The steroid dexamethasone is preferred to prednisone because of the high glucocorticoid activity and less significant mineralocorticoid effect.[14]

For a longer term strategy, bisphosphonates may be an option. Moderate relief of the pain can be seen about 12 weeks after onset of treatment.[15] In addition to pain control, they may prevent skeletal events, which may help preserve function in someone with a prognosis of more than a few months.

Short-acting opioids like morphine and oxycodone may be used for breakthrough pain related to movement or incidental pain, but their onset of action is often too long compared with the severe but temporary increase in pain. If a patient is tolerant of short-acting opioids, and they do not seem to adequately relieve the pain, introducing long-acting opioids may help prevent severe incidental pain. Despite concerns about diversion and addiction, when prescribed appropriately and with close follow-up, opioids may be critical tools, especially near the end of life.

External beam radiation works slightly faster than bisphosphonates, with many patients noticing a difference in as little as 1 month. There is growing evidence to suggest that 1 or 2 fractions of radiation may prove as beneficial as 10 or more fractions.[16] Because travel is often complex for these patients, fewer visits for radiation can make a meaningful improvement on their quality of life. It is important to work closely and proactively with local radiation oncologists to ensure a treatment plan that works for each patient.

Instability of bone may be an indication for interventional techniques, which are rapidly evolving. Several different approaches are now available, based on the basic concept of a vertebroplasty, in which cement is injected into the metastasis. Checking on the expertise and experience of local interventionists is the first step in ensuring that patients get the right care. Other considerations for bone pain include surgery, transcutaneous electrical nerve stimulation units, and physical and occupational therapy. Many of these are based on availability and coverage, which, along with their limited efficacy, may make them secondary options to consider in bone pain.

Pelvic Pain

Pelvic pain can have numerous different causes related to anatomic structures or neuropathic disorder, a full discussion of which is beyond the scope of this article. Understanding the cause of the pelvic pain and determining whether there is any reversible component is key. However, for most people with advanced illness and near the end of life, major interventions are limited because of frailty. After ruling out bladder spasm based on the characteristics of the pain (discussed later), opioids, NSAIDs, and steroids are the likely medications to address this challenging symptom. In select cases, injection of steroids or analgesic nerve blocks and other interventional modalities may offer relief, but access may vary widely by institution.

Delirium

Delirium is a common symptom near the end of life, but it is not always clear whether it is caused by an underlying reversible medical condition or part of the dying process. A good history, discussion with the nurses, and in certain cases a diagnostic straight catheter helps to rule urinary retention in or out as a potential reversible cause of delirium. Some of the medications that are often used to treat urinary incontinence, including steroids, opioids, anxiolytics, and anticholinergics, can increase the risk for delirium.

Hematuria

Degree of bleeding does not correlate with seriousness of underlying condition. It is more common in malignancies of the urinary tract. However, in patients who may have recently taken cyclophosphamide or ifosfamide, a urinary metabolite called acrolein can cause severe inflammation and hemorrhagic cystitis. Clot retention leading to bladder distention may require bladder irrigation or endoscopic intervention for clot evacuation. Suprapubic catheters are unlikely to be of sufficient diameter to clear a blood clot from a bladder. Continuous bladder irrigation (CBI) can be implemented using a 3-way indwelling catheter. Because of discomfort associated with CBI or manual bladder irrigation from the bladder distention, short-term analgesia may be necessary. Hematuria may also result in significant anxiety on the part of patient, family, and staff. Clear communication and a plan can help alleviate some of this stress, but, if necessary, anxiolytics for the patient may occasionally be necessary in severe cases of hematuria-induced anxiety. For refractory hematuria there are other rarely used options, but it is best to consult with a urologist and possibly a palliative care physician to come up with a more detailed plan.

Sudden Urinary Stoppage

Recognizing that people near the end of life have a tapering of their urinary output as they take in less fluids, wise clinicians need to recognize when there is a more acute stoppage in output. Depending on the history, especially if there is any urologic disorder, it may be possible to identify that a lower urinary tract (bladder neck, prostate, urethra) or upper urinary tract (ureter or kidney) obstruction is present. With lower-tract obstruction, a full bladder may be palpable on examination. A close examination of the genitals is important to identify meatal stenosis, scarring, tumor formation, or trauma from catheter placement. For patients with a history of prostate disorder, a rectal examination to assess any change in the prostate may help identify the location of the obstruction.

If a lower-tract obstruction is highly suspected or identified, insertion of a urinary catheter is the first-line treatment. If the urinary catheter is unable to be placed, a suprapubic catheter may be an acceptable method of relieving pressure on the bladder, which may help relieve pain and delirium.

Upper tract obstructions usually do not result in sudden urinary stoppage unless it occurs to both ureters or the patient has a known single functioning kidney with a single obstructed ureter. Because of the direct effect on the kidneys, signs of acute renal failure may also be present, in addition to flank pain, or colic typically found in nephrolithiasis. For patients with a prognosis of several weeks to months, ureteral stents or percutaneous nephrostomy tube placement may be a reasonable option if it fits with the overall goals of care. If a patient has a prognosis of days to a few weeks, medical symptom management may be preferable by patient and family. Assessing the patient's values in situations like this is critical to choosing the correct therapy.

Fistula

There are multiple types of fistula that may be associated with the hollow viscus of the urinary tract, including vesicoenteric, vesicocolonic, vesicovaginal, rectovaginal, rectourethral, and urethrocutaneous. This article does not discuss these individually but instead focuses on the overall care approach to patients. These fistulas can result in bothersome symptoms and substantial negative effects on quality of life for most patients. The role of definitive therapy, which often requires reconstructive surgery, must be placed in the overall context of goals of care.

Urinary Tract Symptoms in Patients near the End of Life

Patients with primary urologic disease as the underlying cause of symptoms both systemic and localized to the kidneys, bladder, and prostate were discussed earlier. Here, this article discusses common urinary tract symptoms found in patients with a variety of terminal illnesses at the end of life.

Diseases such as multiple sclerosis, amyotrophic lateral sclerosis, spinal cord injury, and stroke, which affect the nervous system, often have significant impacts on urologic health for patients. It is important for providers to concentrate on a good history and physical examination for these patients to best understand the impact of urologic issues.

SYMPTOMS
Renal Colic and Flank Pain

Often brought on by an acute obstruction, such as a stone, clot, or occasionally a malignancy, the mechanism of pain is capsular distention of the kidney. A good history and examination may direct the clinician to the likely source without the immediate need for imaging, which may be especially important for patients in hospice settings, where the preferred imaging approach may be technically challenging to obtain.

Bladder Pain/Bladder Spasm

The mechanism of bladder spasm is from severe contractions of the detrusor muscle. The trigone is sensitive to expansion and, as the bladder fills and expands, the trigone sends signals to the brain to empty the bladder, therefore resulting in contraction. The 2 main categories of bladder pain have obstructive and irritative causes. Obstructive bladder pain presents with bladder distention and overflow incontinence. Chronic obstruction may be painless, whereas acute obstruction can cause severe lower abdominal pain, restlessness that can manifest as anxiety and/or delirium, and frequent requests to use the bathroom. Bladder outlet obstruction is common in the dying process, related to natural changes in the body or to anticholinergic side effects of medications commonly used to treat other symptoms at end of life. The primary treatment is removal of offending agents if possible, or relief with a urinary catheter.

Irritative bladder pain is caused by inflammation from various causes and is characterized by excessive urinary frequency, dysuria, and urgency incontinence. More common causes include external radiation, chemotherapeutic agents such as cyclophosphamide, tumors either intrinsic to or external to the bladder, irritation from indwelling catheters, and bladder calculi. Treatment is focused on removing any offending agent or treating any local disease, in addition to considering placement of a urethral or suprapubic catheter.

Polyuria

Polyuria is a rare problem in patients with advanced illness because it is more typical to see a reduction in urine output with the natural decreased intake as the body shuts down. Urinary tract infections should be ruled out as the most common cause. Occasionally, patients do present with polyuria (typically more than 3 L/d), which may be diabetes insipidus (DI). Trauma, hypoxia, and ischemia may be the root causes of central or neurologic DI, commonly caused by the decreased production of antidiuretic hormone. Nephrogenic DI is likely to be caused by progressive renal failure with inability to concentrate urine and retain water, hypercalcemia, or chronic lithium use.

Infection

Infections present a unique dilemma to patients, families, and clinicians at the end of life. Infections cause unpleasant symptoms and may be reversible with a short course of antibiotics without much side effect. In contrast, infections are becoming more difficult to eradicate and may present as a false-positive, making treatment ineffective or unnecessary. Classic signs and symptoms of urinary tract infections include fever, dysuria, increased urinary frequency and urgency, and occasionally pelvic pain. Having an indwelling or suprapubic catheter does increase the risk for bacterial infections, and 50% of patients are bacteriuric by 10 to 14 days.[17]

Change in Urine Appearance

A common question that families observing a loved one near the end of life ask is, "Why does the urine look different?" As a patient is dying, numerous factors may lead to a change in the color and appearance of the urine. Many of the changes, such as decreased urine output with darkening of the urine, may be related to the dying process, including decreased fluid intake and impaired renal function. However, there are also other identifiable causes of change in urine appearance (**Table 1**).

Catheters

Recently there has been a strong push in health care to drastically reduce the use of bladder catheters because of the high incidence of catheter-associated urinary tract infections (CAUTIs).[18] When patients have advanced disease, and especially when they are near the end of life with a prognosis of a few weeks or less, the risk/benefit ratio may need to be thoughtfully considered. Often people want to be cared for in their homes, with the bulk of care by family or friends. A bladder catheter may reduce the need for briefs and uncomfortable situations, which may preserve the dignity of the patient and reduce the caregiver burden. If a patient does develop a CAUTI, then consideration of removal of the catheter may be prudent after discussion with the patient and family.

Sexual Intimacy at the End of Life

Patients facing a terminal illness may still desire sexual intimacy with their partners. This intimacy may occur via sexual intercourse or in a variety of other intimate settings. It is important for medical providers to address these issues and provide opportunities for discussion to serve their patient's needs.[19]

Psychological challenges with sexual intimacy, such as changes in self-image or anxiety, may be addressed with counseling by a provider trained in these issues. In addition, in cases of physical challenges related to weakness, prosthetic or amputated limbs, stroke, or other nonurologic primary causes, it is appropriate to work with occupational and physical therapists who can help with methods and even positioning for such encounters.

In addition, a person may be faced with sexual dysfunction related to their disease. In many cases, medications used to treat such dysfunction in the general population may be used. In other cases, prosthetics and other devices are a safer option with a lower side effect profile. Like all treatments in the geriatric population, the risks and benefits of each intervention must be carefully weighed.

In patients with urinary catheters because of bladder dysfunction or outlet obstruction from their disease process, there are several possible approaches. People who are functionally able can be trained by a medical provider to remove the catheter for sexual intercourse and then reinsert it later. However, if the disease process

Table 1 Common changes in urine appearance	
Changes in Color	**Common Causes**
Red	Hematuria, rifampin, phenazopyridine (Pyridium), senna laxatives
Orange	Sulfasalazine, phenazopyridine (Pyridium), liver or bile duct obstruction or other disease, dehydration
Blue/green	Amitriptyline, indomethacin, propofol (Diprivan)
Dark brown	Liver or kidney disease, urinary tract infection, metronidazole (Flagyl), nitrofurantoin, senna laxatives, methocarbamol (Robaxin)
Sediment or floating material	Protein crystallization, urolithiasis, tissue shedding, or blood clots

prevents this, there are a couple of options for sexual intercourse to occur with a catheter in place. In the case of a woman, with some cautious positioning she or her partner may be able to secure the catheter to her leg without obstructing her vaginal orifice. It is more challenging for men, but one recommended option is to use a large condom over the penis and catheter, leaving plenty of extra tubing at the end of the condom so as not to remove the catheter. This technique can also be helpful if there are additional issues with erectile dysfunction preventing penetration because the catheter tubing might support the penile shaft.

It is also important to recognize that sexual intimacy does not always require intercourse and, particularly in end of life, may be expressed in physical touch, cuddling, and intimate conversation.

Caregiver Burden

It is widely known that caregivers experience increased burden and decreased psychological well-being as urinary incontinence worsens for the patient. This burden may be related to increased trips to the toilet, increased laundry and clothing changes, or increased cost of incontinence pads or medications. The burden is so great that patients with dementia are significantly more likely to be institutionalized, and interventions to treat incontinence in dementia have often been unsuccessful.[20]

In the setting of chronic disease other than dementia, caregiver burden may be lessened with methods that either prevent or contain the incontinence episodes. Options include a bedside commode, briefs, scheduled voiding, or medications. Importantly, clinical providers must support not only patients but their caregivers. Referral to a local support group or other resources may be helpful and should be considered as needed.

Integrating Palliative Care into Urologic Practice

Palliative care specialists and geriatricians can provide valuable aspects of care with patients near the end of life. However, all interested health care providers can gain skills in this area, and can play an important role in the care of these patients. Recent research has shown that incorporation of palliative care concepts into urologic practice can be done efficiently, and can enhance clinical experiences for both patients and providers.[21] A variety of educational options exist that can be used to enhance knowledge about palliative care for specialists in other areas of medicine, and increase their comfort and ability to include this as part of their regular care practice.[22]

Professional Coping

Caring for people near the end of life can be challenging for clinicians, especially when they have developed close relationships with the patients and their families. Becoming aware that a physician's value to a patient does not entirely depend on the ability to offer a new treatment, but instead being present and listening to the wishes, concerns, and goals of a patient can be a difficult transition for even seasoned clinicians. Talking with professional peers and other team members is a valuable method to debrief and gain insight in caring for this unique patient population. Other methods of self-reflection and self-care, such as journaling, meditation, exercise, or creative outlets such as art and music may be beneficial for professionals providing this type of care for patients and their families. Although provision of palliative and end-of-life care can be challenging for health care professionals, it can also be an extremely rewarding aspect of clinical practice.

SUMMARY

When assisting people with advanced illness, whether from primary urologic disorders or other organ failure, a palliative care approach may be most helpful to align patient values and goals with the most effective but least burdensome therapies. Being clear about expected life expectancy, time to benefit of any proposed therapy, and advanced care planning is of great help in developing a treatment plan around geriatric urology issues. Families and patients often appreciate honest, direct communication delivered with a compassionate approach. When working toward a comfort care plan, more invasive approaches are still potentially available but they should not necessarily be the default approach as might be expected in people with less advanced disease. However, it is important to consider the full range of options available and match them with the patient's informed goals.

REFERENCES

1. Howlader N, Noone AM, Krapcho M, et al. In: Tatalovich Z, Mariotto A, Lewis DR, et al, editors. SEER cancer statistics review, 1975-2012. Bethesda (MD): National Cancer Institute; 2015. Based on November 2014 SEER data submission, posted to the SEER Web site. Available at: http://seer.cancer.gov/csr/1975_2012/.
2. Christakis NA, Lamont EB. Extent and determinants of error in doctors' prognoses in terminally ill patients: prospective cohort study. BMJ 2000;320(7233):469–72.
3. Mei AHY, Jin WLC, Hwang MKY, et al. Value of the palliative performance scale in the prognostication of advanced cancer patients in a tertiary care setting. J Palliat Med 2013;16(8):887–93.
4. Moss AH, Lunney JR, Culp S, et al. Prognostic significance of the "surprise" question in cancer patients. J Palliat Med 2010;13(7):837–40.
5. Maltoni M, Caraceni A, Brunelli C, et al. Prognostic factors in advanced cancer patients: evidence-based clinical recommendations–a study by the Steering Committee of the European Association for Palliative Care. J Clin Oncol 2005; 23(25):6240–8.
6. Lunney JR, Lynn J, Foley DJ, et al. Patterns of functional decline at the end of life. JAMA 2003;289(18):2387–92.
7. Nelson JE, Puntillo KA, Pronovost PJ, et al. In their own words: patients and families define high-quality palliative care in the intensive care unit. Crit Care Med 2010;38(3):808–18.
8. Barrio-Cantalejo IM, Simón-Lorda P, Molina-Ruiz A, et al. Stability over time in the preferences of older persons for life-sustaining treatment. J Bioeth Inq 2013; 10(1):103–14.
9. Hancock K, Clayton JM, Parker SM, et al. Truth-telling in discussing prognosis in advanced life-limiting illnesses: a systematic review. Palliat Med 2007;21(6):507–17.
10. Bischoff KE, Sudore R, Miao Y, et al. Advance care planning and the quality of end-of-life care in older adults. J Am Geriatr Soc 2013;61(2):209–14.
11. Hennessy JE, Lown BA, Landzaat L, et al. Practical issues in palliative and quality-of-life care. J Oncol Pract 2013;9(2):78–80.
12. Greer JA, Pirl WF, Jackson VA, et al. Effect of early palliative care on chemotherapy use and end-of-life care in patients with metastatic non-small-cell lung cancer. J Clin Oncol 2012;30(4):394–400.
13. Laird BJA, Walley J, Murray GD, et al. Characterization of cancer-induced bone pain: an exploratory study. Support Care Cancer 2011;19(9):1393–401.
14. Twycross R, Wilcock A, editors. Hospice and palliative care formulary USA. 2nd edition. Nottingham (United Kingdom): Palliativedrugs.com, Ltd; 2008.

15. Wong R, Wiffen PJ. Bisphosphonates for the relief of pain secondary to bone metastases. Cochrane Database Syst Rev 2002;(2):CD002068.
16. Wu JS, Whelan T, Bezjak A, et al. Meta-analysis of single-fraction versus multi-fraction radiotherapy trials for palliation of painful bone metastases. Int J Radiat Oncol Biol Phys 2001;51(3):53.
17. Sedor J, Mulholland SG. Hospital-acquired urinary tract infections associated with the indwelling catheter. Urol Clin North Am 1999;26(4):821–8.
18. Zimlichman E, Henderson D, Tamir O, et al. Health care-associated infections: a meta-analysis of costs and financial impact on the US health care system. JAMA Intern Med 2013;173(22):2039–46.
19. Lemieux L, Kaiser S, Pereira J, et al. Sexuality in palliative care: patient perspectives. Palliat Med 2004;18(7):630–7.
20. Torti FM, Gwyther LP, Reed SD, et al. A multinational review of recent trends and reports in dementia caregiver burden. Alzheimer Dis Assoc Disord 2004;18(2):99–109.
21. Bergman J, Ballon-Landa E, Lorenz KA, et al. Community-partnered collaboration to build an integrated palliative care clinic: the view from urology. Am J Hosp Palliat Care 2014. [Epub ahead of print].
22. Bergman J, Lorenz KA, Ballon-Landa E, et al. A scalable web-based module for improving surgical and medical practitioner knowledge and attitudes about palliative and end-of-life care. J Palliat Med 2015;18(5):415–20.

Index

Note: Page numbers of article titles are in **boldface** type.

United States Postal Service

Statement of Ownership, Management, and Circulation
(All Periodicals Publications Except Requestor Publications)

1. Publication Title	2. Publication Number	3. Filing Date
Clinics in Geriatric Medicine	0 0 0 - 7 0 4	9/18/15

4. Issue Frequency	5. Number of Issues Published Annually	6. Annual Subscription Price
Feb, May, Aug, Nov	4	$320.00

7. Complete Mailing Address of Known Office of Publication (Not printer) (Street, city, county, state, and ZIP+4®)

Elsevier Inc.
360 Park Avenue South
New York, NY 10010-1710

Contact Person
Stephen R. Bushing
Telephone (Include area code)
215-239-3688

8. Complete Mailing Address of Headquarters or General Business Office of Publisher (Not printer)

Elsevier Inc., 360 Park Avenue South, New York, NY 10010-1710

9. Full Names and Complete Mailing Addresses of Publisher, Editor, and Managing Editor (Do not leave blank)

Publisher (Name and complete mailing address)

Linda Belfus, Elsevier Inc., 1600 John F. Kennedy Blvd., Suite 1800, Philadelphia, PA 19103

Editor (Name and complete mailing address)

Jessica McCool, Elsevier Inc., 1600 John F. Kennedy Blvd., Suite 1800, Philadelphia, PA 19103-2899

Managing Editor (Name and complete mailing address)

Adrianne Brigido, Elsevier Inc., 1600 John F. Kennedy Blvd., Suite 1800, Philadelphia, PA 19103-2899

10. Owner (Do not leave blank. If the publication is owned by a corporation, give the name and address of the corporation immediately followed by the names and addresses of all stockholders owning or holding 1 percent or more of the total amount of stock. If not owned by a corporation, give the names and addresses of the individual owners. If owned by a partnership or other unincorporated firm, give its name and address as well as those of each individual owner. If the publication is published by a nonprofit organization, give its name and address.)

Full Name	Complete Mailing Address
Wholly owned subsidiary of	1600 John F. Kennedy Blvd, Ste. 1800
Reed/Elsevier; US holdings	Philadelphia, PA 19103-2899

11. Known Bondholders, Mortgagees, and Other Security Holders Owning or Holding 1 Percent or More of Total Amount of Bonds, Mortgages, or Other Securities. If none, check box ☐ None

Full Name	Complete Mailing Address
N/A	

12. Tax Status (For completion by nonprofit organizations authorized to mail at nonprofit rates) (Check one)
The purpose, function, and nonprofit status of this organization and the exempt status for federal income tax purposes:
☐ Has Not Changed During Preceding 12 Months
☐ Has Changed During Preceding 12 Months (Publisher must submit explanation of change with this statement)

13. Publication Title	14. Issue Date for Circulation Data Below
Clinics in Geriatric Medicine	August 2015

15. Extent and Nature of Circulation			Average No. Copies Each Issue During Preceding 12 Months	No. Copies of Single Issue Published Nearest to Filing Date
a. Total Number of Copies (Net press run)			448	351
b. Legitimate Paid and/or Requested Distribution (By Mail and Outside the Mail)	(1)	Mailed Outside-County Paid/Requested Mail Subscriptions stated on PS Form 3541. (Include paid distribution above nominal rate, advertiser's proof copies and exchange copies)	170	137
	(2)	Mailed In-County Paid/Requested Mail Subscriptions stated on PS Form 3541. (Include paid distribution above nominal rate, advertiser's proof copies and exchange copies)		
	(3)	Paid Distribution Outside the Mails Including Sales Through Dealers And Carriers, Street Vendors, Counter Sales, and Other Paid Distribution Outside USPS®	88	94
	(4)	Paid Distribution by Other Classes of Mail Through the USPS (e.g. First-Class Mail®)		
c. Total Paid and or Requested Circulation (Sum of 15b (1), (2), (3), and (4))			258	231
d. Free or Nominal Rate Distribution (By Mail and Outside the Mail)	(1)	Free or Nominal Rate Outside-County Copies included on PS Form 3541	75	64
	(2)	Free or Nominal Rate In-County Copies included on PS Form 3541		
	(3)	Free or Nominal Rate Copies mailed at Other classes Through the USPS (e.g. First-Class Mail®)		
	(4)	Free or Nominal Rate Distribution Outside the Mail (Carriers or Other means)		
e. Total Nonrequested Distribution (Sum of 15d (1), (2), (3) and (4))			75	64
f. Total Distribution (Sum of 15c and 15e)			333	295
g. Copies not Distributed (See instructions to publishers #4 (page #3))			115	56
h. Total (Sum of 15f and g)			448	351
i. Percent Paid and/or Requested Circulation (15c divided by 15f times 100)			77.48%	78.31%

* If you are claiming electronic copies go to line 16 on page 3. If you are not claiming Electronic copies, skip to line 17 on page 3.

16. Electronic Copy Circulation	Average No. Copies Each Issue During Preceding 12 Months	No. Copies of Single Issue Published Nearest to Filing Date
a. Paid Electronic Copies		
b. Total paid Print Copies (Line 15c) + Paid Electronic copies (Line 16a)		
c. Total Print Distribution (Line 15f) + Paid Electronic Copies (Line 16a)		
d. Percent Paid (Both Print & Electronic copies) (16b divided by 16c X 100)		

☐ I certify that 50% of all my distributed copies (electronic and print) are paid above a nominal price

17. Publication of Statement of Ownership
If the publication is a general publication, publication of this statement is required. Will be printed in the November 2015 issue of this publication.

18. Signature and Title of Editor, Publisher, Business Manager, or Owner

Stephen R. Bushing
Stephen R. Bushing – Inventory Distribution Coordinator

Date: September 18, 2015

I certify that all information furnished on this form is true and complete. I understand that anyone who furnishes false or misleading information on this form or who omits material or information requested on the form may be subject to criminal sanctions (including fines and imprisonment) and/or civil sanctions (including civil penalties).

PS Form 3526, July 2014 (Page 3 of 3)

PS Form 3526, July 2014 (Page 1 of 3 (Instructions Page 3)) PSN 7530-01-000-9931 PRIVACY NOTICE: See our Privacy policy in www.usps.com

Printed and bound by CPI Group (UK) Ltd, Croydon, CR0 4YY

03/10/2024

01040496-0004